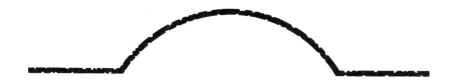

# Eat, Drink and Be Healthy

# Eat, Drink and Be Healthy

## A Guide to Healthful Eating and Weight Control

**Janet M. Chiavetta**
in collaboration with
Carolyn J. H. Barrett, R.D., M.S., M.P.H.
Stephen V. Chiavetta, M.D.

Fulcrum Publishing
Golden, Colorado

Cataloging-In-Publication Data

Chiavetta, Janet M.
    Eat, drink, and be healthy : a guide to healthful eating and weight control / Janet M. Chiavetta, in collaboration with Carolyn J. H. Barrett, Stephen V. Chiavetta.
        p.      cm.
    Includes bibliographical references and indexes.
    ISBN 1-55591-199-4
    1. Nutrition.    2. Low-fat diet—Recipes.    I. Barrett, Carolyn J. H.
II. Chiavetta, Stephen V.  III. Title.
RA784.C475          1994
613.2—dc20                                                      94-11611
                                                                CIP


Printed in the United States of America
0 9 8 7 6 5 4 3 2 1

Fulcrum Publishing
350 Indiana Street, Suite 350
Golden, Colorado 80401-5093
800/992-2908

*Dedicated with love*
*to my sons, Stephen and John.*
*This book should enable them and others*
*to enjoy the pleasures of good foods,*
*while at the same time, protecting their health.*

# Contents

# *Preface*

*"… and yet the true creator is necessity, which is the mother of our invention."*

— Plato (circa 375 B.C.)

This maxim is as true today as it was over 2,000 years ago. This cookbook and guide to healthful eating was created because of our family's *need* to change our diet. Because of my own struggle to learn what constitutes a healthy diet, I saw the need for a practical, comprehensive book on healthy eating. I also realized the need for a collection of tasty low-fat recipes that would appeal to typical American families.

Our family's need to change our diet became evident 8 years ago when my husband's cholesterol measured 330. We were shocked because we thought we were following a healthy diet. Furthermore, he was at his ideal body weight and jogged four miles a day. It was only after I did considerable research — on the amount of fats in foods, learned how misleading

food labels could be, and found out that all the so-called "heart-healthy" fats can also contribute to heart disease — that I realized our diet was indeed not so healthy after all.

In the beginning, my main priority was to significantly reduce the fat in our diet, especially saturated and hydrogenated fats. The results were very promising. After less than three months on our new diet, my husband's cholesterol dropped over 100 points to 210. At that time, I decided I would write a book on what I had learned through my research and our own personal experience, hoping others would benefit from it.

More research led to more questions. Why did the American Heart Association recommend a diet of less than 30% of calories from fat? Why not 25% or 20%? What foods constitute a diet of 20% or 30% of calories from fat? Can one consume too little fat, and not get enough essential nutrients? If so, can this increase the risks for cancer or other diseases? What exactly constitutes a healthy, balanced low-fat diet? How important are exercise and other life-style factors?

After months of reading and research, and after studying nutrition at a nearby college, the answers to these questions and others began to unfold. While writing the book, I consulted on a regular basis with Carolyn Barrett, clinical assistant professor of nutrition at the University of North Carolina at Chapel Hill. My husband, a physician, was also invaluable to me as a consultant. The information presented in the book is medically and nutritionally sound and includes the most current scientific data on diet and life-style as a form of preventive medicine—not just for heart disease, but for cancer, stroke and intestinal disorders.

After learning what constituted a healthy low-fat diet, I was ready to begin compiling a recipe collection that met the approval of my family, which included two teenage sons. Since my teenagers were hooked on high-fat junk food like others their age, it was a real challenge. The recipes needed to meet the approval of the entire family, or be discarded or altered until they met the test. Friends and members of my extended family also tested recipes.

My goal was to produce a collection of recipes with enough variety to meet the needs of all anticipated occasions. Now, I am able to entertain formally or casually, plus prepare foods for my family, using only this cookbook. All the recipes have been tested at least twice and most of them many more times. I hope your families and friends will be as fond of these recipes as mine are.

# *Acknowledgments*

I would like to express my gratitude to a number of people who were a tremendous help to me in preparing this book. Without their assistance, this book would not have been possible. To begin with, my sister Delaine Moe, a dietitian, has been an invaluable resource and an enthusiastic supporter. Her firsthand experiences with diet counseling and promoting wellness was most helpful.

I would also like to thank Kaye Lasater, Harriet Hill, Fran Preston and Barbara Smith for critiquing the information portion of the book, offering comments and suggestions to make the text more readable.

Testing more than 240 recipes was made easier and more enjoyable with the help of my sister Joanne Johnson and friends Mary Scarantino and Betty Vogel. Mary also provided me with some of her own family recipes, which have been included in the book and are among my favorites. A special thank you to my sister Jerie Moe Jacobsen for her wonderful whole-grain bread recipes.

My husband, Steve Chiavetta, M.D., and Carolyn Barrett, R.D., M.P.H., provided their valuable assistance, which helped ensure that the information presented is both nutritionally and scientifically sound. My son John assisted in typing and entering nutritional data into the computer. His computer experience was a real asset.

Finally, a special thank you to the members of my immediate family, Steve, Stephen and John, for their patience, helpful comments and support in testing all these recipes.

# Introduction

Many health-conscious Americans are changing the way they eat. They are especially concerned with reducing saturated fat and cholesterol in their diet to lower blood cholesterol levels. They also are paying closer attention to monitoring their blood pressure and are taking the time to exercise regularly. For many, these efforts are paying off. The death rate from heart disease has decreased by nearly 30% since 1978.

Still, based on current statistics, one-third of Americans will suffer a heart attack, stroke or blockage of an artery in a leg before the age of 65. Eventually, slightly over half of us will die as a result of heart disease.

One of the problems is that many Americans still are not aware of the *extent* of dietary changes necessary to make a significant difference in health risks — not only for heart disease, but also for cancer and other diseases. A recent national food survey shows that many Americans who are trying to eat "right" are making unhealthy food choices without realizing it. Many have cut down on red meats and high-fat dairy products, or added more fish to their diet. But, are they doing enough? Are *you* doing enough to reduce your risks for heart disease and cancer? In many cases, the answer may be no. The diet changes mentioned above clearly are beneficial, but the diet still may be too high in cholesterol, fat or salt, and too low in fiber.

This book will show you how the typical American diet plays a major role in many common diseases. It will help you achieve a healthier diet by giving you a better idea of how much fat, cholesterol, salt, sugar and fiber is optimum for you. You will learn obvious as well as hidden sources of these food components. Knowing this, you can monitor the amounts in your diet more closely. You will learn about different kinds of fat and how to read food labels. Sample daily menus will demonstrate tasty, healthy meal planning.

Once you know and understand the importance of certain foods to your body, and the bad effects of other foods, changing to a healthier diet becomes much easier. Finally you have the *motivation* to make gradual and permanent diet changes, knowing that it will reduce your risks for a wide array of the most common diseases.

Other life-style changes to promote good health will also be addressed, including weight control and exercise. All these changes together will significantly reduce your risks for heart disease, cancer, high blood pressure and intestinal diseases. Perhaps, even more important, these diet and life-style changes, by helping you maintain better health, should improve the *quality* of your life during your middle and later years.

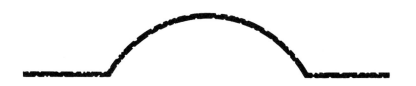

# PART ONE

*A Guide to
Healthful Eating
and Weight Control*

# ONE

## The Relationship Between Diet and Disease

### ATHEROSCLEROSIS, HEART DISEASE AND STROKE

These three terms—atherosclerosis, heart disease and stroke—are closely related. Atherosclerosis occurs when plaque, made up primarily of cholesterol, is formed on artery walls. This restricts the opening of the arteries and causes a dangerous impediment to blood flow. One of the most common sites for this to occur is in the three pencil-thin coronary arteries which carry blood to the heart. When atherosclerosis affects these arteries, the term coronary heart disease (CHD) or coronary artery disease is used. If one of these arteries is severely blocked, a small clot can totally cut off the blood supply to the heart, resulting in a heart attack. If this happens in a clogged artery leading to the brain, a stroke results. A coronary artery spasm, often a result of severe stress, can also damage the heart by temporarily reducing or shutting off blood flow.

Sometimes when a coronary artery becomes severely blocked, smaller arteries upstream from the blockage open up and take over, actually bypassing the blockage. This is referred to as collateral circulation. Circulation to the heart is maintained, but with less than ideal blood flow. This phenomenon is what enables some people to function fairly normally with nearly total blockage of one or more coronary arteries. Figure 1.1 shows the cross-section of a coronary artery with no atherosclerosis, and progressive stages of the disease.

Atherosclerosis and its related diseases cause 51% of all the deaths in the United States each year—more than all other diseases and accidents combined! Each year 1.5 million Americans have heart attacks and over one-third of these die as a result of their first heart attack. Over 750,000 suffer strokes, which account for approximately 250,000 deaths annually. Many survivors do not fully recover—71% of stroke victims and 24% of heart attack victims find themselves

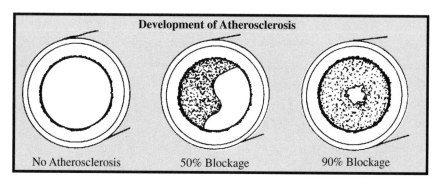

**Development of Atherosclerosis**

No Atherosclerosis    50% Blockage    90% Blockage

Figure 1.1 The cross-section of a coronary artery showing the progression of atherosclerosis.

with physical or mental limitations. Even more distressing is the fact that 16% of stroke victims and 11% of heart attack victims are left incapacitated.

Heart disease develops silently, over a period of many years. Often no symptoms appear until one of the coronary arteries is over 90% closed. In most cases, a physical exam will not disclose the disease until it is in its advanced stages. A resting EKG (electrocardiogram), for example, often records a "normal" pattern unless there is a blockage greater than 90%. A vigorous stress treadmill EKG test usually picks up coronary artery disease earlier, but not until a blockage obstructs about 65 to 90% of an artery.

## ATHEROSCLEROTIC CHANGES BEGIN IN EARLY LIFE

Atherosclerotic changes begin to develop at a much earlier age than most people are aware. In 1,600 autopsies conducted by the Louisiana State University School of Medicine, it was found that fatty streaks (the earliest visible sign of atherosclerosis) were found in all children over three years old. Plaque deposits were present in some individuals in the second decade of life and were more frequent in the third decade, with males having greater evidence of disease than females. By the end of the fourth decade (age 39), plaque deposits of varying degrees were present in a *majority* of subjects, both male and female. It was found that our population cannot be divided into those individuals having or not having atherosclerosis, but rather, it must be divided according to the degree of severity of the disease.

Autopsy studies done on American soldiers who died in Korea and Vietnam also demonstrate the early onset of this disease. In 1953, Dr. William Enos published the results of his studies on 300 American soldiers killed in the Korean War. The autopsies showed that 77% of the men had evidence of coronary artery disease, ranging from minimal thickening to total closure of one or more of the three main coronary arteries. Three percent of these men had complete closure of one or more

coronary vessels. Their average age was 22. In autopsies performed on soldiers killed in action in Vietnam, it was found that 5% had severe atherosclerosis.

## CHOLESTEROL LEVELS—KEY INDICATORS OF CORONARY HEART DISEASE

Cholesterol levels have proven to be reliable indicators of the extent of atherosclerosis present in the body. Autopsy studies have shown a direct correlation between elevated cholesterol levels and the degree of atherosclerosis. Cholesterol levels are also excellent predictors of the likelihood of developing heart disease; the higher the levels, the greater the chance of suffering a heart attack or other heart related problems.

On the other hand, reducing cholesterol levels lowers the risk for heart disease. In 1984, after a 10-year study, an advisory panel of the National Institutes of Health came to this conclusion: "For every 1% reduction in blood cholesterol, there is a 2% reduction in the risk of coronary heart disease." Thus, if you lower your blood cholesterol level by 25% and maintain it (using diet, drugs or a combination of both), you will lower your risk of heart attack and other complications of heart disease by 50%. Dr. Daniel Steinberg, chairman of the advisory panel, stated that if Americans would change their diets to reduce cholesterol levels by just 10%, then ultimately 100,000 fewer would die each year. Changes at any point in life are beneficial, but the earlier the changes are made, the better. Figure 1.2 shows the relationship of blood cholesterol levels to an increased risk of coronary heart disease, based on the reputable Framingham Heart Study.

Population studies, comparing the mean cholesterol levels and fat intake between nations, further verify the relationships between cholesterol lev-

Figure 1.2 Risk of coronary heart disease (includes heart attack or angina resulting from physical exertion or excitement) over a six year period, in men aged 30 to 49 years, based on total cholesterol levels.

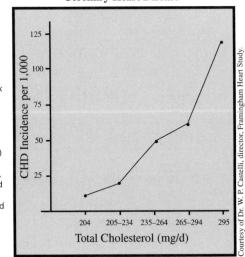

**Relationship of Blood Cholesterol Levels to Increased Incidence of Coronary Heart Disease**

Courtesy of Dr. W. P. Castelli, director, Framingham Heart Study.

els, diet and the risk of CHD. Western countries, where the majority of people consume a high-fat diet (approximately 40% of calories from fat), have higher cholesterol levels and are at greater risk for heart disease. Oriental countries and Third World nations, where a low-fat diet is the norm (10 to 20% of calories from fat), have low cholesterol levels and lower incidence of heart disease. The mean cholesterol level for adults in Japan is 163 milligrams per deciliter (mg/dl), while in the United States, it is 250. Our incidence of heart disease is 10 times greater than in Japan. Eastern Finland has the world's highest mortality rate from heart disease and its mean cholesterol level is 270. Its people consume a very high-fat diet (40+% of calories from fat) and much of the fat is highly saturated. Other population studies further document this relationship.

## SIGNIFICANCE OF DIET VS. GENETICS

In an attempt to see if genetics played a role in the wide discrepancies in cholesterol levels between nations, Dr. Ancel Keys of the University of Minnesota studied three groups of Japanese—each living in a different environment, with totally different diets. The first group lived in Japan and consumed a low-fat Asian diet consisting of about 10% of calories from fat. The second group lived in Hawaii and had a combination of the oriental diet and the American diet. The third group lived in Los Angeles and ate a typical American diet of about 40% of calories from fat. The blood cholesterol levels and incidence of heart attack rose with each group. The Japanese living in Los Angeles suffered 10 times as many heart attacks as those who lived in Japan! Their incidence of heart attack became the same as the average American.

According to the Journal of the American Medical Association, 80% of middle-aged men in America probably run a sizable risk of dying prematurely from heart disease because the cholesterol level in their blood is too high. Research has indicated that *over 50% of all middle-aged adult males in the United States have a serious blockage of one or more of their coronary arteries*. A woman's development of heart disease is slower than a man's, due in part to her production of estrogen during the reproductive years. Estrogen is a sex hormone produced by the ovaries which seems to lower blood cholesterol and the risk of coronary artery disease. However, shortly after menopause when estrogen production decreases, women experience heart attacks at approximately the same rate as men.

The most promising news is that by reducing blood cholesterol levels, we not only lower the risk of suffering from heart disease, but, in some cases, can actually *reverse* the disease process. Lowering cholesterol levels can reduce plaque deposits and increase blood flow to the heart in some individuals. This fact was announced in June 1987, by David Blankenhorn and colleagues at the University of Southern California, when they released the results of their two-year study. They reported that by lowering total blood cholesterol levels (an average of 26%) with diet and drugs over a two-year period, vessel disease was decreased in 16.2% of the men studied. The others receiving the drug/diet therapy showed significantly less progression of disease than the control group (no treatment).

In another study published in 1990, 82% of a small group of heart patients (28 patients) experienced reversal of disease (a slight reduction in plaque deposits) after following a strict vegetarian diet in combination with comprehensive lifestyle changes. This reversal occurred after just one year's time and without the use of cholesterol-lowering drugs.

The participants in this study, conducted by Dr. Dean Ornish of the University of California at San Francisco, followed a diet containing less than 10% of calories from fat and 5 milligrams of cholesterol per day. In addition, they refrained from smoking and drinking caffeinated beverages; exercised moderately 30 minutes per day, six days a week; and participated in stress management training (including yoga and meditation) at least one hour a day. Salt was restricted only for those who had hypertension. Cholesterol levels were lowered significantly, in some cases by as much as half. Chest pains disappeared in nearly all those who had complained of them prior to the study.

More recent studies have shown that disease reversal also can be accomplished, although to a lesser extent, with less restrictive diets. One study, published in 1992 in *Circulation*, reported that 32% of a group of 56 men who had partially blocked coronary arteries, experienced a reversal of blockages after one year on a moderately restrictive low-fat diet. The diet consisted of less than 20% of calories from fat, less than 7% of calories from saturated fat and less than 200 mg cholesterol per day. The participants also took part in an exercise program for at least 30 minutes per day.

In studies with Rhesus monkeys, severe coronary artery disease was produced through feeding these animals a high-fat, high-cholesterol diet. (Extensive disease was found in all the monkeys fed this diet. Ordinarily, these animals consume a low-fat diet and heart disease is rare.) On the other hand, after three years of feeding the monkeys a low-fat, cholesterol-free diet, the arterial blockages were reduced from 60% to only 20%.

From these studies, it becomes apparent that diet is a two-sided coin — It can either work for you or against you, depending on the choices made. The best research to date has shown that if cholesterol levels are kept below 150 (mg/dl) throughout a lifetime, heart attacks are virtually nonexistent. From 150 to 180, significant atherosclerosis and related diseases are extremely rare. From 180 to 200, the incidence of heart disease increases only slightly; and above 200, it increases more dramatically (See Figure 1.2). The National Institutes of Health recommends that all adults over 20 should strive to keep cholesterol levels below 200. Children's cholesterol levels should be less than 170.

Since most people are not willing to follow a diet as restrictive as in the Ornish study, prevention should be the primary goal. For most, this can be accomplished with a lifelong program of following a low-fat diet consisting of 20% of calories from fat and adopting other aspects of a healthy life-style. Additional information on cholesterol appears in Chapters 2, 3 and 8.

## HIGH BLOOD PRESSURE

High blood pressure, or hypertension, as it is sometimes called, occurs when the heart is forced to pump harder to move the blood throughout the body. Its causes are not fully understood, but the main factors affecting the disease are age, stress, genetics and diet. The most important dietary factors are too much sodium (found in greatest concentration in table salt and other condiments and processed foods), obesity, too little potassium and calcium, and too much alcohol.

High blood pressure increases the risk for heart disease, heart attacks and strokes. When the blood is pumped with greater pressure through the blood vessels, it gradually weakens them or causes cracks to develop in the lining of the vessels. Cholesterol, circulating in the bloodstream, is deposited in these cracks. Smooth muscle tissue develops at these sites, and together with the cholesterol, form atherosclerotic plaque. Thus, the atherosclerotic process is accelerated when hypertension is accompanied by high cholesterol. In addition, the damaged arteries are more susceptible to forming blood clots, increasing the risk of a heart attack or a stroke. The heart muscle itself weakens and enlarges as a result of hypertension, causing greater stress to the heart. Figure 1.3 shows how the risk factors for heart attack are cumulative. For each additional risk factor—smoking, high cholesterol and high blood pressure—the overall risk increases significantly.

Hypertension, like high cholesterol, can go unnoticed for years because there are no symptoms until the damage is excessive. Nearly 25% of the adult population over the age of 40 has high blood pressure. The incidence increases with age, affecting more than 50% of Americans over the age of 65.

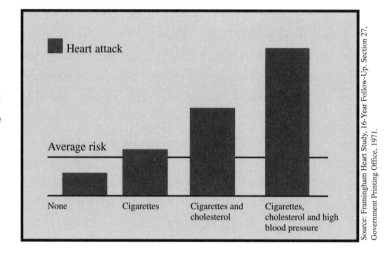

Figure 1.3 The danger of heart attack increases with the number of risk factors present (using the example of a 45-year-old male). Numbers represent the incidence per 100,000 population.

Source: Framingham Heart Study, 16-Year Follow-Up. Section 27, Government Printing Office, 1971.

## DIETARY INFLUENCES ON BLOOD PRESSURE

Numerous studies have indicated a definite link between a high-salt diet and the incidence of high blood pressure. Cultures that consume high amounts of salt, such as in Northern Japan (20,000 milligrams of sodium or about 9 teaspoons of salt per day),* have the highest incidence of elevated blood pressure, and societies such as the Alaskan Eskimos, who eat very little sodium (less than 2,000 milligrams per day), have almost no hypertension. The same correlation was found by Dr. Lot Page of Harvard, who studied six primitive tribes in the Solomon Islands. Three of the tribes ate a high-salt diet and it was only in these three that high blood pressure existed. The other three tribes consumed a low-salt diet (less than 2,000 milligrams of sodium per day) and had virtually no hypertension.

Researchers have found that high blood pressure among adults is rare when sodium consumption throughout a lifetime is less that 2,000 milligrams per day.

* One teaspoon salt contains approximately 2,300 milligrams sodium.

The average American consumes 3,000 to 6,000 milligrams daily, equivalent to one-and-a-half to three teaspoons of salt. The Recommended Dietary Allowance (RDA) for sodium is a minimum of 500 milligrams and a maximum of 2,400 milligrams per day, well below the average American intake. The RDA includes sodium from all sources—table salt, processed foods and the sodium that occurs naturally in foods. (The sodium present naturally in foods accounts for only 10% or less of total sodium intake.)

High blood pressure also has been produced in laboratory animals by feeding them a high-salt diet. Some strains of animals are more susceptible, suggesting genetic factors. This is also the case with humans, because about half are not salt-sensitive; that is, their blood pressure is not adversely affected by salt consumption.

Obesity can also contribute to high blood pressure. Obese adults (weight greater than 20% above desired weight) have double the incidence of high blood pressure as non-obese individuals. Overweight people with high blood pressure who lose 50% of their excess weight often experience a significant reduction in blood pressure.

Studies have also shown a steady increase in blood pressure as alcohol consumption increases. More than one or two drinks per day, or about an ounce of alcohol, causes blood pressure to rise in some individuals. Those who have high blood pressure, therefore, should be careful to limit their alcohol intake.

## CANCER

Cancer accounts for 20% of all deaths in the United States each year. Dr. Peter Greenwald, director of the National Cancer Institute (NCI), estimates that diet is a significant factor in about one-third of all cancers. Other researchers have estimated the figure to be even higher—from 40 to 60%.

*The main factors in the diet that lead to an increased incidence of cancer are excessive fat, inadequate intake of fruits and vegetables and too little fiber.* Added substances such as preservatives and pesticides are also a concern, but food substances such as fat cause an estimated 35 times as much disease as added substances, according to a report by Tufts University Nutrition Department.

In both animal experiments and population studies it has been shown that the higher the intake of fat, the greater the likelihood of malignant tumors; especially of the colon, prostate and breast. Fiber intake primarily affects colon cancer rates; populations that eat a high-fiber diet have a lower incidence of colon cancer.

One of the most convincing population studies linking cancer with fat intake involves a comparison of breast cancer rates between Japanese and American women. Both groups live in highly industrialized societies with similar amounts of environmental pollution, which eliminates pollution as a probable cause of the discrepancies. Nevertheless, Japanese women have less than one-quarter the incidence of breast cancer as American women. Prior to World War II, their incidence was only one-tenth that of Americans. At that time, their fat consumption was only about 12% of total calories, but now it is about 24%, compared to our approximately 40%.

In addition, when Japanese migrate to the United States, the second generation's breast cancer death rate equals the rate of Americans. This suggests that the differences are not due to genetics. Other international studies show that although there may be large differences in the incidence of cancer between nations, after one or more generations, the migrant groups experience the same cancer rate as the host country. A change in dietary habits is considered the primary reason for this occurrence.

Even within a country, studies have shown that as fat intake increases, so does the incidence of cancer. Since World War II, there have been dramatic increases in cancer rates in Japan, Greece and Iceland, which coincides with an increase in fat consumption. Figure 1.4 shows the relationship between breast cancer rates and fat consumption of 40 different countries.

High-fat diets also produce more malignant tumors in laboratory animals than low-fat diets. In at least 25 different studies in different countries, it was shown that animals fed a low-fat diet (10 to 20% of calories), exhibited one-third to one-half fewer breast tumors than those fed a high-fat diet (40% of calories.) This is the case regardless of the type of fat used.

## COLON CANCER: EXCESSIVE FAT & INSUFFICIENT FIBER

Colon cancer is linked to *both* excessive fat and insufficient fiber in the diet. Recent population studies suggest that the concentration of bile acids in the feces (body's waste products) is the most significant factor in predicting the incidence of colon cancer in population groups. The higher the fat intake, the higher the amount of bile acids in feces, and consequently, the greater the incidence of cancer. Bile acids are made in the liver, stored in the gall bladder, and are secreted into the intestines to help digest fat.

Dietary fiber, researchers say, helps protect against cancer by increasing the volume of feces and thereby diluting the concentration of bile acids in the stool. It is not known whether the bile acids irri-

## The International Fat–Breast Cancer Link

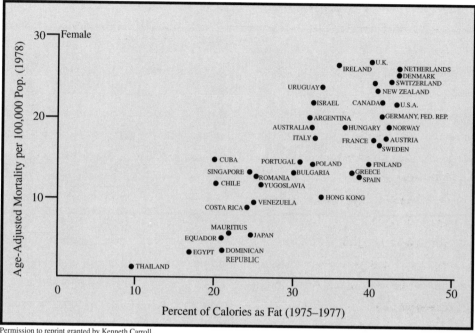

Figure 1.4 A high-fat diet, in countries such as the U.S., is associated with higher rates of death from breast cancer.

tate the colon wall, leaving it more vulnerable to cancer-causing agents, or if the bile acids are converted into carcinogens by fecal bacteria.

Whatever the case, epidemiologic studies have shown that fat is a stronger cancer promoter than fiber is a protector. For example, the Finnish diet is high in fat and fiber, and Finns have half the colon cancer rate of Americans. Japanese, on the other hand, consume a low-fat, low-fiber diet and their colon cancer rate is only one-fourth that of the United States.

## DIETARY FACTORS TO LOWER RISK OF CANCER

Just as choosing high-fat foods can increase the risk of developing certain types of cancer, making wise dietary choices can decrease risk. Foods which have demonstrated a protective effect against cancer are whole grain foods, which are good sources of fiber, and fruits and vegetables, especially the cruciferous vegetables and those that contain the antioxidants vitamin C and beta carotene. Beta carotene, found in deep green and yellow fruits and vegetables, is a "pre-vitamin," which is converted to vitamin A during digestion. Vitamin C is found in a wide variety of fruits and vegetables, especially citrus fruits.

Cruciferous vegetables, which include broccoli, cauliflower, cabbage,

Brussels sprouts and others, contain a substance called *indoles* that triggers production of special enzymes in the liver. These enzymes appear to break down cancer-promoting agents.

Looking at a combination of animal, laboratory and human studies suggests that there are many different components in fruits and vegetables that inhibit cancer. At this point, though, beta carotene has produced the most conclusive evidence of a specific food component's ability to fight cancer. Smokers who consume a lot of beta-carotene-rich foods have half the rate of lung cancer as those who consume few of these foods.

Beta carotene also has been shown to inhibit tumors in animals. Animals, exposed to a carcinogen and subsequently given beta-carotene injections, did not develop mouth tumors as did the control group not treated with beta carotene. Dr. Gerald Sklar, of the Harvard School of Dental Medicine, has stated that beta carotene and vitamin E are the first nontoxic agents that have been shown to both prevent and reverse cancer in experimental animals. (Drug-level doses of vitamin E, also an antioxidant, have been shown to enhance the immune systems of older adults, and may reduce the risk for heart disease. For information on vitamin supplements, including vitamin E, refer to Chapter 8.)

*Foods* which are good sources of fiber, beta carotene, vitamin C and indoles—not supplements—have produced the most compelling evidence of their effectiveness in reducing the risk of disease. Antioxidant supplements also may be beneficial, but they will never be an adequate substitute for eating whole grain foods, fruits and vegetables. See Chapter 6 for more information on cruciferous vegetables, and the fruits and vegetables that contain the antioxidants vitamins C and beta carotene.

## How Antioxidants Fight Disease

Oxidation is considered a major factor in the development of cancer and heart disease. Before you can understand how antioxidants work, that is, how they prevent oxidation, it is necessary to understand the oxidation process. Oxidation reactions occur because of the presence of unstable molecules called "free radicals." Free radicals are created in the body during the normal process of metabolizing foods or as a result of smoking, chemicals, viruses or certain types of radiation.

These free radicals try to create stability or electrical balance by raiding another atom or molecule, taking from that atom or molecule what it needs to achieve its own balance. This process is called oxidation. Sometimes the "raid" can damage the DNA in the cell, causing it to become cancerous. With regard to heart disease, free radicals oxidize cholesterol, which in turn draws other cells to the site to repair the "injury." These cells gobble up the oxidized cholesterol and become foam cells, which are considered to be the beginning of atherosclerotic plaque.

The antioxidants work by attaching to these potentially harmful free radicals, rendering them harmless. For this reason, they are called antioxidants because they prevent harmful oxidation from occurring, just as a rust-preventive prohibits rusting, another form of oxidation.

## INTESTINAL DISORDERS

A low-fiber diet contributes to a number of intestinal disorders in addition to colon cancer. These include diverticulosis, irritable bowel syndrome, constipation and hemorrhoids.

Fiber's role in disease prevention first became apparent early in this century. British physicians Denis Burkitt and Hugh Trowell found that rural Africans, consuming a diet of unprocessed, unrefined foods, were virtually free of the intestinal disorders that plagued Western cultures. Decades after the Africans moved to the cities and changed to a more refined diet, their incidence of these diseases rose significantly. Numerous studies on other population groups have confirmed the relationship between a high-fiber diet and low incidence of intestinal disorders.

Intestinal diseases are common in the United States. Colon cancer is the second most prevalent type of cancer and the number one cause of cancer death in people who do not smoke. Constipation and diverticulosis were rare in Western cultures 60 years ago—before refined grains replaced whole-grain products; when meat consumption was lower; and when beans, fruits and vegetables were consumed in greater quantities. Now diverticulosis affects one in three U.S. adults over the age of 60, and constipation is common among all ages but especially among older adults. Irritable bowel syndrome, which causes abdominal pain, accompanied by either diarrhea or constipation, affects nearly 15 to 20% of the adult population. Hemorrhoids affect approximately one-half of all adults over the age of 50.

Fiber is the indigestible portion of plant food. There are two kinds—insoluble and soluble, and both play an important role in the body's health. Insoluble fiber, found primarily in wheat bran, beans, and the peelings of fruits and vegetables, helps prevent constipation. It does this by adding bulk to the feces and attracting water into the digestive tract, which helps move it through the colon at a faster rate. Because fiber attracts water, it is very important to drink an adequate amount of liquid to allow fiber to work properly. (Eight cups of liquid per day is recommended.) The increased volume from fiber and water dilutes the bacteria and bile acids present in feces.

Diets low in insoluble fiber produce firm fecal material within the large intestine, which is difficult to propel through the colon. This often results in constipation. It is thought that chronic constipation leads to diverticulosis. This occurs when excess pressure, exerted to move the fecal matter, builds up within the bowel and causes small pouches (diverticula) to form in the weakened walls of the colon. Diverticulitis occurs when these pouches become inflamed and cause intestinal pain. Hemorrhoids are also a common result of constipation.

Soluble fiber is a special type of fiber that is water soluble and found primarily in oat bran, beans and certain fruits and vegetables. It is beneficial to the body in two ways. First, it binds fatty compounds, including cholesterol, and carries them out of the body with the feces. This lowers blood cholesterol concentration and helps reduce the risk of heart disease. Soluble fiber also has a positive effect on the body's response to glucose. It delays the absorption of nutrients from the intestine, causing a gradual increase in blood sugar rather than a rapid one. This is especially important for people with diabetes.

## OBESITY

Obesity is a serious health problem in our country. Fifteen per cent of the American population, or 34 million people, are 20% or more over their "ideal" body weight. An additional 10 to 15% are overweight to a lesser degree. "Ideal" body weights are based on the 1983 Metropolitan Life Insurance Company table of desirable body weights. (See Table 1.1, page 15.)

According to a study by the Provident Mutual Life Insurance Company of male policyholders, it was found that mortality rates increased with weight. The more overweight, the more likely to die prematurely. "The weights asso-

## 1983 Metropolitan Height and Weight Tables for Men and Women
## According to Frame, Ages 25–59

Weight in Pounds (in indoor clothing)*

| Height (in Shoes)† | | Small Frame | Medium Frame | Large Frame |
|---|---|---|---|---|
| Feet | Inches | | **Men** | |
| 5 | 2 | 128–134 | 131–141 | 138–150 |
| 5 | 3 | 130–136 | 133–143 | 140–153 |
| 5 | 4 | 132–138 | 135–145 | 142–156 |
| 5 | 5 | 134–140 | 137–148 | 144–160 |
| 5 | 6 | 136–142 | 139–151 | 146–164 |
| 5 | 7 | 138–145 | 142–154 | 149–168 |
| 5 | 8 | 140–148 | 145–157 | 152–172 |
| 5 | 9 | 142–151 | 148–160 | 155–176 |
| 5 | 10 | 144–154 | 151–163 | 158–180 |
| 5 | 11 | 146–157 | 154–166 | 161–184 |
| 6 | 0 | 149–160 | 157–170 | 164–188 |
| 6 | 1 | 152–164 | 160–174 | 168–192 |
| 6 | 2 | 155–168 | 164–178 | 172–197 |
| 6 | 3 | 158–172 | 167–182 | 176–202 |
| 6 | 4 | 162–176 | 171–187 | 181–207 |
| | | | **Women** | |
| 4 | 10 | 102–111 | 109–121 | 118–131 |
| 4 | 11 | 103–113 | 111–123 | 120–134 |
| 5 | 0 | 104–115 | 113–126 | 122–137 |
| 5 | 1 | 106–118 | 115–129 | 125–140 |
| 5 | 2 | 108–121 | 118–132 | 128–143 |
| 5 | 3 | 111–124 | 121–135 | 131–147 |
| 5 | 4 | 114–127 | 124–138 | 134–151 |
| 5 | 5 | 117–130 | 127–141 | 137–155 |
| 5 | 6 | 120–133 | 130–144 | 140–159 |
| 5 | 7 | 123–136 | 133–147 | 143–163 |
| 5 | 8 | 126–139 | 136–150 | 146–167 |
| 5 | 9 | 129–142 | 139–153 | 149–170 |
| 5 | 10 | 132–145 | 142–156 | 152–173 |
| 5 | 11 | 135–148 | 145–159 | 155–176 |
| 6 | 0 | 138–151 | 148–162 | 158–179 |

Table 1.1

* Indoor clothing weighing 5 pounds for men and 3 pounds for women.
†Shoes with 1-inch heels

Source of basic data: *Build Study*, 1979 (Society of Actuaries and Association of Life Insurance Medical Directors of America, 1980).
Copyright 1983 Metropolitan Life Insurance Company.

ciated with the greatest longevity, according to the National Institutes of Health, are *below the average* weights of the population, as long as such weights are not associated with illness."

"Obesity is as powerful a risk factor as any that we know, including smoking and high blood pressure," according to Dr. William Castelli, a highly respected medical researcher and director of the Framingham (Massachusetts) Heart Study. Obesity is an added risk factor for all the diseases discussed previously — cardiovascular disease, hypertension, and cancer. In addition, it contributes significantly to the development of adult-onset diabetes mellitus.

Obesity is a major problem in cultures where a high percentage of calories come from fat. It is a rarity in countries where fat intake is 20% or less. The reason for this is fairly simple. Protein and carbohydrates provide 4 calories per gram. Fat yields 9 calories per gram. That means that you can eat *twice* as much in quantity of protein and carbohydrate than you can fat, and still ingest the same number of calories. On a 20% fat diet, 1,000 calories provides the same amount of bulk as 1,600 calories in a diet of 40% fat. This bulk, without excess calories, provides you with a feeling of fullness or satisfaction, making it easier to maintain an ideal body weight. If the typical American diet were composed of approximately 20% fat, far fewer people would be overweight. In Chapter 3, we will show you how to plan a diet of *either* 10%, 20% or 30% of calories from fat.

## SUMMARY

Diet truly does play a crucial role in overall health. By eating the right foods, we *can* greatly reduce the risk of dying prematurely from heart disease or cancer. We can also reduce the chances of being plagued by intestinal disorders. We have greater control over our health than many people are aware, as the numerous research studies have shown.

If we exercise this control by eating right, we practice "preventive medicine." The food we consume will be nourishing our body and helping to prevent disease, rather than clogging our arteries, adding excess fat, or promoting high blood pressure, cancer and intestinal diseases.

Necessary changes are not difficult to make, but first you need to know *what* you are eating. To do this, you must understand some basics; in particular, the different types of fat, and how to read and interpret food labels. These topics will be explained in the next chapter.

# TWO

## Understanding the Basics: Types of Fat and Reading Food Labels

### THE DIFFERENT TYPES OF FAT

#### CHOLESTEROL

Cholesterol is a special type of fat present only in foods of animal origin — red meats, fish, poultry and dairy products. Vegetables and vegetable products do not contain cholesterol. Cholesterol is a vital component in the body's production of cell membranes, hormones and bile acid, which is needed for fat digestion.

Despite its important role in the body, there is no *dietary* need for cholesterol; that is, we do not need to eat foods containing cholesterol. Whatever cholesterol the body needs is manufactured in the liver. The health problems associated with cholesterol occur when too much is present in the blood and the excess is deposited on the artery walls forming atherosclerotic plaque.

#### HOW CHOLESTEROL TRAVELS IN YOUR BLOODSTREAM

Cholesterol is transported through the bloodstream in special protein packages called lipoproteins. (Lipo (fat) + protein = lipoprotein.) Since cholesterol is a type of fat, it is insoluble in water, and therefore must have a water-soluble material to carry it through the bloodstream. Water-soluble protein molecules surround cholesterol and other fat particles, and carry them via the bloodstream to all parts of the body. The two lipoproteins that are the principal trans-porters of cholesterol are: *high-density lipoproteins*, also referred to as HDL or "good" cholesterol, and *low- density lipoproteins*, commonly referred to as LDL or "bad" cholesterol.

HDL cholesterol moves cholesterol out of the body, transporting it from the blood vessels and tissues to the liver. There, much of it is converted to bile acids to aid in fat digestion, and later excreted in the stools. The higher the HDL levels in the blood, the lower the risk of developing heart disease.

LDL cholesterol, on the other hand, moves cholesterol in the opposite direction—from the liver to the various organs and tissues, including the artery walls. High levels of this cholesterol promote atherosclerosis. Although heredity plays some role in the level of LDL in the blood, the high-fat American diet is the principal reason that so many Americans (over 50% of the adult population) have high cholesterol levels. (Additional information on cholesterol, medical tests and ways to improve blood cholesterol levels appears in Chapter 9.)

## SATURATED, POLYUNSATURATED AND MONOUNSATURATED FATS

All the fats and oils we consume contain a combination of saturated, polyunsaturated and monounsaturated fats. The fat may be visible, such as cooking oils and butter, or "hidden" in the foods we eat, such as in peanuts, meats and baked goods.

Although all the fats in our diet contain a combination of these three types, they are generally classified by the primary type of fat present. For example, the fat of sirloin steak is commonly referred to as saturated fat. This fat is indeed highly saturated (52%), but it also contains monounsaturated fat (44%) and polyunsaturated fat (4%). A "highly polyunsaturated" oil such as corn oil contains 61% polyunsaturated, 26% monounsaturated and 13% saturated fat.

These three types of fats have different chemical structures which give them different characteristics. Saturated fats are harder at room temperature and far more stable chemically. The greater stability means that the fats will not spoil or turn rancid for a much longer period of time.

Polyunsaturated fats are less stable chemically which makes them vulnerable to attack by oxygen. When this happens, the oils become rancid, causing the foods made with them to spoil. The more unsaturated a fat, the more liquid it is at room temperature.

Monounsaturated fats differ in chemical structure from polyunsaturated fats, but their characteristics are similar. They are liquid at room temperature and have a shorter shelf life than saturated fats.

Highly saturated fats are the ones responsible for elevating blood cholesterol levels, which can lead to atherosclerosis, heart attack or stroke. The research to date shows that monounsaturated and polyunsaturated fats do not raise blood cholesterol levels.

Knowing that all fats and oils are a combination of the three types of fats is important, especially when trying to lower cholesterol levels. If you *substitute* highly polyunsaturated fat for highly saturated fat, e.g., substitute margarine for butter, your cholesterol levels should drop to some degree because you are consuming less saturated fat. But, the important point to remember is that all the highly monounsaturated and polyunsaturated fats and oils contain some saturated fats. Therefore, the most effective way to lower blood cholesterol levels is to reduce *total fat* intake.

Recent studies have shown that the monounsaturated oils (olive, canola and peanut oils), are preferable to polyunsaturated oils in regard to cholesterol levels. When used instead of saturated fats, both oils lowered LDL cholesterol about the same. However, the monounsaturated oil did not lower the HDL or "good cholesterol," whereas the polyunsaturated oil did slightly. In addition, monos are less susceptible to oxidation, a key element in the formation of plaque deposits; and monos do not promote tumors in animals as polyunsaturated oils do. Considering all these factors, it is advisable to use monounsaturated oils whenever suitable. Olive oil is excellent with stir-fry dishes and on salads; while canola oil, with a milder flavor, works well in baking.

Our bodies have no nutritional need for saturated fat. The only fat essential to our diet is polyunsaturated fat. In order to meet the minimum daily requirement for polyunsaturated fat (3 to 6 grams), you should consume at least 12 to 15 grams of total fat per day, from all sources including the fat already present in foods. If you eat a well-balanced diet with a variety of foods, you will be sure to meet the minimum requirement. The majority of Americans consume from 80 to 130 grams (16 to 26 teaspoons) of fat per day.

## HYDROGENATED FATS

Hydrogenated fats are polyunsaturated fats that have been transformed to more highly saturated fats. Chemists found a simple way to do it: in a large processing vat, liquid oil is bombarded with hydrogen atoms, and the result is shortening—a man-made saturated fat!

Why do manufacturers do this? Remember the commercial advantage of saturated fat just mentioned—a much longer shelf life. The cookies and potato chips on grocery store shelves will stay fresh much longer—for weeks, months, and in some cases years. This greatly reduces the chances of dissatisfied customers returning spoiled merchandise.

Another advantage is that hydrogenated fats have a higher smoking point, which means foods don't scorch as easily at the high temperatures used for frying. This results in significant monetary savings to the food service industry, especially for fast-food restaurants, which don't have to change the grease as often in their deep-fat fryers.

The down side is that the hydrogenation process produces trans fatty acids. This is a unique type of fat that appears to raise cholesterol levels to approximately the same degree as saturated fats. Our diet, though, contains much less trans fats than saturated fats. It is estimated that one-third to one-half of the fat we eat is saturated, whereas less than one-tenth is trans fats.

The foods that contain hydrogenated fats, such as margarine and shortening, do raise cholesterol levels to a greater extent than previously thought. However, margarine is still a better choice than butter because it has *fewer* cholesterol-raising fats. The bottom line is to go light on all fats, margarine included, and select the softer margarines (in a tub) because they are less hydrogenated, or even better yet, use liquid vegetable oils.

## ANIMAL VS. VEGETABLE FAT

Many people think of vegetable fat as liquid and heart-healthy, and animal fat as the type responsible for clogging arteries. The distinction between these two is not that simple, however. Most vegetable fats are indeed liquid at room temperature and highly polyunsaturated or monounsaturated, but some are hard at room temperature and highly saturated. Highly saturated vegetable oils include palm oil, palm kernel oil, coconut oil, cocoa butter and some hydrogenated vegetable oils. See Figure 2.1 for a classification of vegetable oils.

On the other hand, most animal fats are more highly saturated, which means they are more solid at room temperature. The degree of saturation varies, with poultry fat less saturated, and beef fat and butter fat much more so. Fish oil, an unusual animal fat, is in a class by itself. It is less saturated than poultry fat, (most varieties range from 15 to 25% saturated) and in addition, it contains a unique type of polyunsaturated fat, called

Figure 2.1 Vegetable oils are classified by the type of fat most prominent in their chemical composition. Actually all fats and oils include a combination of polyunsaturated, monounsaturated and saturated fats.

| Types of Vegetable Oils | | |
|---|---|---|
| **Highly Polyunsaturated** | **Highly Monounsaturated** | **Highly Saturated*** |
| Corn oil | Olive oil | Coconut oil |
| Safflower oil | Peanut oil | Palm oil |
| Sunflower oil | Canola oil | Palm kernel oil |
| Sesame oil | Cocoa butter | |
| Soybean oil | | |
| Cottonseed oil | | |
| *Have greatest cholesterol-raising effect. | | |

**Comparison of Dietary Fats**

| Dietary Fat | Fatty Acid Content Normalized to 100% | | |
|---|---|---|---|
| Canola oil | 6% | 32% | 62% |
| Safflower oil | 10% | 77% | 13% |
| Sunflower oil | 11% | 69% | 20% |
| Corn oil | 13% | 62% | 25% |
| Olive oil | 14% | 9% | 77% |
| Soybean oil | 15% | 61% | 24% |
| Peanut oil | 18% | 33% | 49% |
| Margarine | 19% | 32% | 49% |
| Cottonseed oil | 27% | 54% | 19% |
| Vegetable shortening* | 28% | 28% | 44% |
| Chicken fat | 31% | 22% | 47% |
| Lard | 41% | 12% | 47% |
| Beef fat | 52% | 4% | 44% |
| Palm oil | 52% | 10% | 38% |
| Cocoa butter | 61% | 5% | 34% |
| Butter (fat) | 66% | 4% | 30% |
| Palm kernel oil | 86% | 2% | 12% |
| Coconut oil | 92% | 2% | 6% |

Saturated Fat    Polyunsaturated Fat    Monounsaturated Fat

Figure 2.2 Breakdown of dietary fats into percentage of saturated, polyunsaturated and monounsaturated fats.

*Crisco shortening

Source: *Agriculture Handbook* No. 8-4. Washington, D.C., U.S. Department of Agriculture.

omega-3 fatty acids. Fish oil actually has been shown to have a *protective* effect against heart disease, but only if it is used *in place of* highly saturated fats. (See next section on fish oils.)

Refer to Figure 2.2 for a breakdown of the percentage of saturated, polyunsaturated and monounsaturated fats in various vegetable and animal fats/oils.

## FISH OILS

Fish oils contain a unique type of polyunsaturated fat known as omega-3 fatty acids. (It is sometimes sold in health-food stores under a specific name or abbreviation, such as EPA for eicosapentaenoic acid or DHA for docosahexaenoic acid.) These fish oils, *when consumed in large quantities in place of* *saturated fat*, have been shown to lower both LDL cholesterol levels and triglycerides. (Triglycerides are other fats circulating in the blood, which may also contribute to heart disease.) In addition, fish oils affect the blood in a similar way to aspirin — they "thin" the blood, making the blood platelets less sticky and thus less likely to form blood clots. They also appear to inhibit the formation of atherosclerotic plaque, which reduces the risks of heart attack and stroke.

These beneficial properties of fish oils first came to light through studies with the Greenland Eskimos. Scientists were puzzled by their low incidence of heart disease. Even though their diet was very high in animal fat from seal meat, fish and whale blubber, their incidence of heart attack was about 100 times lower than in the United States.

When these same Eskimos moved to Denmark and ate the typical Western diet, their incidence of heart disease rose dramatically, to match that of the Danes and other Western Europeans. It was determined that it was the specific *type* of polyunsaturated fat in the fish oil that made the difference. The effectiveness of these fish oils as a protective influence against heart disease was further verified in studies with Japanese fishermen and with animals in the laboratory.

Does this mean that we should eat one pound of fish per day as the Eskimos do, or its equivalent of over two tablespoons of fish oil supplements per day? The answer is no, because of the associated health hazards and because more research still needs to be done to determine what, if any, are *safe and effective* doses of the supplements. Although the Eskimos have an extremely low incidence of heart disease, they have other health problems resulting from their high consumption of fish oils. They bruise easily, have frequent nosebleeds, and have prolonged bleeding times, which can lead to a variety of health problems.

Taking supplements of cod-liver oil or other fish oils in quantities of a tablespoon a day or more could lead to problems similar to those mentioned above. In addition, some fish oil supplements (cod-liver oil, especially) can cause vitamin A and D toxicity, because these vitamins are stored in the body and the amounts build up over time. Toxic levels of these vitamins cause serious side effects, and may even cause death.

Because of uncertainties regarding the safety and effectiveness of fish oil supplements, omega-3 oils should be obtained by *eating* fish, rather than taking supplements. Fish is an excellent low-fat protein source; and the type of fat present in fish may actually help reduce the risk of heart disease.

Because of the small amount of total fat in fish (the highest-fat fish have about the same total fat as the leanest red meats), and the beneficial effects of fish oil, the recommended fish portion per day (4 to 6 ounces) is greater than that of meats (3 to 4 ounces). (See Figure 7.1, page 87, for the recommended daily servings and guidelines of the "Food Guide Pyramid.")

| Content of Omega-3 Fatty Acids of Selected Seafood (in 5.25 ounces of fish, uncooked) | |
| --- | --- |
| **Food Item** | **Omega-3 Oil Content** |
| Mackerel, Atlantic | 3.8 g |
| Mackerel, king | 3.3 g |
| Herring, Pacific | 2.6 g |
| Herring, Atlantic | 2.4 g |
| Trout, lake | 2.4 g |
| Tuna, bluefin | 2.4 g |
| Sturgeon, Atlantic | 2.3 g |
| Anchovies | 2.2 g |
| Sabelfish | 2.1 g |
| Tuna, Albacore | 2.1 g |
| Whitefish, lake | 2.0 g |
| Bluefish | 1.8 g |
| Salmon, sockeye | 1.8 g |
| Mullet | 1.7 g |
| Salmon, pink | 1.5 g |
| Halibut, Greenland | 1.4 g |
| Bass, striped | 1.2 g |
| Oysters | 0.6 to 1.2 g |
| Smelt, rainbow | 1.1 g |
| Pompano | 0.9 g |
| Mussels, blue | 0.8 g |
| Trout, rainbow | 0.8 g |
| Rockfish | 0.8 g |
| Shrimp | 0.3 to 0.8 g |
| Halibut, Pacific | 0.6 g |
| Haddock | 0.3 g |
| Lobster, Maine | 0.3 g |
| Perch, Ocean | 0.3 g |
| Red Snapper | 0.3 g |
| Swordfish | 0.3 g |
| Scallops | 0.3 g |

Source: *Journal of The American Dietetic Association,* June, 1986.

Table 2.1

Table 2.1 lists the amount of omega-3 oils present in selected seafood. Other excellent sources of omega-3 fatty acids are cooked beans, especially soybeans.

## SIMPLESSE—THE FAT SUBSTITUTE

Available to the public only since February 1990, Simplesse is a fat substitute made of egg whites and milk protein. These two ingredients are cooked and blended into a smooth thick fluid that resembles the creamy texture of fat.

The Food and Drug Administration (FDA) classified this new fat substitute as (GRAS) "generally regarded as safe," when it was released for public use. It can only be used in products that do not require heating, such as sour cream, mayonnaise, yogurt and ice cream, since baking or frying destroys its creamy texture.

The fat and calorie savings with Simplesse, as with other low-fat and nonfat foods, can be substantial. For example, an 8-ounce serving of ice cream (11% fat) has about 14 grams of fat and 270 calories, while a similar serving of nonfat ice cream made with Simplesse has less than 1 gram of fat and only 144 calories. A tablespoon of regular mayonnaise has 6 grams of fat and 65 calories, compared to less that one gram of fat and only 9 calories in mayonnaise made with Simplesse.

Simplesse makes it possible to enjoy the creamy textures of ice cream and other foods without the high fat and high calories. Still, it is best to reserve these foods for occasional use, and to choose primarily nutritious foods that do not need a rich texture to taste good, like fruits, vegetables and whole-grain products.

## INTERPRETING FOOD LABELS

In May 1994, new food labeling regulations went into effect, marking the first major overhaul of food labels in 20 years. The labels were designed to help consumers choose more healthful foods and to encourage food companies to improve the nutritional quality of their products.

The nutrition information provided on food labels includes the amount per serving of those nutrients that are of greatest importance to today's health-conscious consumer. The information is prominently displayed under the title "Nutrition Facts." (See Figure 2.3.)

Previously, only about half of all packaged foods had nutrition labels; now 90% provide this information. The exceptions are few: foods that contain no significant amounts of nutrients, such as coffee, tea and spices; ready-to-eat foods prepared primarily on site, such as deli and bakery items; foods that are produced by very small businesses; and packaged foods too small for a label to fit: for example, Life Savers candy. In the latter case, a phone number must be listed on the package, so the consumer may call to request the nutrition information.

Nutritional claims that appear on the front of food packaging, e.g. "light," "low-cholesterol" and "low-calorie," have been more carefully defined, to curb deceptive marketing. Now you can be assured that these claims have met strict guidelines and are legitimate.

**Sample Food Label**

| **Nutrition Facts** | |
|---|---|
| Serving Size 1 cup (228g) | |
| Servings Per Container 2 | |

| **Amount Per Serving** | |
|---|---|
| **Calories** 260 Calories from Fat 120 | |

| | **% Daily Value*** |
|---|---|
| **Total Fat** 13g | **20%** |
| Saturated Fat 5g | **25%** |
| **Cholesterol** 30mg | **10%** |
| **Sodium** 660mg | **28%** |
| **Total Carbohydrate** 31g | **10%** |
| Dietary Fiber 0g | **0%** |
| Sugars 5g | |
| **Protein** 5g | |

| Vitamin A 4% | • | Vitamin C 2% |
|---|---|---|
| Calcium 15% | • | Iron 4% |

\* Percent Daily Values are based on a 2,000 calorie diet. Your daily values may be higher or lower depending on your calorie needs:

| | Calories: | 2,000 | 2,500 |
|---|---|---|---|
| Total Fat | Less than | 65g | 80g |
| Sat Fat | Less than | 20g | 25g |
| Cholesterol | Less than | 300mg | 300mg |
| Sodium | Less than | 2,400mg | 2,400mg |
| Total Carbohydrate | | 300g | 375g |
| Dietary Fiber | | 25g | 30g |

Calories per gram:
Fat 9 • Carbohydrate 4 • Protein 4

← Heading "Nutrition Facts" signals a new label.

← Serving Size—Similar food products have similar serving sizes.

← Calories from Fat—Helps you better understand how much fat is in a food.

← % Daily Value—Shows how a food fits into the overall daily diet; helpful for comparison shopping.

← Nutrients shown on nutrition panel are those most important to the health of today's consumers.

← Daily Values Footnote—provides reference values on which the % Daily Values are based. Some labels show values for both a 2000- and 2500-calorie diet.

← Calories per Gram Footnote—Gives the approximate number of calories in a gram of fat, carbohydrate and protein.

Figure 2.3
Sample Food
Label

## NUTRITION LABEL FORMAT

The nutrients listed on the sample label are all mandatory, including calories, calories from fat, total fat, saturated fat, cholesterol, sodium, total carbohydrate, dietary fiber, sugars, protein, vitamins A and C, calcium and iron. In addition, they must appear in the order shown, although a horizontal format is acceptable for small containers. (Exception: Certain foods that do not contain significant amounts of nutrients, such as a can of cola, can display a simplified label.)

Food companies can voluntarily list several other dietary components. These include a further breakdown of fat into polyunsaturated and monounsaturated fat, a breakdown of fiber into soluble and insoluble, and additional essential vitamins and minerals.

In response to the health concerns associated with fat intake, especially saturated fat, food labels now provide more complete information on the fat content of foods. Labels not only list the amount of total fat and saturated fat, but also the calories derived from fat. This makes it much easier to determine if the food is indeed a high-fat food.

Important information missing from food labels is the amount of trans fats in foods. These fats, created when oils are hydrogenated, raise cholesterol levels to approximately the same extent as saturated fats, according to several studies conducted in the early 1990s. (This information was not known when the regulations governing food labels were drawn up.)

Therefore, if you see "partially hydrogenated oil" in the list of ingredients, be aware that the amount of cholesterol-raising fat is greater than the number of grams listed for saturated fat. In most cases, the amount of trans fats present is about the same or slightly less than the saturated fat listed. So, simply double the figure listed for saturated fat to get a truer picture of the amount of cholesterol-raising fat.

*The main objective is to reduce all fats and oils.* As a general rule, a food item can be considered low-fat if it has two or fewer grams of total fat per 100 calories. This means it would have less than 20% of its calories from fat. (For an example of how to compute the percentage of fat calories a food item has, see Figure 2.4.) Not all the foods you eat need to be low-fat. What's most important is your average intake over a period of time, not what you eat in a single food or even a single meal.

Figure 2.4 Using the sample label as an example, you can easily determine the percentage of calories from fat by dividing the calories from fat by total calories. (120 ÷ 260 = .46 or 46%) At 46% of calories from fat, this represents a high-fat food, and a health-conscious consumer would either avoid it or eat it in limited quantities.

| Computing Percentage of Fat Calories | | |
|---|---|---|
| Calories from Fat ÷ Total Calories | = | Percentage of Fat |
| 120 ÷ 260 | = | .46 or 46% |

## % DAILY VALUES

At first glance, the % Daily Value column of numbers makes the label appear more complicated than before. This needn't be the case once you become accustomed to it. It will actually make comparison shopping easier.

The % Daily Value was designed to help you understand how each particular food item fits into the context of a total daily diet. The numbers represent the percentage (per serving) of a day's total recommended intake of each nutrient; or upper limit, in the case of total fat, saturated fat, cholesterol and sodium.

The % Daily Values are based on a 2,000-calorie diet, with less than 30% of calories from fat. Therefore, you may want to adjust the values slightly to fit your own calorie intake or desired fat intake levels. (In Chapter 3, you will learn how many grams of fat you should target for the day based on your calorie intake and whether you want to consume 10%, 20% or 30% of calories from fat.)

The % Daily Values are not intended to tell you what amounts of nutrients you should eat every day, but rather to provide a rough estimate of daily dietary needs. They can serve as a signal of whether the foods are too high in the nutrients you want to restrict, or good sources of the vitamins and minerals you want to increase. As a general rule, foods that have a % Daily Value of 20% or more can be considered "high" in that nutrient, and those that have 5% or less are "low."

Percent Daily Values also can be helpful for comparison shopping. For instance, one frozen turkey dinner meal might list the % Daily Value for fat as 18% and another brand as 34%. Obviously, the one whose fat content is 18% of the Daily Value would be a much better low-fat choice than the one that is 34%. Also, if you are looking for foods high in vitamin C, vitamin A, iron or calcium, the % Daily Value will make it much easier to choose the better sources.

## SERVING SIZE

Serving sizes have been standardized for the same types of food, and they more realistically represent what people actually eat in a single serving. For example, all ice creams and frozen yogurts have a serving size of a half cup. This makes it much easier to compare different brands. If the serving size you consume is larger than that given on the label—for example, if you consume one cup of frozen yogurt—you simply double the number of calories, fat grams and other nutrients listed.

## SUGARS PRESENT IN FOODS

Food labels can be helpful if you are trying to decrease your sugar intake. Listed in grams, the sugar content includes sugars that are present naturally in foods (including lactose in milk and fructose in fruit), as well as added sugars. As a result, foods like unsweetened yogurt, milk and fruit juices will appear relatively high in sugar, even though they may have no added sugars.

To determine if sugars have been added to foods, check the list of ingre-

dients. Terms such as "sugar (sucrose),"
"fructose," "maltose," "lactose," "honey,"
"syrup," "corn syrup," "high-fructose
corn syrup," "molasses" and "fruit juice
concentrate" are used to describe sweeteners added to foods.

A food is likely to be high in added
sugars if one of these terms is listed first
or second in the list of ingredients, or if
several of them are listed. As a frame of
reference, 4 grams of sugar equals 1 teaspoon of table sugar.

## DAILY VALUES FOOTNOTE

The % Daily Values footnote,
marked by an asterisk which appears
near the bottom of the label, states that
the % Daily Values are based on a 2,000-
calorie diet. Nutrition labels on larger
packages also include a chart listing the
recommended daily amounts of selected
nutrients for both a 2,000- and a 2,500-
calorie diet. These figures represent either the upper limit, as with fat (*less than*
65 grams), or recommended intakes, as
with fiber (25 grams).

The figures under the 2,000-calo-
rie column are the reference values on
which the % Daily Values are based.
Some labels also state, as shown on the
sample label, the number of calories
per gram of fat (9 calories), carbohydrate (4 calories), and protein (4 calories). These are the three energy nutrients that supply all our food calories. (Alcohol also supplies calories, 7
per gram, but is not considered a
food.)

## HEALTH CLAIMS

Food packages may now carry
health claims, but only under very strict
guidelines. A health claim is a statement
that describes the relationship between
a nutrient and a disease or health-related
condition.

There are seven relationships in
which health claims are allowed: calcium
and a reduced risk of osteoporosis; sodium
and an increased risk of high blood pressure; dietary saturated fat and cholesterol
and an increased risk of heart disease; dietary fat and an increased risk of cancer;

fiber-containing grain products, fruits and
vegetables and a reduced risk of cancer;
fruits, vegetables and grain products that
contain fiber, particularly soluble fiber,
and a reduced risk of coronary heart disease; and fruits and vegetables and a reduced risk of cancer.

Foods bearing health claims must
not contain any nutrient or food substance in an amount that increases the
risk of a disease. In other words, for a
food to make a health claim, it must meet
the standards for "low saturated fat,"

"low cholesterol," and "low-fat." For example, whole milk may not carry the calcium and osteoporosis claim, because the fat content is too high to meet the "low-fat" standard.

In stating the diet-disease relationship, health claims may only say the substance "may" or "might" reduce the risk. They also must indicate the disease depends on many factors. In some cases, the claim must mention other factors that affect the benefit, such as regular exercise in calcium-osteoporosis claims.

---

### Tighter Reigns on Label Claims

Nutrition claims, prominently displayed on package fronts, such as "light," "no cholesterol" or "lean," have been carefully defined, so the conscientious food shopper can take them seriously. The following provides an explanation of the most commonly used terms and the principal regulations that govern the use of these words:

**Calorie Free:** fewer than 5 calories per serving.

**Low Calorie:** 40 calories or less per serving.

**Light or Lite:** One-third fewer calories, half the fat or half the sodium; if more than half the calories are from fat, fat content must be reduced by 50% or more.

**Fat Free:** less than 0.5 grams of fat per serving.

**Low-Fat:** 3 grams of fat or less per serving.

**% Fat Free:** product must meet the definition for low fat to state "% fat free," since consumers expect that these claims imply low fat.

**Cholesterol Free:** less that 2 milligrams cholesterol *and* 2 grams or less saturated fat per serving (saturated fat also raises blood cholesterol).

**Low Cholesterol:** 20 milligrams or less cholesterol *and* 2 grams or less saturated fat per serving.

**Sodium Free:** less that 5 milligrams sodium per serving.

**Low Sodium:** 140 milligrams or less sodium per serving.

**High Fiber:** 5 grams or more fiber per serving.

**Lean:** food (meat, poultry, seafood or game meats) has less than 10 grams of fat, less than 4 grams of saturated fat and less than 95 milligrams of cholesterol per serving and per 100 grams (3.5 ounces).

**Extra Lean:** food (meat, poultry, seafood or game meats) has less than 5 grams of fat, less than 2 grams of saturated fat and less than 95 milligrams of cholesterol per serving and per 100 grams (3.5 ounces).

**Enriched, Fortified:** food must contain at least 10% more of the "fortified" or "enriched" nutrient than what was originally present in the food, or than the reference food that it resembles.

**High:** each serving must contain 20% or more of the Daily Value for that nutrient.

**Good Source:** each serving contains 10 to 19% of the Daily Value for the nutrient.

---

## INGREDIENT LABELING

A list of ingredients is required on all food labels. The ingredients are given in descending order according to weight; that is, the item listed first is the most abundant ingredient, and so on. Manufacturers must be specific in listing certain color additives, flavorings, spices and preservatives, particularly those that are known to cause allergic reactions or sensitivities in some people.

Fruit juices must declare the total amount of juice in a beverage. If a beverage is flavored with a fruit juice, the percentage of juice must be given in a 5% range, for example, flavored with 2 to 7% raspberry juice.

## NUTRITION INFORMATION FOR PRODUCE, FISH AND MEATS

Comprehensive nutrition information pertaining to raw fruits, vegetables and fish is now available in a majority of supermarkets at the produce and fish counters. As part of the Food and Drug Administration's (FDA) *voluntary* point-of-purchase nutrition information program, at least 60% of grocery stores must supply this information, or the program will become mandatory. The FDA first checked compliance in 1992 and will continue to check every two years by surveying 2,000 food stores nationwide.

The nutrition information must include serving size; calories per serving; amount of protein, carbohydrates, total fat and sodium per serving; and percent of the U.S. Recommended Dietary Allowance (USRDA) for iron, calcium and vitamins A and C per serving. Grocers have some flexibility in how the information is conveyed. Posters, brochures, leaflets or stickers may be used, as long as the materials are available in the appropriate food department. The information is only required for the 20 most frequently eaten raw fruits, vegetables and fish.

A similar program, providing nutrition information for raw meat and poultry, has been set up by the U.S. Department of Agriculture. As with the FDA program, at least 60% of grocers must comply or the program will become mandatory. Compliance will be checked every two years beginning in 1995.

The nutrition information required for meats and poultry is the same as that required on the "Nutrition Facts" label for processed foods.

With this comprehensive information now available on food labels and at the meat, poultry, fish and produce counters, health-conscious consumers are in a much better position to make healthy food choices at the supermarket. The guesswork is finally being taken out of food shopping.

# THREE

## Pursuing a Healthy Diet: Reducing Fat and Cholesterol

### CONSUMPTION OF FAT AND CHOLESTEROL

One of the most important steps toward a healthier diet is to eat less fat, especially saturated fat and cholesterol. Consuming too much fat and cholesterol increases the risks for heart disease, cancer and obesity. As mentioned previously, the minimum amount of fat adults need is very small—only 12 to 15 grams a day from all sources, or less than 10% of total calories. Children, however, need about 20% of calories from fat to achieve optimum nutrition during their growth years.

### RECOMMENDATIONS ON FAT CONSUMPTION

The National Committee on Diet, Nutrition and Cancer and the American Heart Association recommend a diet in which *no more than* 30% of calories comes from fat. Furthermore, *no more than* 10% of total calories should come from saturated fat. The American Heart Association recommends a greater reduction in saturated fat—to *less than* 7% of total calories—if blood cholesterol levels remain above 200 (mg/dl). Keep in mind that these recommended levels are not targets, but *ceilings.*

Today, many leading nutritionists in diet and health research recommend a 20% fat diet (20% of total calories from fat) for everyone, regardless of cholesterol levels, because it is a practical prevention diet in which the whole family can thrive. The 20% fat diet has demonstrated success in reducing the risk of heart disease, in combating obesity, and in decreasing the risks of some cancers. (Note: Children below the age of two need additional fat because of the tremendous growth that takes place during the first two years. Follow the advice of your pediatrician or dietitian for this age group.)

In a study sponsored by the National Institutes of Health (NIH), a 20% fat diet was found to be an approachable goal for typical Americans accustomed to a much higher fat diet. The 233 families who took part in the NIH study were educated about the merits of a lower-fat diet. Eighty per cent of them remained in the study for the full five years. During that time, they gradually reduced their fat intake to between 20% and 30% of total calories. They made the necessary changes and stuck with them. By the end of the study, most had decided to make the lower-fat diet a permanent part of their lifestyle.

Some adults have gone even further with fat reductions, following the recommendations of Dean Ornish, M.D., and the late Nathan Pritikin. Both recommend a very stringent diet consisting of approximately 10% of calories from fat, and very low salt and sugar. Many of these adults have experienced drastic reductions in cholesterol levels, and when exercising care in eating a balanced diet, have managed to be well nourished at the same time. Although very effective in reducing cholesterol levels, these diets are not recommended for children of any age because they need more fat to achieve their full growth potential.

Later in this chapter, simple guidelines are listed which show how to limit fat to approximately 20% of total calories. A chart showing total daily fat intakes (based on calorie consumption) for diets of 10%, 20% and 30% of calories from fat also is provided.

## RECOMMENDATIONS ON CHOLESTEROL CONSUMPTION

The American Heart Association recommends that adults and children consume no more than 300 milligrams of cholesterol per day. For those with high cholesterol levels (above 200), their recommendation is less than 200 milligrams per day. Some leading nutritionists recommend only 100 milligrams of cholesterol per day for everyone, as a preventive measure, regardless of blood cholesterol levels.

The main point to keep in mind is that the less cholesterol you eat in foods, the lower your blood cholesterol levels should be and the lower your risk of heart disease. Several studies suggest that eating foods with cholesterol increases your risk of heart disease, regardless of how much it raises your blood cholesterol levels.

Since most foods high in saturated fat are also high in cholesterol, if you eat less saturated fat, you will also consume less cholesterol. The guidelines listed near the end of this chapter for the 20% fat diet will keep cholesterol intake to approximately 100 to 150 milligrams per day, provided whole eggs are not used. It should

also keep saturated fat intake to less than 7% of total calories.

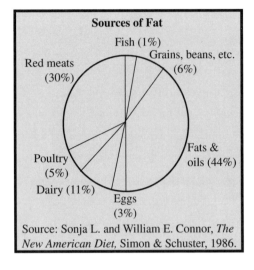

Source: Sonja L. and William E. Connor, *The New American Diet*, Simon & Schuster, 1986.

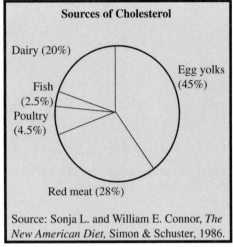

Source: Sonja L. and William E. Connor, *The New American Diet*, Simon & Schuster, 1986.

(left)
Figure 3.1
The sources of dietary fat in a typical American diet.

(right)
Figure 3.2
The sources of cholesterol in a typical American diet.

## STEP 1—IDENTIFY SOURCES OF FAT AND CHOLESTEROL

Before you can effectively reduce fat and cholesterol in your diet, it is necessary to know the sources—both the obvious and the "hidden." Figure 3.1 identifies the sources of fat in the typical American diet. The largest amount (44%) comes directly from fats and oils, with half (22%) from visible fats added at the table in the form of spreads and dressings; and the other half (22%) from baked goods and cooking oils used in food preparation. The next largest amount is from red meats (30%), followed by dairy (11%), poultry (5%), eggs (3%), grains, beans, fruits and vegetables (6%), and fish (1%).

From this chart, it is evident that fat consumption can be reduced most

effectively by limiting the fats and oils used in baking, cooking, in spreads and salad dressings, and by cutting down on fats from red meats and dairy products.

Figure 3.2 shows the sources of cholesterol in the typical American diet. The largest percentage comes from egg yolks (45%) with approximately half from visible eggs (2 to 3 per week), and half from eggs used in food preparation. The next largest percentage is from red meat (28%), followed by dairy products (20%). Cholesterol in dairy products comes from the following: 9% from milk, 5% from cheese, 4% from butter and 2% from ice cream. Poultry contributes 4.5% of the dietary cholesterol, and fish contributes 2.5%.

Referring to Figure 3.2, it is easy to see that eliminating whole eggs would reduce cholesterol from foods by nearly one-half. The other major sources of cholesterol are red meats and dairy, which are also high-fat sources, as shown previously. Therefore, if you cut down on red meats and high-fat dairy products, both fat and cholesterol will be reduced.

## CHOLESTEROL-SATURATED FAT INDEX FOR FOODS

Since *both* saturated fat and cholesterol are responsible for elevating blood cholesterol levels, the Cholesterol-Saturated Fat Index (CSI) for foods was devised, taking into account both these factors. The higher the number, the greater the cholesterol-raising effect; and conversely, the lower the number, the less tendency to raise blood cholesterol levels. The CSI is particularly effective in making comparisons between foods from the same food group. See Table 3.1.

## COMPARISONS OF MEAT, FISH AND POULTRY

In comparing the CSI of meat, fish and poultry, the better choices are obvious—fish, including shellfish, and poultry without skin, are preferable to red meats. That does not mean that red meats should necessarily be avoided, but definitely reduced. When eating red meats, be sure to choose the leaner cuts and trim the visible fat. Check with your butcher to find the leanest cuts. Also, on the days you eat red meat, make sure most of your other foods are lower in fat.

You may have heard in the past that shrimp and lobster are high in cholesterol and therefore should be avoided. It is true that they are relatively high in cholesterol, but the saturated fat content is so small that their CSI is similar to poultry without skin.

How does the presence of skin and manner of cooking affect the fat content of poultry? With the skin, the fat in poultry is roughly doubled. (To achieve the fat savings effect, the skin can be removed either before or after cooking.) If the poultry is dipped in batter with the skin on and deep fried, a common practice in many fast-food restaurants, the fat content is approximately tripled, because of the extra fat absorbed by the batter. This means that a fried chicken breast from a fast-food restaurant may contain as much, or more fat, than a large hamburger.

## PROCESSED POULTRY PRODUCTS

Many processed foods made with chicken or turkey are now available in supermarkets. These include chicken and turkey hot dogs, turkey bologna and ground turkey. Are these any better than those made with beef and pork? One of the best ways to determine this is to compare the grams of fat on the food labels.

If this information is not available, the following guidelines should be helpful. On the average, chicken and turkey dogs have 30% less fat than regular hot dogs. But this still does not put them in a low-fat category. They contain about 9 grams of fat for a 2-ounce hot dog, as compared with 14 grams of fat for their beef or pork counterparts. Turkey burgers have about one-fourth less fat than "lean" ground-beef burgers. Again, however, the total fat is still quite high—11 grams per 3-ounce patty. The fat content is high because the visible fat from the turkey is included when the meat is ground. If you grind your own turkey at home after removing the skin and visible fat, the same amount of ground turkey (3 ounces) has about 6 grams of fat for the dark meat, and only 2.5 grams for the light meat.

### COMPARISONS OF FATS AND OILS

Comparing the CSI of fats and oils in Table 3.1 makes it apparent that there are vast differences in their effects on the heart and blood vessels. All of the highly polyunsaturated vegetable oils (CSI of 4) are far better than the highly saturated vegetable oils including coconut oil, palm oil, and cocoa butter (CSI of 24). So don't be fooled again by the claim "all vegetable oil"—find out what kind of vegetable oil! Even bacon grease is only half as harmful as the highly saturated vegetable oils.

These comparisons also show that, whenever possible, it is better to use soft margarines, which have a CSI of 5, than hard-stick margarines which have a CSI of 8. Mayonnaise has a CSI of 5, but there are tasty lower-fat substitutes available, including those advertised as "light." Many of these have fewer calories and consequently less fat because they are more highly whipped, and therefore partly filled with air. Still, watch the quantity—a thin scraping is best.

Peanut butter should be used in moderation because 50% of its calories come from fat. It is fine to use in a sandwich as a protein source instead of meat or cheese, but if you eat large quantities as a snack, you will be consuming too much fat. The "partially hydrogenated" peanut butters available at the super market are not very hydrogenated (about 20%) and are therefore still very unsaturated. Some peanut-butter lovers have found a way to reduce the fat in peanut butter, and still enjoy the peanut taste. They buy natural peanut butter, with the oil separated on the top, and pour this off, removing much of the fat. Some find this too dry, but others find it satisfies their peanut craving.

## The Cholesterol-Saturated Fat Index (CSI) and Calorie Content of Selected Foods

| Fish, Poultry, Red Meat (3 1/2 ounces, cooked) | CSI | Calories |
|---|---|---|
| White fish (snapper, perch, sole, cod, halibut, etc.), shellfish (clams, oysters, scallops), water-pack tuna | 4 | 91 |
| Salmon | 5 | 149 |
| Shellfish (crab, lobster) | 5 | 100 |
| Poultry, no skin | 6 | 171 |
| Shrimp | 7 | 105 |
| Pork tenderloin; beef top round, lean | 7 | 180 |
| Beef, Pork and Lamb: | | |
| 10% fat (ground sirloin, flank steak) | 9 | 214 |
| 15% fat (ground round) | 10 | 258 |
| 20% fat (ground chuck, pot roasts) | 13 | 286 |
| 30% fat (ground beef, pork, and lamb steaks, ribs, pork and lamb chips, roasts) | 18 | 381 |

| Cheeses (3 1/2 ounces) | | |
|---|---|---|
| Low-fat cottage cheese, tofu (bean curd), pot cheese | 1 | 98 |
| Cottage cheese, Lite-line, Lite n' Lively, Weight Watchers, part-skim ricotta | 6 | 139 |
| Cheddar, Roquefort, Swiss, Brie, Jack, American, cream cheese, Velveeta, cheese spreads (jars) and most other cheeses | 26 | 386 |

| Eggs | | |
|---|---|---|
| Whites (3) | 0 | 51 |
| Egg substitute (equivalent to 2 eggs) | <1 | 91 |
| Whole (2) | 29 | 163 |

| Fats (2 tablespoons) | | |
|---|---|---|
| Peanut butter | 3 | 177 |
| Most vegetable oils | 4 | 265 |
| Mayonnaise | 5 | 216 |
| Soft vegetable margarines | 5 | 216 |
| Hard-stick margarines | 8 | 216 |
| Soft shortenings | 8 | 265 |
| Bacon grease | 12 | 271 |
| Very hydrogenated shortenings | 14 | 265 |
| Butter | 19 | 215 |
| Coconut oil, palm oil, cocoa butter (chocolate) | 24 | 265 |

| The Cholesterol-Saturated Fat Index (CSI) and Calorie Content of Selected Foods (cont'd) | | |
|---|---|---|
| **Frozen Desserts (1 cup)** | **CSI** | **Calories** |
| Water ices, sorbets | 0 | 245 |
| Sherbet, low-fat frozen yogurt | 2 | 290 |
| Ice milk | 6 | 214 |
| Ice cream, 10% fat | 13 | 272 |
| Rich ice cream, 16% fat | 18 | 349 |
| Specialty ice cream, 22% fat | 34 | 684 |
| | | |
| **Milk Products (1 cup)** | | |
| Skim Milk, (0.1 %), skim-milk yogurt | <1 | 88 |
| 1% milk, buttermilk | 2 | 115 |
| 2% milk, plain low-fat yogurt | 4 | 144 |
| Whole milk, (3.5% fat), whole-milk yogurt | 7 | 159 |
| Liquid nondairy creamers: Mocha Mix, Poly Rich | 4 | 326 |
| Liquid nondairy creamers: store brands, Cereal Blend, Coffee Rich | 22 | 344 |
| Sour cream | 37 | 468 |
| Imitation sour cream (IMO) | 43 | 499 |

< = less than.

Source: Adapted from Sonja L. and William E. Connor, *The New American Diet*, Simon & Schuster, 1986.

Table 3.1 The Cholesterol–Saturated Fat Index (CSI) is a numerical value which shows the relative effect of particular foods in raising blood cholesterol levels. It takes into account both the cholesterol and saturated fat in foods. The higher the number, the greater the cholesterol-raising effect. (The CSI is calculated by using the following formula: 1.01 x Saturated Fat (gm) + 0.05 x Cholesterol (mg) = CSI)

## COMPARISON OF CHEESES

Cheese has become an integral part of the American diet. We put it on hamburgers, in sandwiches and casseroles and sprinkle it on pasta dishes. It is probably the most common appetizer served with crackers at a cocktail party or dinner party. The unfortunate thing about cheese, however, is that most of our favorites are loaded with saturated fat and cholesterol. Ounce for ounce, they have a cholesterol-saturated fat index well above the fattiest red meat—a CSI of 26 for cheese vs. 18 for the highest-fat red meats (See Table 3.1.) Just one ounce of these high-fat cheeses contains between 7 and 10 grams of fat, or about 2 teaspoons of fat. *Approximately 90% of their calories come from fat.*

There are several ways to reduce the fat intake from cheese. One way is to eat lower fat cheese. There are many choices currently on the market, some of which are listed in the first two columns of Figure 3.3. Some find these to be satisfactory substitutes, while others complain that they "miss the mark" for flavor. Another is to find tasty alternatives to cheese. For example, instead of cheese and crackers as an appetizer, serve Hummous, Tabouli or Artichoke Relish (see recipes) with toasted pita chips or low-fat crackers. Seedless grapes or other fresh fruits complement these appetizers nicely.

For casseroles or side dishes, grated Parmesan cheese is an excellent choice. It has a sharp, distinct flavor, so a little bit goes a long way. Using 1/4 cup in a casserole dish for a family of four amounts to just 1 tablespoon per person. One tablespoon has only 1.5 grams of fat—not much when compared to 1 ounce of the non-grated varieties (7 to 10 grams of fat). It is also very tasty sprinkled on pasta dishes.

Low-fat cottage cheese (1% milk fat) is another good choice, either eaten alone, or served with fruit or baked potatoes. It can also be mixed in a 1:1 ratio with a processed cheese spread to reduce the fat calories of the cheese spread by nearly one-half. The cheeses can be mixed by hand, or if a smooth mixture is preferred, in a food processor.

**Cholesterol-Saturated Fat Index (CSI) of Selected Cheeses**
**(1-ounce portions unless otherwise indicated)**

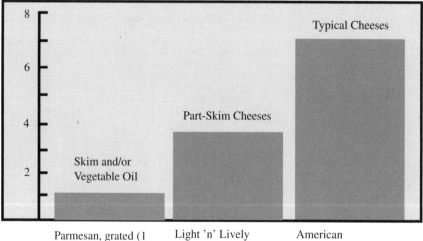

Figure 3.3 The Cholesterol-Saturated Fat Index (CSI) of selected cheeses.

| Parmesan, grated (1 Tbsp.) | Light 'n' Lively | American |
| Cottage cheese 1% fat (1/2 c) | Mozzarella, part skim | Blue cheese |
| Imitation mozzarella | Ricotta, part skim | Cheddar |
| Heart Beat | Cream cheese, light | Colby, Swiss |
| | Kraft Light Naturals | Cream cheese |
| | Cottage cheese, creamed | Ricotta, whole milk (1/4 c) |

Source: Adapted from Sonja L. Connor, *Journal of the American Dietetics Association,* June, 1989.

A salad is not necessarily a low-fat food item. It can become a high-fat entree or side dish with the addition of salad dressings. This can be prevented either by using a smaller amount of dressing or by choosing a low-fat or nonfat variety.

The *quantity* of salad dressing can only be monitored if you add it yourself. Therefore, if you are eating out, be sure to ask for the dressing to be served on the side. Add just enough to lightly flavor the greens and vegetables. At a salad bar, be mindful that the small ladles usually hold about 2 tablespoons of dressing. This amounts to 150 or more calories if using the regular Blue Cheese, Italian or Thousand Island dressings.

In addition to being mindful of the quantity, it is just as important to be aware of the cholesterol-saturated fat content of dressings. The great differences in the CSI of the various salad dressings is due to the *amount* and *type* of fat in the dressings. The low-calorie commercial salad dressings generally have less than one-quarter of the fat and calories of the higher-fat varieties. The no-oil dressings have negligible fat content and often have fewer than 12 calories per 2-tablespoon serving. Read labels to make comparisons.

Low-fat salad dressings can also be made at home by using low-fat or nonfat mayonnaise, yogurt or sour cream bases. A comparison of the cholesterol-saturated fat index of some popular salad dressings is provided in Figure 3.4.

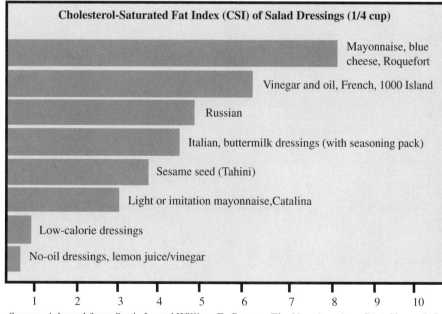

**Cholesterol-Saturated Fat Index (CSI) of Salad Dressings (1/4 cup)**

Mayonnaise, blue cheese, Roquefort

Vinegar and oil, French, 1000 Island

Russian

Italian, buttermilk dressings (with seasoning pack)

Sesame seed (Tahini)

Light or imitation mayonnaise, Catalina

Low-calorie dressings

No-oil dressings, lemon juice/vinegar

1  2  3  4  5  6  7  8  9  10

Figure 3.4 The Cholesterol-Saturated Fat Index (CSI) of selected salad dressings. The lower the CSI number the less cholesterol and saturated fat.

Source: Adapted from Sonja L. and William E. Connor, *The New American Diet,* Simon & Schuster, 1986.

# STEP 2—HOW MUCH FAT IS RIGHT FOR YOU?
## DETERMINING THE AMOUNT OF FAT FOR YOUR DIET

To determine the specific amount of fat for your diet, you must first decide if your goal is to consume a diet of 10%, 20% or 30% of calories from fat. A diet of 20% of calories from fat is optimum for most adults, because it is a practical diet that is effective in reducing the incidence of cancer, heart disease and obesity. Those who have suffered a recent heart attack, have known coronary artery disease or are having difficulty losing weight may want to come closer to the 10% fat level. On the other hand, a diet of closer to 30% may be more workable for some. Less than 30% of calories from fat is still within the guidelines of the American Cancer Society and the American Heart Association.

An important point to remember is that most preferences for certain types of food are acquired, and therefore it takes time to get used to different foods. Many people, after becoming accustomed to a lower-fat diet, actually grow to prefer the lighter fare. They feel better and have lost the craving for many high-fat foods.

Once you have decided on your goal, you need to determine your average daily calorie consumption. From this, you can figure how many grams of fat you should consume per day.

## ESTIMATE DAILY CALORIE INTAKE

Estimating how many calories you eat in a day can be done in one of two ways. First, you can refer to Table 3.2, which gives the average calorie consumption based on age and sex. You can adjust the number of calories higher or lower, depending on your size, your level of exercise, and your eating habits. Looking at the Table, if you are an average-size 30-year-old woman, you fall into the second category and probably consume about 2,000 calories per day.

For a more accurate measure of your total calorie intake, keep an exact record of everything you eat and drink for three consecutive days (representative of your usual eating habits). Give this information to a dietitian, who can figure your average daily calorie consumption for you.

If you have access to a calorie chart, you can figure it yourself. You simply add up all the calories from the food and drinks you have recorded for the three-day period, and divide this total by 3 to get the average number of calories you eat per day. Keep in mind that if you want to lose weight, you should set a goal of fewer calories than what you are now consuming.

| Average Daily Calorie Intake | |
|---|---|
| | No. of Calories |
| Women (19 to 22 years) | 2100 |
| Women (23 to 50 years) | 2000 |
| Women (51 to 75 years) | 1800 |
| Men (19 to 22 years) | 2900 |
| Men (23 to 50 years) | 2700 |
| Men (51 to 75 years) | 2400 |
| Children (7 to 10 years) | 2400 |
| Girls (11 to 18 years) | 2150 |
| Boys (11 to 18 years) | 2750 |

Table 3.2 U.S. RDA table showing average recommended calorie intakes for men, women, and children based on age. The usual calorie variation for maintaining weight at any age is ± 400 calories.

### DETERMINE GRAMS OF FAT PER DAY

After you know the approximate number of calories you eat in a day, you can refer to Table 3.3 to determine how many grams of fat you should consume, depending on the percentage of fat in your diet. To use the chart, first locate the number of calories you consume per day. Next, look in the appropriate column to the right to find the grams of fat for your preferred diet. Using 2000 calories as an example, you see that you can consume 22 grams of fat per day in a 10% fat diet, 44 grams per day in a 20% fat diet, and 67 grams per day in a 30% fat diet.

## STEP 3—COUNTING GRAMS OF FAT IN FOODS

As you may have guessed, knowing the amount of fat (in grams) to include in your diet is useless, unless you also know the amount of fat in the foods

| Recommended Fat Consumption Based on Daily Caloric Intake | | | |
|---|---|---|---|
| Total Calories | Grams of Fat/Day Fat=10% of Calories | Grams of Fat/Day Fat=20% of Calories | Grams of Fat/Day Fat=30% of Calories |
| 1200 | 14 | 27 | 40 |
| 1400 | 16 | 31 | 47 |
| 1600 | 18 | 36 | 53 |
| 1800 | 20 | 40 | 60 |
| 2000 | 22 | 44 | 67 |
| 2200 | 25 | 49 | 73 |
| 2400 | 27 | 53 | 80 |
| 2600 | 29 | 58 | 87 |
| 2800 | 31 | 62 | 93 |
| 3000 | 34 | 67 | 100 |
| 3200 | 36 | 71 | 107 |
| 3400 | 38 | 76 | 113 |

Table 3.3 Grams of fat per day in diets of 10%, 20% and 30% of calories from fat, based on daily caloric intakes of 1200 to 3400 calories.

you eat. For example, if you have decided to set a target of 36 grams of fat for your diet, you need to know what foods constitute that amount of fat.

This is not as difficult as it seems. The grams of fat per serving are listed on most food labels, and are included with recipes in some cookbooks. By reading labels and also becoming familiar with the grams of fat in many basic foods, you can closely estimate the quantity of fat in the foods you eat and in the recipes you prepare. In a short period of time, you will become accustomed to what you can eat and what you should avoid in order to stay within your limit. Counting grams of fat will no longer be necessary.

The fat content of many of our most commonly eaten foods is listed in Table 3.4. As you can see from this, almost all fruits and vegetables without added sauces and most breads have little or no fat.

Comparing the grams of fat in various types and cuts of meats, trimmed and untrimmed, shows the wide differences in their fat content. The white meat of turkey and chicken are by far the lowest and the highest are the untrimmed red meats, especially ribs.

Dairy products also have great variations in fat content. Skim milk has all the calcium and protein of the higher fat milk, but without most of the fat. It's fairly easy to get used to, if you do it gradually—from whole milk, to 2% milk, to 1% milk and then to skim. If you can't get accustomed to skim, 1% or 2% is preferable to whole milk. Ice milk, low-fat frozen yogurt, sherbet and nonfat ice cream are good substitutes for regular ice cream. Different brands vary in fat content and flavor. Shop around until you find the one(s) that best suit your family's preferences. If you crave the creamy taste of ice cream but prefer less fat, try the ice creams made with the fat substitute "Simpless," which taste creamy, but contain almost no fat.

### FAT CONTENT IN FAST FOODS

Since fast foods play such an important part in the typical American diet, it is important to be aware of the amount of fat in these foods. It is a rare family indeed that doesn't make an occasional stop at McDonald's, Hardee's, Burger King, Taco Bell, etc. Table 3.5 lists the fat content of a sampling of foods available at several fast food restaurants.

Many of the foods from fast-food restaurants are high in fat. However, this does not mean that these restaurants should be avoided entirely. There are wide variations in the fat content of foods that each restaurant serves. One simply has to learn which ones are the lowest in fat and order these when eating out. (Several fast-food restaurants have nutrition

## Fat Content of Selected Foods

| Fruits and Vegetables | Fat(g) | Cal. |
|---|---|---|
| Fruits and vegetables, canned, frozen or fresh, with no added sauces (except avocado) | 0.1 | 50–100 |
| **Breads** | | |
| Wheat, raisin, rye, white, pumpernickel, etc. (1 slice) | 1.0 | 50–80 |
| **Poultry (per 3 oz. cooked, 4 oz. uncooked)** | | |
| Turkey, light, without skin | 2.7 | 135 |
| Turkey, dark, without skin | 6.2 | 160 |
| Chicken, light, without skin | 3.3 | 127 |
| Chicken, dark, without skin | 7.1 | 150 |
| Duck, without skin | 9.6 | 172 |
| Ground turkey, commercial | 10.5 | 183 |
| Chicken hot dog (2 oz.) | 8.8 | 116 |
| **Beef (per 3 oz. cooked, 4 oz. uncooked)** | | |
| Top round, trimmed,* braised | 4.9 | 176 |
| Eye of round, trimmed, choice, roasted | 5.7 | 156 |
| Round tip, trimmed, roasted | 5.4 | 153 |
| Top sirloin, trimmed, broiled | 6.6 | 170 |
| Tenderloin (filet mignon), broiled | 8.6 | 180 |
| Beef chuck pot roast, trimmed, braised | 8.8 | 199 |
| Rib eye, trimmed, choice, broiled | 9.9 | 191 |
| Rib eye, untrimmed, choice, broiled | 17.7 | 250 |
| T-bone steak, trimmed, choice, broiled | 8.8 | 182 |
| T-bone steak, untrimmed, choice, broiled | 20.9 | 276 |
| Ground beef, lean, broiled | 16.2 | 234 |
| Beef ribs, untrimmed, braised | 35.7 | 400 |
| Beef bologna (1 oz.) | 6.6 | 72 |
| Hot dog, beef (2 oz.) | 16.3 | 180 |
| **Veal (per 3 oz. cooked, 4 oz. uncooked)** | | |
| Veal cutlet, trimmed, braised | 4.3 | 172 |
| Veal loin chop, trimmed, roasted | 5.9 | 149 |
| Veal sirloin, untrimmed, braised | 11.2 | 214 |
| Veal sirloin chop, trimmed, braised | 5.5 | 173 |
| Veal rib roast, trimmed, choice | 6.3 | 151 |
| **Lamb (per 3 oz. cooked, 4 oz. uncooked)** | | |
| Leg of lamb, trimmed | 6.6 | 162 |
| Leg of lamb, untrimmed | 14.0 | 219 |
| Lamb loin chop, trimmed, choice, broiled | 8.2 | 183 |
| **Pork (3 oz. cooked, 4 oz. uncooked)** | | |
| Pork tenderloin, trimmed | 4.1 | 141 |
| Center loin chop, trimmed, broiled | 8.9 | 196 |
| Center loin chop, untrimmed, pan-fried | 25.9 | 318 |
| Ham, boneless, regular (11% fat) | 7.7 | 151 |
| Ham, boneless, lean (5% fat) | 4.7 | 123 |
| Bacon, 3 slices | 9.4 | 109 |
| Pork sausage (2 oz.) | 16.2 | 184 |

Table 3.4 Fat and calorie content of selected foods.

## Fat Content of Selected Foods (cont'd)

| Seafood (3 oz. cooked w/no extra fat) | Fat(g) | Calories |
|---|---|---|
| Flounder and sole | 1.3 | 99 |
| Orange roughy | 6.0 | 107 |
| Perch, ocean | 1.8 | 103 |
| Salmon, pink | 5.1 | 118 |
| Salmon, sockeye or red | 9.3 | 183 |
| Swordfish | 4.4 | 132 |
| Clams | 1.7 | 126 |
| Scallops | 0.8 | 88 |
| Shrimp | 0.9 | 84 |
| **Dairy Products** | | |
| Cheese (1 oz.)** | 8–10.0 | 105 |
| Parmesan cheese (1 tbsp.) | 1.5 | 23 |
| Cottage cheese, regular (1/2 cup) | 5.1 | 117 |
| Cottage cheese, 1% fat (1/2 cup) | 1.2 | 82 |
| Mozzarella, park skim (1 oz.) | 4.5 | 72 |
| Heavy cream (2 tbsp.) | 11.2 | 104 |
| Sour cream (2 tbsp.) | 5.0 | 52 |
| Milk, whole (1 cup) | 8.2 | 150 |
| Milk, 2% fat | 4.7 | 121 |
| Milk, 1% fat | 2.4 | 104 |
| Milk, skim | 0.4 | 86 |
| Buttermilk (1 cup) | 2.2 | 99 |
| Eggnog (1 cup) | 19.0 | 342 |
| Ice Cream, 10% fat (1 cup) | 14.3 | 269 |
| Ice Cream, rich, 16% fat (1 cup) | 23.7 | 349 |
| Ice milk, hard (1 cup) | 5.6 | 184 |
| Sherbet (1 cup) | 3.8 | 270 |
| **Fats, Oils** | | |
| Butter, cooking oils (1 tsp.) | 4–5 | 40 |
| Whipped margarine (1 tsp.) | 2.5–3 | 23–27 |
| Mayonnaise (1 tbsp.) | 10 | 100 |
| Light mayonnaise (1 tbsp.) | 5 | 50 |
| Salad dressings, regular (2 tbsp.) | 12–18 | 140–170 |
| Salad dressings, low-cal. (2 tbsp.) | 2–5 | 30–50 |
| **Desserts** | | |
| Brownies (2" square) | 6–8 | 150–170 |
| Cookies, homemade (4 cookies) | 10 | 180 |
| Fruit pies, homemade (1/8 pie) | 12–14 | 280–300 |
| Pecan pie, homemade (1/8 pie) | 23 | 431 |
| Cake (from mix): chocolate, white, Yellow (1/12 cake) | 10–12 | 250–300 |
| Muffins, homemade or from mix | 3–4 | 100–120 |

*Trimmed indicates all visible fat has been removed.

**Includes provolone, Swiss, cheddar, American, Roquefort, Brie, etc.

Source: U.S. Dept. of Agriculture Handbooks No. 8-5, 8-10, 8-13, 8-15, 8-17, and *Bowes and Church's Food Values of Portions Commonly Used*, 15th Edition, revised by Jean A. T. Pennington. Harper & Row, New York, 1989.

Table 3.4
(cont'd)

information available upon request for all the foods they serve.) Some of the best meat choices are the regular hamburgers and grilled chicken breast sandwiches (preferably without mayonnaise or cheese), and chicken tacos. Chunky Chicken Salad (from McDonald's), is low in fat, whereas the Taco Salad (from Taco Bell) is high, so do not assume salads are always low-fat. The strawberry shake from McDonald's is made with ice milk so the grams of fat are not as high as one might expect—a good choice for an occasional treat for a child (or an adult who is not calorie conscious) because of the calcium content. A soft drink, however, would have no fat and fewer calories, so may be preferable if watching fat

| Fat Content in Selected Foods from Fast-Food Restaurants | | |
|---|---|---|
| **McDonalds** | **Fat(g)** | **Calories** |
| Regular Hamburger | 9 | 255 |
| Big Mac | 26 | 500 |
| Filet of Fish | 18 | 370 |
| Quarter Pounder with Cheese | 28 | 510 |
| McGrilled Chicken Sand. | 12 | 390 |
| Chunky Chicken Salad | 4 | 150 |
| French Fries (medium) | 17 | 320 |
| Apple Pie | 15 | 260 |
| Strawberry Low-fat Shake | 5 | 340 |
| **Kentucky Fried Chicken** | | |
| Original Recipe (breast) | 15 | 283 |
| Extra Crispy (drum & thigh) | 44 | 610 |
| Cole Slaw (one serving) | 7 | 119 |
| Mashed Potatoes with Gravy | 2 | 71 |
| **Burger King** | | |
| Whopper | 36 | 614 |
| Whopper, Double | 53 | 844 |
| Hamburger | 11 | 272 |
| BK Broiler Chicken Sand. | 8 | 267 |
| Saus. Egg, Cheese Crossanwich | 40 | 534 |
| **Taco Bell** | | |
| Bean Burrito with red sauce | 14 | 447 |
| Beef Burrito with red sauce | 21 | 493 |
| Taco, hard shell, beef | 11 | 183 |
| Soft Taco, Chicken | 10 | 213 |
| Taco Salad, without shell | 31 | 484 |
| **Domino's Pizza (16", 2 slices)** | | |
| Cheese Pizza | 10 | 376 |
| Pepperoni Pizza | 17 | 460 |
| Deluxe Pizza | 20 | 498 |

Table 3.5 Fat and calorie content of selected foods from fast-food restaurants.

Source: Michael F. Jacobson and Sarah Fritschner, *The Completely Revised and Updated Fast Food Guide*, 2nd Edition, Workman Publishing, New York, 1991.

and calories very closely. (See Appendix for more complete nutrition information on a wide variety of foods served at fast-food restaurants.)

## HIGH-FAT DINNERS ARE NOT LIMITED TO FAST FOODS

High-fat meals are not limited to fast-food restaurants. Let's analyze a menu from a typical steak-house meal to demonstrate this point. (See Figure 3.5.) The menu includes the following:

*T-Bone Steak, 10 Ounces, Trimmed*
*Baked Potato with Butter and Sour Cream*
*Tossed Green Salad with Italian Dressing*
*Hot Roll with Butter*
*Coffee with Cream*
*Cheesecake*

Figure 3.5 The fat and calorie content of a typical steak dinner. Most of the total calories (61%) come from fat.

| Fat Content of Typical Steak Dinner | | | |
|---|---|---|---|
| **Food** | **Serving Size** | **Fat (g)** | **Calories** |
| T-bone steak | 10 oz | 50 | 769 |
| Baked potato | 1 large | 0 | 145 |
| Butter | 2 tsp | 8 | 72 |
| Sour cream | 2 tbsp | 5 | 52 |
| Tossed green salad | 2 cups | 0 | 20 |
| Italian dressing | 3 tbsp | 27 | 252 |
| Dinner roll | 1 | 2 | 80 |
| Butter | 1 tsp | 4 | 36 |
| Coffee | 1 cup | 0 | 0 |
| Cream | 1 tbsp | 5 | 44 |
| Cheesecake | 1 piece | 16 | 257 |
| **Totals** | | **117 g.** | **1727 cal.** |

Figure 3.6 Fat and calorie content of lower-fat steak dinner. The percentage of calories from fat was reduced from 61% to 28%.

| Fat Content of Adjusted Steak Dinner | | | |
|---|---|---|---|
| **Food** | **Serving Size** | **Fat (g)** | **Calories** |
| Beef tenderloin | 4 oz | 11 | 233 |
| Baked potato | 1 large | 0 | 145 |
| Margarine | 1 tsp | 4 | 36 |
| Nonfat sour cream | 2 tbsp | 0 | 20 |
| Carrots, steamed | 1/2 cup | 0 | 35 |
| Zucchini, steamed | 1/2 cup | 0 | 14 |
| Tossed green salad | 2 cups | 0 | 20 |
| Low-fat dressing | 2 tbsp | 2 | 40 |
| Whole wheat bread | 1 slice | 1 | 70 |
| Margarine | 1/2 tsp | 2 | 18 |
| Coffee | 1 cup | 0 | 0 |
| Sugar | 1 tsp | 0 | 15 |
| **Totals** | | **20 g.** | **646 cal.** |

The grams of fat are listed to show the amount of fat in each food item. As you can see, this one meal contains over 1,700 calories, and 61% of the calories come from fat. Furthermore, the majority of the fat comes from foods high in saturated fat.

The menu can be altered to bring the fat content down to a much healthier 27% of calories. (See Figure 3.6.) It is important to keep in mind that this meal is a typical evening meal, including more meat and thus probably more fat than the other two meals of the day. Therefore, the *percentage* of fat calories for the *day* could be less, provided low-fat food selections were made at breakfast and lunch. Four ounces of meat per day is more than adequate to supply protein needs.

A low-fat salad dressing was used to keep the fat calories down. The margarine allotted for the bread (1/2 teaspoon) and baked potato (1 teaspoon) is limited, but should be adequate. Nonfat sour cream was added to the potato to provide additional flavor without increasing the fat.

## TIPS FOR REDUCING THE FAT IN YOUR DIET

Now that you know the sources of fat and cholesterol, and the number of fat grams you should have targeted for your daily limit, you are ready to begin cutting down. The best and easiest way to begin is simple substitution. Figure 3.7 lists suggested lower-fat/lower-cholesterol substitutions.

### SAMPLE DAILY MENU—FAT LIMITED TO 20% OF TOTAL CALORIES

It's not difficult to follow a diet in which only 20% of the calories come from fat. To demonstrate this, let's examine a sample day's menu of about 1,600 calories. Refer to Figure 3.8. The total fat must be limited to 36 grams to stay within 20% of the calories. The fat content of foods is shown in grams.

The total fat for the day is 33 grams, which is within the desired goal of 36 grams of fat, or 20% of total calories. If you wanted to limit fat to 10% of 1,600 carlores, your daily target would be 18 grams of fat; and at 30% of calories, fat consumption would be limited to 53 grams per day. (The majority of recipes in this book are low enough in fat that they may be successfully incorporated into a 10% fat diet.)

This sample daily menu, where fat intake is kept to just 20% of total calories, demonstrates several things:

1. Greater quantities of food can be eaten when fat is kept to a minimum. This sample menu includes three fairly large meals and two snacks, but contains just 1,600 total calories. The quantity of food would be significantly greater for

2,000 to 3,000 calories, which is what most men consume daily.

2. It is important to choose lower-fat food items in order to keep the fat allowance within the limits—for example, choosing skim milk (0 grams fat), instead of whole milk (8 grams fat/cup); and choosing a broth-based soup, such as minestrone (2 grams fat/cup) instead of a cream-based soup, such as cream of mushroom soup (11 grams fat/cup). Whole milk (1 7/8 cup) would have added 14 grams

Figure 3.7 Suggested substitutions to reduce fat and cholesterol in your diet. The grams of fat in each food item are given to show you the fat savings that result from the substitutions.

| **Suggested Substitutions** | | | | | |
|---|---|---|---|---|---|
| **Instead of . . .** | | | **Use . . .** | | |
| | **Serving Size** | **Fat(g)** | | **Serving Size** | **Fat(g)** |
| Sour cream | 1 cup | 48 | Plain yogurt (low-fat) | 1 cup | 1 |
| Butter* | 1 tbsp. | 12 | Margarine (whipped) | 1 tbsp. | 7 |
| 1 whole egg | 1 egg | 6 | 2 egg whites or 1 egg substitute | 2 whites | 1 |
| 2 whole eggs | 2 eggs | 12 | 3 egg whites or 2 egg substitutes | 3 whites | 1 |
| Milk, whole | 1 cup | 8 | Milk, 2% | 1 cup | 5 |
| Milk, 1% | 1 cup | 1 | Milk, skim | 1 cup | 0 |
| Evaporated milk (canned) | 1 cup | 17 | Evaporated skim milk | 1 cup | 1 |
| Whipped cream (over fruit, desserts) | 1/4 cup | 5 | Vanilla yogurt (low-fat) | 1/4 cup | 1 |
| Ice cream | 1/2 cup | 7 | Ice milk, 1% fat | 1/2 cup | 2 |
| Yogurt, plain (whole milk) | 1 cup | 7 | Yogurt, plain (skim milk) | 1 cup | 1 |
| Cream (in coffee) | 1 tbsp. | 2 | Skim milk, Powdered milk, | 1 tbsp. | 0 |
| Cinnamon Danish | 1.3 oz. (1) | 9 | Raisin & honey bagel | 1 bagel | 1 |
| Croissant | 1 oz. (1) | 6 | Whole wheat bread | 2 slices | 2 |
| Cr. of Mushroom Soup | 10 oz. | 11 | Minestrone soup | 10 oz. | 2 |
| Bologna | 1 oz. | 7 | Ham slice, 5% fat | 1 oz. | 1 |
| Italian dressing | 2 tbsp. | 16 | Italian dressing (reduced calorie) | 2 tbsp. | 0 |
| Mayonnaise | 1 tbsp. | 11 | Light mayonnaise | 1 tbsp. | 5 |
| Tuna, in oil, drained | 3 oz. | 10 | Tuna, in water | 3 oz. | 1 |
| Butter or margarine (on potatoes or vegetables) | 1 tsp. | 4 | *Butter Buds* or *Molly McButter* (powdered) | 1/2 tsp. | 0 |

*Even when the trans fats in margarine are included as saturated fat, butter is still more saturated than margarine (66% vs. 29%).

of fat and the cream of mushroom soup would have added 9 grams of fat. Just these two changes would have increased the fat content by 23 grams, or almost 5 teaspoons of additional fat. Even 2% milk (1 7/8 cups) would have added 8.5 grams of fat.

3. It is essential to *avoid very high-fat foods*. For example, McDonalds "Big Mac" contains 26 grams of fat, a doughnut con-

| Breakfast | Fat(grams) | Calories |
|---|---|---|
| 6 oz. orange juice | 0 | 75 |
| 1/2 cup Shredded Wheat n' Bran | 1 | 90 |
| 1/2 cup skim milk | 0 | 5 |
| 1 1/2 tbsp. raisins | 0 | 40 |
| Whole wheat toast (2 slices) | 2 | 120 |
| 1 teaspoon margarine (1/2 t./slice) | 5 | 35 |
| **Total breakfast** | **8 grams** | **405 calories** |
| | | |
| **Snack** | | |
| 1 apple | 0 | 80 |
| | | |
| **Lunch** | | |
| Minestrone soup (1 cup) | 2 | 226 |
| Ham sandwich: | | |
|    Lettuce leaf | 0 | 0 |
|    Tomato slice | 0 | 8 |
|    Ham (1 slice) | 1 | 25 |
|    Mustard | 0 | 5 |
|    2 slices whole wheat bread | 2 | 120 |
| Skim milk (8 oz.) | 0 | 90 |
| **Total lunch** | **5 grams** | **474 calories** |
| | | |
| **Snack** | | |
| Rye Crisp Bread (2 crackers 2 1/2" X 4 1/2") | 0 | 50 |
| | | |
| **Dinner** | | |
| Beef tenderloin (4 oz.) | 12 | 220 |
| Baked potato (1 large) | 0 | 140 |
| Margarine, whipped (1 teas.) | 4 | 35 |
| Carrots, steamed (1/2 cup) | 0 | 25 |
| Green beans, steamed (1/2 cup) | 0 | 25 |
| Mixed green salad (1 cup) | 0 | 0 |
| French dressing, reduced cal. (2 Tbsp.) | 2 | 40 |
| Coffee (1 cup) w/ skim milk (2 tbsp.) | 0 | 11 |
| Fresh strawberries (1 cup) mixed w/ | 1 | 55 |
|    1/4 cup low-fat strawberry yogurt | 1 | 58 |
| **Total dinner** | **20 grams** | **609 calories** |
| | | |
| **DAILY TOTALS** | **33 grams** | **1618 calories** |

Figure 3.8 A daily meal plan in which fat is limited to 20% of total calories.

tains 10 grams of fat, and a medium order of French fries contains 17 grams of fat. These three items alone would bring you well over the fat limit on a 1,600-calorie diet. The main point is to avoid the highest-fat items entirely and choose the lower-fat foods, whether you are eating at home or in a restaurant. Also, if you choose a moderately high-fat item at one meal, be especially careful the rest of the day to choose low-fat or nonfat foods.

## GUIDELINES FOR LIMITING FAT TO 20% OF TOTAL CALORIES
### BREAKFAST AND LUNCH

Limit breakfast and lunch to about 10 grams of fat per meal, unless total calories are *much* higher than 1,600 calories. In that case, eat low-fat foods, but increase the quantity. For example, eat two lower-fat sandwiches or 2 cups of broth-based soup, rather than one thick hamburger or one cup of a cream-based soup. There is a great variety of breakfasts and lunches that remain within these limits. Some examples are shown in Figures 3.9 and 3.10.

| Sample Low-Fat Breakfasts | |
|---|---|
| **Breakfast I** | **Grams of Fat** |
| Pancakes (3) | 6 |
| 1 teaspoon whipped margarine | 3 |
| Syrup (2 T.) | 0 |
| Orange juice (6 oz.) | 0 |
| Skim milk (8 oz.) | 0 |
| **Total** | **9 grams fat** |
| | |
| **Breakfast II** | |
| Egg substitutes (2 Eggbeaters) | 0 |
| fried in 1 teas. whipped margarine | 3 |
| Toast (2 pieces) | 2 |
| with 1 teas. whipped margarine | 3 |
| Cantaloupe (1/4 cantaloupe) | 0 |
| Coffee (1 cup) | 0 |
| **Total** | **8 grams fat** |
| | |
| **Breakfast III** | |
| 2 whole bagels | 2 |
| with 2 teas. light cream cheese | 2 |
| Cantaloupe (1/2 cantaloupe) | 0 |
| Coffee (1 cup) | 0 |
| **Total** | **4 grams fat** |

| Sample Low-Fat Lunches | |
|---|---|
| **Lunch I** | **Grams of Fat** |
| McDonald's Regular Hamburger | 9 |
| Apple | 0 |
| Tossed Green Salad | 0 |
| With No-oil dressing | 0 |
| Skim milk or coffee | 0 |
| **Total** | **9 grams fat** |
| | |
| **Lunch II** | |
| Minestrone Soup (1 cup) | 2 |
| Turkey or Ham Sandwich | |
| 1 slice lean ham or turkey | 1 |
| Whole wheat bread (2 slices) | 2 |
| Mustard (1 teas.) | 0 |
| Orange (1) | 0 |
| Skim milk or coffee | 0 |
| **Total** | **5 grams fat** |

Figure 3.10 Two sample lunches where fat is limited to 10 grams or less per meal.

Figure 3.9 Three sample breakfasts where fat is limited to 10 grams or less per meal.

1. Determine your remaining fat allowance after subtracting the fat consumed during breakfast and lunch. Plan the dinner meal accordingly. If you are cooking for a family, try to limit the fat for the dinner meal to no more than 30% of total calories. This would be an upper limit of 20 grams of fat for a 600-calorie meal. See sample daily menu, Figure 3.8.

2. Use a low-calorie salad dressing with salads, and *Butter Buds* or another nonfat butter substitute on potatoes (instead of margarine), if this is necessary to keep fat allowance within the limit. It may not be necessary if the other foods served at the meal are low in fat.

3. Steam or microwave vegetables and serve without adding butter or high-fat sauces. Instead, sprinkle with herbs, dry *Butter Buds*, or *Molly McButter*. The butter substitutes provide the natural butter flavor without the added calories. When sprinkled over hot, steaming vegetables, including potatoes, these products appear to melt as butter.

4. Eat breads dry or with a thin scraping of soft-spread tub margarine or olive oil. Measure the amount you use (1/4 teaspoon to 1 teaspoon) to accurately calculate it into your total daily fat intake.

5. Avoid high-fat casseroles. Keep in mind when preparing casseroles for a family of four, that for every 2 tablespoons of fat (including cooking oils, butter and margarine) you add, you are adding 7 grams of fat per person. If serving only two, you would be adding 14 grams of fat per person.

6. Fat used in cooking is not limited to just cooking oils, butter and margarine. It is also present in concentrated amounts in cheese, sour cream, mayonnaise, cream, whole milk, cream-based soups and most salad dressings. Limit use of these foods or substitute with low-fat varieties. Read labels to be aware of the fat you are adding when using these foods.

7. Use low-fat sauces or nonfat gravy with meats or fish. See sauce recipes in this book. For instructions on how to make a nonfat gravy, see recipe for Turkey Gravy, p. 264.

8. Whenever possible, serve fruits for dessert. They contain almost no fat, are low in calories (compared to cakes and pies), and are loaded with nutrients and fiber.

9. Begin to think of meat as a con-

diment at meals instead of the main food to fill up on. Limit meat portions to about 4 ounces, and fish portions to 6 ounces per day. Four ounces of meat is roughly equivalent to the size of a deck of cards. For chicken, a single chicken breast is about 4 ounces, and a leg and thigh together equal about 4 ounces. A list of lower-fat meat choices is provided in Table 3.6.

## CHOOSE THESE MEATS TO REDUCE FAT AND CHOLESTEROL

The meats listed below are good choices (some better than others) when you are limiting fat and cholesterol in your diet. Under each category of beef, pork and poultry, the cuts are listed in ascending order according to fat content, i.e. the lowest fat cuts are listed first. All the figures shown are for 3-ounce cooked servings (4 ounces uncooked), with all visible fat removed. None of the meats was prepared with added fat. (During cooking, meats lose approximately 25% of their weight, mostly in water and fat.)

Table 3.6 Calories, total fat, saturated fat and cholesterol content of selected lower fat meats.

| Name of Cut | Cal. | Fat | Sat. Fat | Chol. |
|---|---|---|---|---|
| **Beef (choice grade)***  | | | | |
| Top Round Steak, braised | 176 | 4.9 | 1.7 | 76 |
| Round Tip, roasted | 153 | 5.4 | 1.9 | 69 |
| Eye of Round, roasted | 156 | 5.7 | 2.0 | 59 |
| Top Sirloin, broiled | 170 | 6.6 | 2.6 | 76 |
| Bottom Round, roasted | 164 | 6.6 | 2.2 | 66 |
| Chuck Arm Pot Roast, braised | 187 | 7.4 | 2.7 | 86 |
| Tenderloin, broiled | 180 | 8.6 | 3.2 | 71 |
| Flank Steak, broiled | 176 | 8.6 | 3.7 | 57 |
| **Pork** | | | | |
| Tenderloin, roasted | 141 | 4.1 | 1.4 | 79 |
| Ham, canned, (4% fat) | 116 | 4.1 | 1.4 | 35 |
| Ham, canned, (5% fat) | 123 | 4.7 | 1.5 | 45 |
| Center Loin Chop, broiled | 196 | 8.9 | 3.1 | 83 |
| **Poultry (roasted)** | | | | |
| Turkey, light meat, no skin | 135 | 2.7 | 0.9 | 59 |
| Chicken breast, no skin | 127 | 3.3 | 0.9 | 62 |
| Chicken, 2 drumsticks, no skn | 152 | 5.0 | 1.3 | 82 |
| Turkey, dark meat, no skin | 160 | 6.2 | 2.1 | 73 |

*The three grades of beef (based on fat content) are prime, choice and select. Prime is the highest in fat, followed by choice and then select.
Source: U.S. Dept. of Agriculture Handbooks No. 8-5, 8-10, and 8-13.
Adapted From: *Mayo Clinic Nutrition Letter*, November 1988.

## TIPS FOR REDUCING THE FAT IN YOUR DIET

• Incorporate more beans into your diet in place of meat as a protein source. For example, when making chili, use less meat and more beans, or totally eliminate the meat. (See recipe, Vegetarian Chili, page 302) Beans are an excellent low-fat protein source, and provide generous amounts of fiber and iron.

- Instead of red meats, use more poultry and fish in the main meal. Limit portions of meat to about 4 ounces per day, and fish portions to about 6 ounces per day.

- Use turkey breast in recipes calling for beef or veal. Raw turkey breast can be sliced thin and used in recipes calling for veal cutlets. It can also be ground and made into meatballs, burgers, etc., preferably after the skin and visible fat have been removed. You can grind it yourself in a food processor, or take it to your butcher to be ground.

- Buy canned fish packed in water rather than oil. If not available, drain oil well.

- Use only lean meats and trim all visible fat before cooking. Roast meat on a rack so that fat can drip off and be discarded.

- Remove skin from poultry before eating. (You can leave it on while baking or roasting to retain moisture. This will not increase fat content because fat does not migrate inward.) If seasonings or sauces, such as barbecue sauce, are used during baking or roasting, remove the skin before cooking, so that the sauce or seasoning flavor is not lost when the skin is removed.

- When browning meat, especially ground meat, spoon off excess fat before adding other ingredients. Blot cooked patties with a paper towel.

- Before making gravy, refrigerate meat drippings so that chilled and hardened fat can be removed from the top and discarded. If time does not permit refrigeration, pour drippings into a tall glass and remove liquid fat from the top with a spoon. Discard the fat. Make nonfat gravy from the remaining juices, following directions for Turkey Gravy, page 264.

- When making tuna or chicken salad, replace the mayonnaise with nonfat mayonnaise, "light" mayonnaise and/or nonfat yogurt. Begin with half "light" mayonnaise and half nonfat mayonnaise and cut the fat further, i.e. increase the proportion of nonfat mayonnaise, if taste permits. Do the same when making potato salads or other mayonnaise-based dishes. Tuna salad also tastes great using no mayonnaise—just nonfat yogurt, pickle relish, and chopped onions with the tuna.

- When selecting frozen dinners or entrees at the supermarket, look for ones with 2 grams of fat or less per 100 calories. These will derive less than 20% of their calories from fat. Supplement these dinners with bread and fresh fruit or fruit salad.

- When opening canned soups, skim fat from the top if it is visible. If making your own soup or stew, do the same.

• Reduce oil (butter, margarine or shortening) in recipes by 25% to 50%. Start with 25% less and reduce it further if taste and texture permit.

• Make hot fruit sauces with no oil. Thicken by adding cornstarch to cool fruit juice mixture. It will thicken when sauce comes to a boil. Fruit sauces are delicious with desserts or served over meat or fish.

• If possible, use non-stick pans for baking. This usually eliminates the need to grease the pan. However, if you still experience some sticking, use a vegetable cooking spray. A small amount prevents sticking more effectively than other oils or shortening.

• When sautéing vegetables, use a non-stick pan, with a small amount of water or vegetable spray. If sticking occurs, add water and steam until water is gone. Watch carefully because water evaporates quickly and burning can occur. The water prevents the vegetables from sticking or burning. When browning meats in non-stick pans, it is usually not necessary to add grease or water.

• Use vegetarian baked beans with no added fat, rather than regular baked beans (with pork). There are several different brands available at most grocery stores.

• Instead of topping baked potato with sour cream, use nonfat sour cream, low-fat yogurt or cottage cheese.

• Use reduced-calorie or fat-free salad dressings instead of regular salad dressings. Many of the reduced-calorie and fat-free dressings have less than two grams of fat per 2-tablespoon serving, while the regular dressings have from 12 to 18 grams of fat per 2-tablespoon serving.

• In fruit salads, such as Waldorf Salad (recipe, page 226), or over fresh fruit, use low-fat vanilla or fruit flavored yogurt rather than mayonnaise or whipping cream.

• Check grams of fat on cereal boxes. Some of those thought to be "healthy," such as granola cereals, are high in both sugar and fat compared to other cereals.

• Make crustless fruit pies for dessert. Most of the fat in fruit pies is in the crust. If served a pie with crust, you can reduce fat calories by not eating the crust.

• Use unsweetened cocoa powder instead of baking chocolate in recipes, since it is *much* lower in fat, especially saturated fat. Baking chocolate is loaded with cocoa butter, one of the highly saturated fats.

• Try substituting applesauce or other pureed fruits in place of half or all the fat in sweet baked goods, including muffins, cakes, brownies and cookies.

• Reduce the fat in cheese spreads by mixing the spread 1:1 with low-fat cottage cheese (1% fat) in a food processor. It will reduce the grams of fat by nearly one-half.

# FOUR

## Sodium and Other Factors Affecting Blood Pressure

### SALT IN THE DIET

No one is born with a craving for salt. Babies respond no differently to salted or unsalted foods, although they do show a definite preference for sweetened foods. Our love of salt is an *ac-* *quired* taste. By eating foods with added salt, we grow to expect the salty taste in foods. That is why when we try to restrict salt, food tastes bland and unappetizing—at least at first.

### DOES EVERYONE NEED TO RESTRICT SALT?

There is not universal agreement on whether everyone should restrict salt because research has shown that less than half the population is salt sensitive, i.e. their blood pressure is affected by the amount of salt in their diet. Nevertheless, restricting salt is still recommended by many physicians and most government advisory committees for *both* the prevention and treatment of high blood pressure. As explained in Chapter 1, population studies show that if sodium intake (one of the components of salt) is low enough (less than 2,000 milligrams per day), hypertension (high blood pressure) rarely develops. On the other hand, in countries with very high consumption of sodium, such as Japan, about 60% of the population develops the disease. It makes sense to limit sodium to reduce the risk of hypertension, especially if this condition runs in your family.

Keep in mind, though, that sodium intake must be kept at a very low level (below 2,000 milligrams per day) to inhibit the development of hypertension. Restricting it to a lesser degree will not necessarily reduce the risk of developing hypertension, but for those who are salt sensitive, it should minimize the rise in blood pressure.

If you have high blood pressure, salt restriction is especially important. Sometimes, reducing salt can eliminate the need for medication, particularly for those whose blood pressure is only slightly elevated. Cutting sodium by 50%

results in an average drop of 5 millimeters of mercury (mm Hg) for systolic pressure (top number) and 4 mm Hg for diastolic pressure (bottom number). For example, a blood pressure of 140/90 would drop, on the average, to 135/86. If diet changes are not sufficient and drugs are still needed, limiting sodium can reduce the amount of medication needed. Also, certain medications work more effectively with fewer negative side effects when sodium is restricted.

If you do not have high blood pressure and choose not to limit sodium in your diet, be sure to have your blood pressure checked annually. This way, if hypertension develops, you can be treated with diet or drugs before major harm is done to your heart and blood vessels. (See Chapter 9 for additional information on medical tests for high blood pressure, normal blood pressure ranges, etc.)

## OTHER FACTORS THAT PLAY A ROLE

Other factors that help lower blood pressure are losing weight (if overweight), regular aerobic exercise, and limiting alcohol to no more than two drinks a day. (The following constitutes one "drink": a 12-ounce beer, a 4- or 5-ounce glass of wine, a 3-ounce glass of sherry, or a 1 1/4-ounce jigger of 80-proof liquor.) Increasing potassium and calcium in the diet also appears to have a positive effect on blood pressure in some individuals.

### POTASSIUM'S ROLE

A diet rich in potassium has shown some promise in helping to reduce hypertension. Studies have shown that some individuals experience a decrease in diastolic blood pressure (bottom number) of 3 to 5 mm Hg by doubling potassium intake from foods, while sodium is kept constant. The amount of potassium that brought about this reduction was 4,000 to 5,000 milligrams per day, or about twice the average American intake of 2,500 milligrams per day. See Table 4.1 for a list of potassium-rich foods. Try to incorporate more of these foods into your diet, especially the fruits, vegetables and beans.

Adding supplements of potassium do not appear to be beneficial, and could result in an overdose, so this is *not* recommended. A study, reported in *The New England Journal of Medicine*, has shown that adding a potassium supplement (potassium chloride) to a low-salt diet had no effect on the blood pressures of those in the study group. Although these

| Choose Potassium-Rich Foods | | | |
|---|---|---|---|
| | Potassium (mg) | | Potassium (mg) |
| **Beans (cooked, 1 cup):** | | **Meat, Fish, Poultry (3 oz):** | |
| Grt. northern beans | 919 | Beef, average, lean | 317 |
| Navy beans | 755 | Pork, average, lean | 300 |
| Baked beans | 907 | Haddock | 296 |
| Red kidney beans | 658 | Snapper | 355 |
| Lentils | 731 | Scallops (6 scallops) | 428 |
| Split peas | 710 | Salmon, sockeye | 332 |
| **Fruits & Fruit Juices:** | | Rainbow trout | 539 |
| Apricots, fresh (3) | 313 | **Vegetables, (cooked):** | |
| Apricot nectar (1 c) | 214 | Lima beans (1/2 c) | 476 |
| Avocado, 1/2 | 651 | Broccoli (1 stalk) | 286 |
| Banana (1 banana) | 451 | Carrot (1 carrot) | 233 |
| Dates, pitted (10) | 541 | Cauliflower (1/2 c) | 200 |
| Fruit cocktail (1 c) | 230 | Collards (1/2 c) | 214 |
| Grapefruit juice (6 oz) | 300 | Potato (1 potato) | 844 |
| Grape juice (6 oz) | 250 | Pumpkin, canned (1/2 c) | 251 |
| Cantaloupe (1/2) | 682 | Spinach, raw (1 c) | 312 |
| Honeydew (1/4) | 935 | Spinach, frozen (1/2 c) | 283 |
| Orange | 250 | Sweet potato (1) | 397 |
| Pear (1 pear) | 208 | Tomato (1) | 254 |
| Pineapple juice (6 oz) | 255 | Tomato juice (6 oz) | 376 |
| Prunes (5 large) | 313 | Mixed vegetables (1/2 c) | 248 |
| **Dairy Products:** | | Brussels sprouts (1/2 c) | 247 |
| Buttermilk (1 c) | 371 | Squash, acorn (1/2 c) | 446 |
| Skim milk (1 c) | 406 | Rutabaga (1/2 c) | 244 |
| Yogurt (1 c) | 531 | Zucchini (1/2 c) | 228 |

Table 4.1 The potassium content of selected foods. All the foods listed here are excellent sources of potassium.

Source: *Bowes and Church's Food Values of Portions Commonly Used,* 15th Edition, revised by Jean A.T. Pennington, Harper & Row, New York, 1989.

studies are not conclusive, adding potassium-rich foods is highly recommended as part of an overall healthy diet.

## PROCESSED FOODS LOSE POTASSIUM, GAIN SODIUM

There's a simple, painless way to increase potassium and decrease sodium in your diet—eat fewer processed foods and more natural foods. An unfortunate change occurs with many foods when they are processed—they gain sodium and lose potassium, and in some cases, not just a little, but a lot. See Table 4.2.

Nature did not intend for us to eat a lot of sodium, since all unprocessed foods—fruits, vegetables, grains and meats are naturally low in sodium. So why do processed foods contain so much? The main reason is that process-

| How Processed Foods Gain Sodium and Lose Potassium | | | | |
|---|---|---|---|---|
| Food | Amount | Potassium (mg) | Sodium (mg) | Ratio |
| Milk | 1 cup | 370 | 122 | 3:1 |
| Chocolate pudding (cooked from mix) | 1 cup | 354 | 343 | 1:1 |
| Chocolate pudding (instant) | 1 cup | 335 | 820 | 1:2 |
| Beef roast (cooked) | 3 oz. | 279 | 42 | 7:1 |
| Corned beef (canned) | 3 oz. | 51 | 803 | 1:16 |
| Chipped beef | 3 oz. | 170 | 3660 | 1:22 |
| Corn (cooked) | 1 cup | 304 | 71 | 4:1 |
| Creamed corn (canned) | 1 cup | 248 | 671 | 1:3 |
| Sugar-coated corn flakes | 1 cup | 27 | 262 | 1:10 |

Table 4.2 When foods are processed, they often lose potassium and gain sodium as indicated by the values in this chart.

Reprinted by permission from *Nutrition: Concepts and Controversies, Third Edition* by Eva May Nunnelley Hamilton, et al.; Copyright © 1985 by West Publishing Company. All rights reserved.

ing often removes the natural flavors of foods, and salt is added to enhance what would otherwise be a bland product. Salt is also added as a preservative for some foods, such as bacon, ham and sausage.

## CALCIUM'S ROLE

Adding calcium to the diet has been shown to lower blood pressure in some individuals, especially those whose calcium intakes are below recommended levels. In a number of studies, adding 800 to 1,500 milligrams of calcium per day (1 glass of milk contains about 300 milligrams of calcium) lowered diastolic blood pressure by about 5 mm Hg in one-third or fewer of the participants.

In a Harvard study of 60,000 nurses, it was found that those who consumed very little calcium and magnesium had a 23% greater chance of developing hypertension than those who consumed the recommended amount. Adding calcium supplements for those who are already consuming sufficient amounts of the mineral has not been shown to lower blood pressure. The main concern should be to get *adequate* amounts of calcium in your diet, so you do not *increase* your risk for hypertension and to protect yourself from osteoporosis. This can be accomplished by eating a balanced diet, as explained in Chapter 7.

## ADVANTAGES AND DISADVANTAGES OF MEDICATION

Medication is an important tool in treating high blood pressure. Some individuals with hypertension do not respond adequately to weight loss, sodium restriction and other dietary measures. Medication is their only choice. In the last 25 years, the use of blood-pressure medication has helped reduce the number of premature deaths due to heart disease and stroke.

However, there are certain drawbacks to taking medication, and therefore, it should be used only if diet modification does not work. Some of the more common negative side effects include the following: Diuretics used in treating high blood pressure can raise cholesterol values 5 to 10% or roughly 20 points in some individuals. Diuretics can also cause blood sugar levels to become elevated and potassium to fall in 1/3 of those taking them. Other medications (beta blockers) can cause HDL, the "good" cholesterol, to decline. Newer drugs, known as ACE (angiotensis converting enzyme) inhibitors and calcium entry blockers, have slightly fewer side effects, but diet and weight reduction are still the best options if they work for you.

## HOW MUCH SODIUM IS IDEAL?

The Recommended Dietary Allowance (RDA) for sodium is a maximum of 2,400 milligrams per day, or roughly 1 teaspoon of salt. (1 teaspoon salt contains about 2,300 milligrams sodium.) Actually, our bodies only need 500 milligrams per day. Keeping sodium levels within the recommended guidelines calls for major changes for most Americans who consume an average of 3,000 to 6,000 milligrams per day.

## WHERE SODIUM COMES FROM

Where does all this sodium come from? Only about 10% occurs naturally in foods. Another 30 to 40% comes from the salt shaker, including salt used at the table (15%) and in cooking (15 to 25%). Finally, the largest percentage (40 to 60%) comes from processed foods, with about 20% of this coming from breads, cereals and other grain products.

For a more specific idea of the sodium content in foods, refer to Table 4.3. Becoming aware of the amount of sodium in the foods you eat enables you to choose your foods more wisely.

Obviously, you could stay well within the suggested guidelines by only eating simple, unprocessed foods, with no added salt. In fact, you could keep

**Sodium Content of Selected Foods**

| | Amount of Sodium (in milligrams) |
|---|---|
| **Naturally Low-Sodium Foods** | |
| Fresh fruits & vegetables | |
| Frozen fruits & vegetables (plain) | |
| Hot cereal, pasta, rice | Generally less than |
| Dry beans, peas, lentils, nuts | 50 mg. per serving |
| Canned or dried fruits, jellies | |
| Spices and herbs (no salt added) | |
| Eggs | |
| **Foods with Low/Moderate Sodium** | |
| Milk (1 cup) | 125 |
| Yogurt (1 cup) | 150 |
| Cottage cheese (1/2 cup) | 450 |
| Cold breakfast cereals (average) | 0–250 |
| Meat, fish, poultry (3.5 oz.), unprocessed | 50–80 |
| Shellfish (3 oz. cooked) (without added salt) | 50–250 |
| Bread (1 slice) | 150–200 |
| Margarine (1 teaspoon, soft) | 35 |
| **Condiments** | |
| Salt (sodium chloride) | 2300/teaspoon |
| Seasoned salt mixtures | 1200/teaspoon |
| Lite salt* | 1100/teaspoon |
| Monosodium glutamate (MSG) | 600/teaspoon |
| Light seasoned salt | 300/teaspoon |
| Baking soda | 800/teaspoon |
| Baking powder | 400/teaspoon |
| Soy sauce | 825/tablespoon |
| Mild or lite soy sauce | 600/tablespoon |
| Steak sauce, chili sauce | 250/tablespoon |
| Mustard, worcestershire, tartar sauce | 200/tablespoon |
| Catsup, BBQ sauce, seafood cocktail sauce | 150/tablespoon |
| Mayonnaise, sweet pickle relish | 100/tablespoon |
| Bouillon, broth, powdered soup base | 900/cup |
| **Processed Foods/Fast Foods** | |
| Frozen chicken TV dinner | 1150 |
| Pot pie | 800 |
| Fried chicken dinner (fast food) | 2250 |
| Small hamburger (fast food) | 500 |
| Large hamburger (fast food) | 1500 |
| Chicken sandwich (fast food) | 700–1200 |
| Large pickle | 1450 |
| Canned beans (3/4 cup) | 550 |
| Lunchmeat (1 oz.) | 300 |
| Cheese (1 oz.) | 250–500 |
| Quick breads | 400 |
| Cake (1 piece), cookies (4), brownies (1) | 100–200 |

*Lite salt contains a mixture of half sodium chloride and half potassium chloride.

Table 4.3

your sodium intake to about 500 milligrams per day, but that is extremely difficult to do and it's not necessary. There is still a place for your favorite condiments and sauces if used in moderation. Keep in mind that the sodium content listed for condiments is in quantities of a teaspoon or a tablespoon. Catsup, for example, is not particularly high in sodium if just one tablespoon is used, but some catsup lovers use far more than that. Worcestershire sauce, BBQ sauce and seafood cocktail sauce are also moderate in sodium content (as well as low in fat). Mustard is only slightly higher, but since it has such a strong flavor, sometimes just a teaspoon is sufficient.

## LITE SALT

Lite salt contains a mixture of half sodium chloride and half potassium chloride. By using it in recipes instead of table salt, you will cut sodium intake in half, provided the same quantity is used. When used in cooking, many report that they cannot tell the difference from regular table salt.

If you are taking medication for high blood pressure, check with your doctor before using a salt substitute containing potassium chloride. Some medications cause the kidneys to retain potassium, in which case potassium should be limited.

## MONOSODIUM GLUTAMATE (MSG)

What about monosodium glutamate and seasoned salt mixtures which contain MSG? Some people (1 to 2%) are allergic to MSG and suffer adverse effects, called Chinese Restaurant Syndrome, when eating foods with this additive. Thus, they should try to avoid it. For the vast majority of people, however, it is "generally regarded as safe," according to the FDA.

MSG is a natural compound, the sodium form of glutamate, an amino acid present in virtually all proteins. Glutamate is also naturally present in high levels in many vegetables, including mushrooms, tomatoes and peas.

MSG and seasoned salt mixtures can be added to foods to enhance their flavors without adding as much sodium as table salt. MSG has 600 milligrams of sodium per teaspoon, while table salt has 2,300 milligrams. Generally speaking, just 1/2 teaspoon of MSG per four servings is an optimal amount for flavor. (It enhances flavor, but doesn't taste salty.) That would be only 75 milligrams of sodium per serving—not bad. A seasoned salt mixture (1,200 milligrams of sodium per teaspoon) also can be effective in reducing sodium if used instead of table salt, since it has only about half the sodium. Light seasoned salt, with just 300 milligrams per teaspoon, is an even better choice.

## FAST FOODS AND PROCESSED FOODS

The majority of fast foods and many processed foods are loaded with sodium. These should be eaten only occasionally if trying to keep sodium within the recommended guidelines. Read labels of processed foods, including canned foods, for sodium content.

Some have low or moderate amounts of sodium. Be aware that there are sometimes great variations in sodium from one brand of food to another, even for the same food item. (See Appendix for sodium content in selected fast-food items.)

# MEAL PLANNING GUIDELINES FOR REDUCING SODIUM

### BREAKFAST: LIMIT SODIUM TO LESS THAN 400 MILLIGRAMS

This amount still enables you to choose a variety of breakfast foods. For example:

- Cereal and milk (Choose cereals with less than 200 milligrams of sodium per serving)
  - 1 egg or egg substitute and toast

(2 pieces) with one teaspoon margarine and/or jelly

- 2 pancakes with a pat of margarine (optional) and syrup

Fruit juices and/or fruits can be added to any of these breakfast choices without adding additional sodium.

### LUNCH: LIMIT SODIUM TO LESS THAN 700 MILLIGRAMS

If eating lunch out, this can be difficult, but not impossible. However, you may want to bring fruit from home to supplement the available food. Some food combinations that stay within this guideline include:

- Cold sandwich made with 1 ounce of lean ham or turkey breast on two slices of bread or a bun, with lettuce, tomato and a thin scraping of mayonnaise or mustard; cup of yogurt, and soft drink

- Fast-food hamburger (small), apple and glass of milk
- Salad with unlimited amount of fresh fruit or vegetables and 2 tablespoons salad dressing (less than 300 milligrams of sodium per 2-tablespoon serving); slice of bread or roll, and glass of milk

Additional fruits and vegetables (no salt added) can be added to any of these lunches without adding sodium. (Salt is usually added to the cooked vegetables served in restaurants and cafeterias. You can request that they make no-salt or low-salt varieties available.)

First consider the foods you always include at dinner and find out their sodium content. For example, it might be an 8-ounce glass of milk (125 milligrams) and one slice of bread (150–200 milligrams), totaling about 300 milligrams of sodium. That means you have 700 milligrams left for the remainder of the meal. Use the majority of that on a meat or casserole dish. Make allowance for dessert or salad dressing if having either one. Supplement with as many fruits and vegetables (no salt added) as desired.

The recipes in this book have moderate levels of sodium, and should help you meet the suggested guidelines. You may choose to further reduce the amount of sodium in some recipes. If so, reduce it gradually, unless you are already used to a low-sodium diet. We chose not to make all the recipes low-salt, because, as mentioned before, unless you gradually reduce salt, some foods will be bland and unappealing. The sodium content of all the recipes is provided for your information.

## TIPS FOR REDUCING SODIUM

It is important to remember that the fondness for salt is an acquired taste. Over the years, we have gradually grown to like salty, and sometimes very salty, foods. This did not happen overnight, and it is easier on almost everyone if the change to less salt is done gradually. It usually takes from 1 to 2 months for taste buds to adjust to a lower level of sodium. So give it a chance for at least that long.

• Reduce the salt (sodium) used in cooking by one-half. There are two relatively easy ways to restrict salt in cooking. The first is to use Lite salt instead of regular salt, which automatically reduces the sodium by one-half (provided the same quantity is used), without sacrificing much of the sodium taste. The second is to reduce regular salt in a two-step process. First, reduce it by 25%, which is hardly noticeable, and continue in this fashion for about a month. Then reduce it by another 25%. After three to four weeks, most people don't miss the extra salt. If they return to the amount of salt they had been using, it usually tastes too salty.

• Reduce or eliminate the salt used in non-yeast baking. With many baked goods, you can eliminate the salt and not miss it at all. When making yeast-raised breads or rolls, some salt is needed to react with the yeast. Still, the amount of salt can usually be reduced by one-third to one-half without making a noticeable difference.

• Decrease dependence on the salt shaker at the table. Start by eliminating salting vegetables, and then reduce the amount used on meat dishes. Use herbs, spices or low/moderate salt condiments in place of salt. Some especially good low-salt choices with lots of flavor are garlic powder, onion powder, salt-free Mrs. Dash, lemon juice, vinegar, chili sauce and Tabasco sauce. In addition, a tablespoon of catsup, BBQ sauce or seafood cocktail sauce adds only 150 milligrams of sodium, enabling you to stay within the guidelines if other foods are not high in sodium.

• Eat more natural foods and fewer processed foods. This is one of the most important steps in a low or moderate sodium diet. In almost all cases, you get more flavor and less sodium with fresh natural foods.

• Use low-sodium soy sauce instead of regular soy sauce. This has only about half the sodium of regular soy sauce.

• When choosing canned or frozen vegetables, choose those with no salt added.

• Choose cereals with less than 200 milligrams of sodium per serving.

• Choose salad dressings with less than 300 milligrams of sodium per 2-tablespoon serving.

• Reduce the salt in canned beans and tuna fish by rinsing for one minute. In an experiment at Duke University Medical Center, it was found that rinsing beans resulted in 40% less sodium, and rinsing tuna brought an 82% decline in sodium (from 418 to 74 milligrams).

• When a recipe calls for liquid from canned foods, use water or home-made stock instead.

• When cooking pasta or hot cereals, do not add salt to the water.

• "Cut" the sodium in prepared spaghetti sauces by adding an equal amount of "no salt added" tomatoes or tomato sauce to the spaghetti sauce mixture. To make 4 cups of sauce, use 2 cups of prepared spaghetti sauce and 1 can (16 oz.) "no salt added" tomatoes, chopped. This will result in about 50% less sodium.

• "Cut" the sodium in canned soups by adding two or three times as much water as it calls for. Add sliced carrots and diced potatoes for extra flavor and thickening. Bean soups work well with these additions. Add vegetables or extra pasta to other soups, such as chicken or turkey noodle soup. Most commercial soups contain 800 to 1,000 milligrams of sodium for a 1-cup serving. Following this suggestion will bring the sodium level to about 400 to 500 milligrams per cup.

• For ready-to-eat soups, add a 16-ounce can of "no-salt-added" stewed tomatoes or whole tomatoes, chopped, to reduce the sodium by roughly one-half.

• Avoid obviously salty foods such as pickles, potato chips, sauerkraut and salted nuts.

• If you eat out frequently, find out if there are low or moderate sodium choices available on the menu. Fast foods are usually very high in sodium, as are most restaurant and cafeteria foods. Sometimes restaurants have menu items that are lower in sodium, and it's up to you to inquire if these choices are available. If you eat out only occasionally, don't worry about the salt content. Pay more attention to the amount of fat.

• When choosing processed foods at the grocery store, look for the sodium content on the label, if given. Choose those food items that enable you to stay within the sodium guidelines for each meal.

In summary, if you have high blood pressure, you should definitely limit your sodium intake to within the recommended level. If you fail to do so, you will be putting your cardiovascular health in jeopardy.

If you do not have high blood pressure, you may or may not decide to limit sodium. It is prudent to do so to reduce the risk of developing hypertension later on. But, if you feel you are at low risk, or if you must eat out in restaurants frequently, it may be more practical for you to concentrate on all the other components of a healthy diet. In this case, be sure to get your blood pressure checked yearly, so if you develop hypertension, you can take the appropriate steps to protect your health.

Even if you do not reduce sodium as low as the RDA suggests, restricting it to some degree is still helpful. First of all, if you are salt sensitive, your blood pressure will not rise as high; and second, if you have to restrict it further because you develop high blood pressure, it will be easier since your taste buds will not be accustomed to as high a level of sodium.

# FIVE

## Sugar — Is It Bad for You?

### SUGAR IN THE DIET

Sugar is the number one food additive today, and its widespread use is a recent phenomenon. We now eat more sugar in a week than our ancestors from the early 1800s ate in a year. Over the last 150 years, the methods of sugar production have improved dramatically, increasing the supply and bringing down the prices. Instead of being a rare commodity enjoyed primarily by the rich, it is affordable in seemingly unlimited quantities to almost everyone.

In the mid-1800s, sugar consumption was just 20 pounds per person per year; by 1913, it was 76 pounds per year; and now, *on the average, we eat about 125 pounds of caloried sweeteners a year.* This represents approximately 20% of our total calories. Even with the increased use of artificial sweeteners in the last 20 years, the use of calorie-containing sweeteners has continued to rise.

### SOURCES OF SUGAR

Most of the concentrated sugar we eat (70%) has already been added to the processed foods we buy at the store. This is not only in the obviously sweet foods, but also in condiments, salad dressings, peanut butter, and many other foods. We add about 24% ourselves in baking or at the table; and about 6% is from institutional sources (restaurants, hospitals, etc.).

Unlike our acquired taste for salt, we have an inborn love of sugar. Anyone who has witnessed a baby's enthu-

siasm when eating fruit for the first time knows this is true. Although we are born with a natural sugar craving, the amount of sugar we desire is conditioned. The more sugar you eat, the more you crave in order to satisfy your "sweet tooth." The opposite is also true. The less you eat, over a long period of time, (at least two or three months), the less you will want. You can reduce the amount of sugar in foods you prepare, and then actually prefer that amount once you condition yourself to it.

## SUGAR—NATURAL VS. CONCENTRATED

Are the natural sugars in fruits healthier than concentrated sugar used as an additive? All the different sugars, from those occurring naturally in fruits, to the concentrated sugar in candy bars, are broken down during digestion to glucose, the basic energy unit of carbohydrates. Even the starch in potatoes, rice and corn is broken down to this same glucose, which serves as the fuel for all the cells in the body. Strictly speaking, the body doesn't treat the natural sugar in fruits any differently than concentrated sugar.

Fruits and vegetables are healthier alternatives for another reason. Their diluted sugars come naturally packaged with vitamins, minerals and fiber, all essential to a healthy body. Also, they have less caloric density, which means that there are fewer calories in relation to the bulk of the food. Because of this, you are less likely to consume too many calories when eating fruit. For example, one apple has just 80 calories; whereas, a piece of apple pie has about 282 calories. You would have to eat three and one-half apples before you would consume as many calories as in that one piece of pie. Most people would feel satisfied after one, or at most, two apples.

Concentrated sugar in candy bars, etc. is also more likely to bring on an insulin response than the diluted sugars in fruits. Initially you feel a burst of energy because the sugar from the candy bar goes quickly into the bloodstream in the form of glucose. This triggers the pancreas to produce insulin to drive the sugar (glucose) from the bloodstream into the cells. In some individuals, this results in an excess of insulin and a deficiency of glucose in the blood, which produces a tired and weak feeling. This occurs shortly after the initial burst of energy. It doesn't cause permanent harm but can keep you from feeling your best.

Recipes for baked goods, which call for concentrated fruit juices instead of granulated sugar, are not necessarily more nutritious. Most of the vitamin C from the juice is destroyed during baking. Vitamin A is not destroyed by baking, but most concentrated juices contain little, if any, of this vitamin. Therefore, follow your taste buds in deciding what sweetener to use. Judge the nutritional value of baked goods by the other ingredients in the recipe, not by the type of sweetener.

## IS TOO MUCH SUGAR HARMFUL?

Is it harmful to your health to derive 20% of your calories from sugar?

A panel of scientists at the Food and Drug Administration (FDA) concluded after extensive study that sugar alone doesn't contribute to any health problems other than dental cavities. That's promising news to everyone who has a strong sweet tooth.

Keep in mind, though, that what accompanies the sugar, in many cases, is harmful. Most candy bars and many desserts are loaded with fat, which can increase our risks for heart disease, cancer and obesity.

There are three factors to consider in determining whether sugar as an additive is detrimental to your health. The first is to look at what accompanies the sugar. If sugar is used to enhance the flavors of nutritious foods, such as low-fat sweetened fruit sauces over lean meat, or a low-fat, low-cholesterol rice pudding, it can indeed be part of a healthy diet. The recipes in this book have combined good nutrition with the use of sugar—they are low in fat and contain other nutritious foods in combination with the sugar.

The second factor to consider is whether you can afford the empty calories in sugar. You may well afford the one teaspoon of sugar (16 calories) in your tea or coffee, but not the 5 teaspoons of sugar (and all the fat) in a chocolate bar. Approximately one in four Americans is overweight, and eating less sugar is a wise way to cut back calories without sacrificing needed nu-

trients. If you limit fat intake and exercise regularly, a moderate amount of sugar should not result in excessive weight gain.

The third consideration is whether the sugar is replacing more nutritious foods. For someone on a low-calorie diet, this can be an especially serious problem. Theoretically, it is estimated that with careful food selection, one needs close to 1,500 calories a day to obtain all the needed nutrients with foods, i.e. without vitamin supplements.

Some teenage girls eat only 1,200 calories a day to maintain their desired body weight. If they are "wasting" 20% or more of these calories on concentrated sugar, they will probably be nutrient deficient in some areas. Anyone on a low-calorie regimen should be extremely careful to eat only the most highly nutritious foods.

On the other hand, teenage boys and girls active in competitive sports may burn 3,000 to 4,000 calories a day. They can well afford some "empty" calories from sugar, if their nutrient needs have already been met.

Also, there are certain health conditions that warrant closer monitoring of sugar. Persons with diabetes, hypoglycemia and high levels of triglycerides in their blood need to watch their sugar intake more carefully.

## TYPES OF SUGAR

Concentrated sugar is listed many different ways on food labels. When trying to limit sugar, it is important to recognize which ingredients represent sugar. Although the names change, the nutritional value of sugars used in processed foods is negligible, except for molasses. Refer to the "Miniglossary of Sugar Terms" for a description of the different types of sugar.

---

### Miniglossary of Sugar Terms

**Brown sugar:** At 51 calories per tablespoon, brown sugar has no significant nutritive value. It is usually made by adding a small amount of molasses to white sugar.

**Confectioner's sugar:** This is finely powdered sucrose (table sugar), 99.9 percent pure.

**Corn syrup:** Corn syrup is made by breaking down corn starch with acids, resulting in a clear, sweet liquid. It is nutritionally equal to white sugar.

**Corn sweeteners:** These include corn syrup and sugars derived from corn.

**Dextrose:** A component of table sugar, dextrose is the technical name for glucose. Hundreds of dextrose (glucose) molecules make up starch molecules, or complex carbohydrates, found in vegetables, beans and grains.

**Fructose:** Fructose is one of several fruit sugars. It is made chemically by splitting sucrose into its components, fructose and dextrose. It does not raise blood sugar levels as much as dextrose and sucrose, and is therefore less of a problem for diabetics.

**Glucose:** One of the simple sugars, glucose is one of the components of sucrose, or table sugar. All carbohydrates are broken down to glucose during digestion.

**High-fructose corn syrup:** This sugar generally contains 42 to 90% fructose, and the remainder dextrose. Because it is inexpensive to make, high-fructose corn syrup, abbreviated HFCS on food and drink labels, is now used in nearly all soft drinks in place of sucrose.

**Honey:** Honey has erroneously been credited with being a healthier alternative to sugar. Actually, it is nutritionally equivalent to table sugar, although somewhat sweeter and more expensive. It causes blood sugar levels to rise more than sucrose (table sugar).

**Lactose:** This is the sugar found naturally in milk and other dairy products. It is less sweet than sucrose.

**Maple sugar:** This sugar is derived from the concentrated sap of the sugar maple tree. Although once a common sweetener, it is now rarely added to foods, and typically has been replaced by sucrose and artificial maple flavoring.

**Molasses:** A by-product of table sugar made from sugar cane, molasses is the only form of sugar that contains substantial amounts of nutrients. One tablespoon of black strap molasses supplies 12% of the U.S. RDA for calcium, and 18% of a woman's RDA for iron (32% of a male's RDA). Light molasses is a diluted form and has about one-third as much of the same nutrients.

**Natural sweeteners:** All of the sugars listed here are natural sugars.

**Raw sugar:** Raw sugar is a less refined version of white table sugar.

**Sucrose:** This is white table sugar, made from sugar cane or sugar beets. It is composed of one fructose molecule and one dextrose (glucose) molecule.

---

# ARTIFICIAL SWEETENERS

The use of artificial sweeteners has skyrocketed since the 1950s when they first became popular in diet drinks. Since that time, there has been a lot of controversy concerning the safety of sugar substitutes. The issue is still not settled, but the available information suggests that they are not harmful to most people. However, they are not recommended for children under the age of two, since their safety for that age group is more questionable.

The two principal artificial sweeteners are saccharin and aspartame. Aspartame is called "Nutra-sweet" in diet drinks, chewing gum, presweetened cereals, etc., and is sold as "Equal" in a powdered form to be used in place of sugar. It is composed of two amino acids that occur naturally in foods, phenylalanine and aspartic acid. The safe daily limit, set by the FDA, is equivalent to about 16 cans of diet drinks (72 packets of Equal) for a 160-pound adult, or 4 cans of diet drinks for a 40-pound child. Most people consume 10% or less of this amount per day. Tests with animals have shown no ill effects when consumption levels are 100 times the acceptable level for humans.

Aspartame can pose a health risk for individuals who have a rare genetic condition called phenylketonuria (PKU). This disease, which is usually diagnosed at birth, involves a sensitivity to the amino acid phenylalanine, one of the components of aspartame. Those with PKU must restrict the amount of phenylalanine they consume. Aspartame may also cause headaches in some individuals.

There is more widespread concern over the use of saccharin than aspartame. It has been banned in Canada, except as a table-top sweetener sold only in pharmacies. The ban was imposed because of a study (March 1977) linking it with an increased incidence of bladder cancer in animals. In the United States, beginning in February 1988, the FDA has required that foods containing saccharin carry a warning label stating that "use of this product may be hazardous to your health." To date, saccharin has not been shown to cause cancer in humans.

Many processed foods contain a combination of both sweeteners. Aspartame is much more expensive than saccharin and it breaks down and loses its sweetness more readily. Therefore, saccharin is added to reduce overall costs and to increase the product's shelf life. Be sure to carefully read the small print on the label if you want to avoid or limit foods sweetened with saccharin.

There are some benefits to using artificial sweeteners. They do not promote tooth decay and they have fewer calories for those who would like to lose weight. Using artificial sweeteners to help lose weight does not work for most people though, since the number of overweight Americans has increased since sugar substitutes were first introduced. Many of them consistently use artificial sweeteners in diet drinks, etc., and use that as a rationalization for eating other high-calorie foods. They may eat several times as many calories in the high-calorie food as they are saving by drinking a diet soda.

## TIPS FOR REDUCING SUGAR CONSUMPTION

Here are some suggestions for reducing the sugar in your diet or your family's diet:

• Reduce the sugar in recipes by one-fourth. When you are accustomed to that taste, try reducing it by another quarter. (Using less sugar in baked goods changes the texture slightly, causing the product to be more dense, less light and airy.)

• Keep fewer candies and desserts in the house and more fresh fruit. When you crave sweets, fruits are more likely to satisfy you when concentrated sweets are not available.

• Use sugar-free or low-sugar jams and jellies.

• Use unsweetened cereals and sweeten them by adding fresh or dried fruits.

• Try to limit high-sugar soft drinks. As an alternative, add spark to unsweetened fruit juices by adding seltzer or club soda.

• Make your own "frozen pops" by freezing fruit juices in plastic pop molds or in small paper cups. Insert stick into cup when juice is partially frozen.

• Choose frozen or canned fruits with little or no sugar added.

# SIX

---

# *Adding Complex Carbohydrates: Fruits, Vegetables and Whole Grains*

## COMPLEX CARBOHYDRATES IN THE DIET

Up to this point we have discussed food components that should be limited in a healthy diet, i.e. fat, cholesterol, salt and sugar. With complex carbohydrates, the opposite is advised. More of these should be *added* to the diet, particularly, more fruits, vegetables and whole-grain products. Calories lost by reducing fat should be replaced, all or in part, by complex carbohydrates. If your goal is to lose weight, then only some of the calories should be replaced, so that total calories are reduced.

## WHY COMPLEX CARBOHYDRATES ARE IMPORTANT

As a whole, complex carbohydrates are low in fat and contain an abundance of natural vitamins, minerals and fiber. Therefore, eating a diet rich in these foods brings many health benefits. It reduces your risks for cancer, heart disease (in part, by replacing the fat) and intestinal disorders. Furthermore, it makes it easier to maintain ideal body weight, since complex carbohydrates (without added fat) are high in bulk, but relatively low in calories. Some complex carbohydrates, particularly beans and grains, are also excellent sources of protein, with only negligible fat. This is in contrast to protein from animal sources, which contains varying amounts of saturated fat.

The components in fruits and vegetables that appear to have a protective effect against cancer are beta carotene (which is converted to vitamin A during digestion), vitamin C, and a non- vitamin compound called *indoles* found in cruciferous vegetables. (See Figure 6.1 for a list of cruciferous vegetables.) Researchers in this field suspect that other components of fruits and vegetables, still unidentified, work in combination with these to produce the overall health benefits. One study showed that the greater the "dose" of produce of any type, the lower the incidence of cancer. The protective effect may be further enhanced if eating more produce means eating fewer fatty foods. Several studies conducted in the early 1990s have shown that beta carotene may also have a protective effect against heart disease and stroke.

The fiber from complex carbohydrates is one of the factors that helps reduce the risk of colon cancer and other intestinal disorders, including diverticulosis, irritable bowel syndrome, constipation and hemorrhoids.

## COMPLEX CARBOHYDRATES ARE NOT FATTENING

Many people are under the mistaken notion that carbohydrates, especially starches, are fattening. Actually, the opposite is true—they are relatively low in calories. Perhaps they have acquired this reputation because of what is added to them. For example, a large, plain baked potato contains only 145 calories. But, if you add two teaspoons of butter or margarine and two tablespoons of sour cream to it, you bring the total calories to 265. Sprinkle on a few bacon bits and one-half ounce shredded cheese and the total reaches 368—a hefty increase from the original 145 calories!

Bread is also relatively low in calories. Most varieties range from 65 to 70 calories per slice. One study demonstrated that a young man's diet could include as many as 12 slices of bread in a day (in addition to other foods to provide a balanced diet) and still allow him to lose more than a pound a week. The 12 slices of bread (780 calories) have about as many calories as just one Wendy's double hamburger with cheese (800 calories).

For many, just eating more fruits and vegetables in place of higher-fat foods enabled them to lose weight without feeling hungry or deprived.

## HOW MANY FRUITS AND VEGETABLES SHOULD WE EAT?

According to National Food Consumption Surveys, most of us fall far short of the number of fruits and vegetables we are advised to eat each day. On any given day, almost a third of Americans report eating no vegetables and about half eat a total of just two or fewer fruits and vegetables per day.

The U. S. Department of Agriculture recommends that we eat three to five serv-

ings of vegetables per day and two to four servings of fruit. A serving is either a half-cup portion or a medium-size fruit or vegetable. Ideally, at least one of the fruits or vegetables should be high in vitamin C, another should be high in vitamin A, and one a cruciferous vegetable. A 6-ounce glass of fruit juice is acceptable as a fruit portion, but the nutrients and fiber in a fresh fruit are superior to those in juice.

Nutritionally, all fruits and vegetables are not created equal. Some are better than others; some are high in one nutrient, but low in another; some have more fiber, etc. For this reason, it is important to vary the fruits and vegetables in your diet to get a balance of all the important nutrients. See Table 6.1 for a comparison of the fiber, vitamin C, vitamin A (beta carotene) and calories in fruits and fruit juices.

Vegetables, like fruits, also vary in the nutrients present. Some are much better sources of vitamin A (beta carotene) and others are high in vitamin C, or fiber. Vary your choices for optimal nutrition. Table 6.2 compares the fiber, vitamin C, vitamin A and calorie content of selected vegetables.

## CRUCIFEROUS VEGETABLES

According to the American Cancer Society, cruciferous vegetables activate enzymes in the liver, which are thought to break down cancer-promoting chemicals. Research indicates that these vegetables reduce the risk of certain types of cancer, including esophageal, stomach, colon, rectal, lung and bladder cancer. Their effectiveness in combating cancer is further enhanced by the fact that they are good sources of vitamins A and/or C. See Figure 6.1 for a list of cruciferous vegetables.

## HOW SAFE IS OUR PRODUCE?

Occasionally, news stories question the safety of our fruits and vegetables, stating that there may be dangerous levels of pesticides or herbicides in supermarket produce. How valid are these concerns? According to the National Research Council (NRC), health risks posed by eating the fruits and vegetables available in supermarkets are very small. However, in 1993, NRC acknowledged that the effects of pesticides in children need to be studied further, because current guidelines may not be strict enough to protect young children. This is because children may eat more of certain foods relative to their size while their bodies are still developing, making them more vulnerable to the potential negative effects.

These media headlines should not overshadow the fact that it is far more harmful to the health of both adults and children to avoid fruits and vegetables than it is to eat them. The recommendation to minimize pesticide or herbicide residues is to wash all fresh produce in plain water, or with a little dishwashing detergent, and either peel it (especially if there is an obvious wax coating) or use a vegetable scrubber. If using soap, be sure

**The Value of Fruits**

| Fruit (serving) | Fiber (grams) | Vit. C (%USRDA) | Vit. A (%USRDA) | Calories |
|---|---|---|---|---|
| Apple (1) | 3.0 | 13 | 1 | 81 |
| Apple, w/o skin | 2.4 | 8 | 1 | 72 |
| Apple juice (6 oz.) | 0.6 | 3* | - | 87 |
| Apricots (3 med.) | 1.4 | 18 | 55 | 51 |
| Banana (1 med.) | 1.8 | 17 | 2 | 105 |
| Blackberries, raw (1/2 c) | 4.7 | 25 | 2 | 37 |
| Blueberries (1/2 c) | 1.7 | 16 | 1 | 41 |
| Cantaloupe (1/4) | 1.1 | 113 | 103 | 57 |
| Cherries (10) | 1.1 | 8 | 3 | 49 |
| Dates, dried (5 dates) | 3.6 | - | - | 114 |
| Grapefruit, pink (1/2) | 0.7 | 78 | 6 | 37 |
| Grapefruit, white (1/2) | 0.7 | 65 | - | 39 |
| Grapefruit juice (6 oz) | 0.4 | 90 | - | 70 |
| Honeydew (1/10) | 0.9 | 77 | 2 | 66 |
| Mango (1) | 3.7 | 95 | 161 | 135 |
| Nectarine (1) | 2.5 | 12 | 20 | 67 |
| Orange (1) | 3.1 | 133 | 5 | 65 |
| Orange Juice (6 oz) | 0.4 | 155 | 7 | 83 |
| Papaya (1/2) | 2.7 | 157 | 61 | 59 |
| Peach (1) | 1.4 | 10 | 9 | 37 |
| Pear (1) | 4.3 | 11 | - | 98 |
| Pineapple (1/2 c) | 1.4 | 20 | - | 39 |
| Plum (1) | 2.5 | 10 | 4 | 36 |
| Prunes, dried (5 prunes) | 3.0 | 3 | 17 | 101 |
| Raisins (1/2 c) | 4.0 | 4 | - | 225 |
| Raspberries (1/2 c) | 4.0 | 26 | 2 | 31 |
| Strawberries (1 c) | 3.9 | 141 | - | 45 |
| Tangerine (1) | 2.0 | 43 | 15 | 37 |
| Watermelon (1 c) | 0.6 | 25 | 11 | 50 |

Table 6.1 Fiber, vitamin C, vitamin A (beta-carotene) and calorie content of selected fruits and fruit juices.

*Fortified apple juice provides 75% of the USRDA for Vitamin C per serving.
(-) less than 1% of the USRDA
(NA) not available.
Sources: *Bowes and Church's Food Values of Portions Commonly Used*, 15th Edition, revised by Jean A. T. Pennington, Harper & Row, New York, 1989; and Human Nutrition Information Service, USDA, Provisional Table on the Dietary Fiber Content of Selected Foods, HNIS/PT-106, 1988.

to rinse thoroughly. The outer leaves of cabbage and lettuce should be discarded. These steps will remove more than 90% of any residues that may be present. Based on sample testing, no more than 2% of domestically grown produce and 4% of imported produce have residues above the legal limits.

| The Value of Vegetables | | | | |
|---|---|---|---|---|
| **Vegetable (serving)** | **Fiber (grams)** | **Vit. C (%USRDA)** | **Vit. A (%USRDA)** | **Calories** |
| Asparagus, raw (1/2 c) | 1.4 | 30 | 15 | 22 |
| Beets (1/2 c) | 1.4 | 9 | - | 26 |
| Broccoli (1/2 c) | 2.0 | 62 | 22 | 23 |
| Brussels sprouts (1/2 c) | 3.4 | 60 | 11 | 33 |
| Cabbage, green (1/2 c shrd) | 0.8 | 28 | - | 8 |
| Carrots (1 raw) | 2.3 | 12 | 405 | 31 |
| Cauliflower (1/2 c) | 1.4 | 57 | - | 15 |
| Celery, raw (1 stalk) | 0.6 | 5 | 1 | 6 |
| Corn, canned (1/2 c) | 2.5 | 10 | 4 | 66 |
| Cucumber (1/2 c sliced) | 0.5 | 3 | - | 7 |
| Eggplant (1/2 c) | 1.2 | - | - | 13 |
| Green beans (1/2 c) | 1.0 | 10 | 8 | 22 |
| Lettuce, Romaine (1/2 c shrd) | 0.5 | 12 | 14 | 4 |
| Lettuce, iceberg (1 leaf) | 0.3 | - | 1 | 3 |
| Mixed vegetables (1/2 c frzn) | 2.1 | 5 | 78 | 54 |
| Mushrooms, boiled (1/2 c) | 1.7 | 5 | - | 21 |
| Onions, raw (1/2 c chopped) | 1.3 | 12 | - | 27 |
| Parsley, raw (1/2 c chopped) | 1.3 | 45 | 32 | 10 |
| Peas (1/2 c) | 2.2 | 13 | 10 | 63 |
| Peppers, sweet (1/2 c chpd) | 0.8 | 106 | 5 | 12 |
| Potato, no skin (baked) | 2.3 | 37 | NA | 88 |
| Pumpkin, canned (1/2 c) | 3.4 | 8 | 538 | 41 |
| Spinach, raw (1/2 c) | 0.7 | 13 | 38 | 6 |
| Spinach, cooked (1/2 c) | 2.0 | 15 | 148 | 21 |
| Squash, all varieties (1/2 c) | 2.2 | 17 | 72 | 13 |
| Sweet potato, mashed (1/2 c) | 3.0 | 47 | 559 | 172 |
| Tomato (1 raw) | 1.6 | 37 | 28 | 24 |
| Turnip, chopped (1/2 c) | 1.2 | 15 | - | 14 |
| Turnip greens, boiled (1/2 c) | 2.2 | 33 | 80 | 15 |
| Watercress, raw (1/2 c chpd) | 0.4 | 12 | 16 | 2 |

Table 6.2 Fiber, vitamin C, vitamin A (beta-carotene) and calorie content of selected vegetables.

(-) Less than 1% of the USRDA
(NA) Not available
Sources: Bowes and Church's *Food Values of Portions Commonly Used*, 15th Edition, revised by Jean A. T. Pennington, Harper & Row, New York, 1989; and Human Nutrition Information Service, USDA, Provisional Table on the Dietary Fiber Content of Selected Foods, HNIS/PT-106, 1988.

## MAXIMIZING THE NUTRITIONAL VALUE OF FRUITS AND VEGETABLES

Many of the vitamins and minerals in fruits and vegetables are susceptible to being lost during the storage or cooking process. However, with proper

| Cruciferous Vegetables | |
|---|---|
| Bok choy | Kohlrabi |
| *Broccoli | Leaf mustard (Chinese spinach) |
| *Brussels sprouts | Radish greens |
| *Cabbage: napa, red, white | Rutabagas |
| *Cauliflower | Sea Kale |
| Chinese kale | Mustard |
| Collards | Spinach |
| Garden cress | Upland cress |
| Horseradish | Watercress |
| Kale, Southern curled | White mustard |

*Animal research has shown that these starred vegetables offer special protection against some forms of cancer. The remaining vegetables, though not yet tested, are members of the cruciferous vegetable family and are expected to offer similar protection.

Figure 6.1 Cruciferous Vegetables.

methods, the majority of these nutrients can be preserved. The following information and suggestions should help you receive the maximum amount of nutrients from fruits and vegetables.

1. In most cases, fresh and frozen produce provide more nutrients than canned fruits and vegetables. Frozen foods may contain more nutrients than fresh fruits and vegetables that have been stored in the produce department for more than a day.

2. Fresh produce contains most nutrients when ripe — not underripe or overripe (soft, wrinkled). To keep fruits and vegetables from becoming overripe and losing nutrients, store in the refrigerator.

3. When selecting citrus fruits, such as oranges and grapefruits, ignore blemishes, scars and outside color. Rather, choose those that are heavy for their size, with smooth skin and no soft spots. The heavier the fruits, the juicier and more nutritious they will be.

4. Cook vegetables over, not in, water. This minimizes the loss of water-soluble vitamins, which include vitamin C and the B vitamins. If cooked in water that is poured down the drain, as much as 50% of these vitamins may be lost, no matter if the food is cooked in 1/4 cup or 4 cups of water.

5. Avoid long cooking times. Cook only long enough to make vegetables "crisp-tender."

6. Cook potatoes with the skins on to preserve nutrients, especially if boiled in water. Nutrients lost in the

water include vitamin C, the B vitamins, potassium, iron and zinc.

7. Try to use the liquid from steamed or boiled vegetables, rather than discarding it, because many water-soluble vitamins and minerals are dissolved in the water. The liquid can be used in soups, in cooking rice, or to moisten casseroles.

8. If you store cut fruits or vegetables, or fruit juices, cover with an airtight wrapper or container and store in the refrigerator. If this procedure is followed for reconstituted orange juice, for example, it will retain 80% of its vitamin C after eight days of storage.

9. Avoid purchasing potatoes that are spongy, wrinkled, or sprouting eyes. If there is a green tinged area, cut it away.

10. Choose broccoli that has dark green, tight florets, with firm, not rubbery stalks. Yellow or enlarged florets are signs of over- maturity.

11. If a banana begins to turn brown, and you are not ready to eat it, refrigerate it. It will slow down the ripening process. Refrigeration causes the peeling to turn an unattractive black color, but that doesn't affect the banana, which will remain fresh inside for several days.

## FIBER

Complex carbohydrates provide the primary source of fiber in the diet. If you are not getting enough fiber, the reason is very simple—you are not eating enough fruits, vegetables and/or whole-grain products.

There are two types of dietary fiber—soluble and insoluble. Both play an important role in overall health. Soluble fiber is needed to remove fatty compounds (including cholesterol) from the body, and to help regulate blood glucose levels. Insoluble fiber is needed to ensure proper elimination of the body's waste products and a healthy digestive system. Soluble fiber is found primarily in oats, oat bran, beans, fruits and vegetables. The main sources of insoluble fiber are whole-grain products, especially wheat bran, beans, and the peelings of fruits and vegetables.

### HOW MUCH FIBER?

The National Cancer Institute and an expert panel convened by the Food and Drug Administration recommend 20 to 30 grams, and no more than 35 grams of dietary fiber per day. The Mayo Clinic Nutrition Department recommends the same minimal level, but with an upper limit of 50 grams of fiber.

This is considerably more than the 10 to 15 grams per day consumed by the average American. The recommendation is considered adequate to reduce the risks for intestinal diseases including colon cancer, diverticulosis and irritable bowel syndrome. It should also be adequate to avoid constipation.

| Dietary Fiber in Selected Foods | | | |
|---|---|---|---|
| | **Fiber (g)** | | **Fiber (g)** |
| **Breads and Rice** | | | |
| Brown rice (1 c) | 3.0 | Pear (1) | 4.3 |
| White rice (1 c) | 1.2 | Strawberries (1 c) | 3.9 |
| Whole wheat bread (1 slice) | 1.6 | **Legumes (cooked)** | |
| White bread (1 slice) | 0.6 | Baked beans (1/2 c) | 6.0 |
| **Cereals (1 oz.)** | | Chickpeas (1/2 c) | 6.0 |
| All-Bran (1/3 c) | 8.5 | Black-eyed peas (1/2 c) | 4.0 |
| Fruit & Fiber (1/2 c) | 4.3 | Lentils (1/2 c) | 4.0 |
| Raisin Bran (1/2 c) | 3.7 | Navy Beans (1/2 c) | 5.0 |
| Shredded Wheat (1 biscuit) | 2.2 | Chestnuts, roasted (3 nuts) | 2.8 |
| Wheat Chex (2/3 c) | 3.7 | **Vegetables** | |
| **Fruits** | | Broccoli, cooked (1/2 c) | 2.0 |
| Apple (1) | 3.0 | Carrot, 1 raw | 2.3 |
| Banana (1) | 1.8 | Lima beans, cooked (1/2 c) | 6.1 |
| Blueberries (1/2 c) | 1.7 | Mixed veg. (1/2 c) | 2.1 |
| Dates, dried (5 dates) | 3.6 | Peas (1/2 c) | 2.2 |
| Mango (1) | 3.7 | Potato w/skin (1 med) | 3.0 |
| Orange (1) | 3.1 | Spinach, cooked (1/2 c) | 2.0 |
| Plum (1) | 2.5 | Sweet potato, (1/2 c) | 3.0 |

Sources: *Bowes and Church's Food Values of Portions Commonly Used*, 15th Edition, revised by Jean A.T. Pennington, Harper & Row, New York, 1989; and USDA Provisional Table on the Dietary Fiber Content of Selected Foods, HNIS/PT-106, 1988.

Table 6.3 Approximate dietary fiber content of selected foods.

An upper limit of 35 to 50 grams per day is suggested because even fiber can have the potential for harm if consumed in excess. Too much fiber can cause mineral losses or dehydration (if you don't drink enough fluids). Mineral losses can occur if foods pass through the body too quickly before some minerals have the chance to be absorbed.

It is best to take in fiber from a variety of sources—whole grains, nuts (in moderation because of high fat content), fruits and vegetables—and to eat it throughout the day, rather than large doses of wheat bran once or twice a day. Not only do you need the nutrients from a wide variety of foods, but cancer studies suggest that the greatest benefits are realized when fiber-rich foods are eaten

| Daily Menus Demonstrating Recommended Fiber Intake | | | |
|---|---|---|---|
| **Day I Menu** | | **Day II Menu** | |
| **Breakfast I** | Dietary Fiber (g) | **Breakfast II** | Dietary Fiber (g) |
| Whole wheat toast (2 slices) | 3.2 | All-bran cereal (1/3 cup) | 8.5 |
| Margarine (1 teaspoon) | - | Milk (1/2 cup) | - |
| Orange juice (6 oz.) | 0.4 | Bagel, plain white | 1.2 |
| Banana | 1.8 | Light cream cheese (2 teaspoons) | - |
| | | Orange | 3.1 |
| **Lunch I** | | | |
| Ham sandwich: | | **Lunch II** | |
|   Hard roll | 1.4 | Salad | |
|   Ham (1 oz.) | - |   Lettuce (1 cup) | 1.0 |
|   Mayonnaise (1 teaspoon) | - |   Tomato | 1.6 |
|   Lettuce | - |   Garbanzo beans (1/4 cup) | 1.4 |
| Baked beans (3/4 cup) | 5.0 |   Salad dressing (2 tablespoons) | - |
| Apple | 3.0 | Whole wheat bread (2 slices) | 3.2 |
| Milk shake | - | Margarine (1 teaspoon) | - |
| | | Apple | 3.0 |
| **Dinner I** | | Iced tea | - |
| Chicken breast (4 oz.) | - | | |
| Whole wheat bread (1 slice) | 1.6 | **Dinner II** | |
| Potato (with skin) | 3.0 | Beef-vegetable stir fry | |
| Broccoli (3/4 cup) | 3.0 |   Beef (3 oz.) | - |
| Tossed salad w/vegetables | 1.5 |   Cauliflower (1/4 cup) | 0.7 |
| Strawberries (1/2 cup) | 2.0 |   Broccoli (1/4 cup) | 1.0 |
| Skim milk (8 oz.) | - |   Green pepper (1/4 cup) | 0.4 |
| **Total Fiber for Day I** | **25.9 (g)** | Brown rice (1 cup) | 3.0 |
| | | French bread (1 slice) | 0.6 |
| | | Frozen yogurt (1 cup) | - |
| | | Skim milk (8 oz.) | - |
| | | **Total Fiber for Day II** | **28.7 (g)** |

Table 6.4 Two daily menus to show different combinations of food that meet the recommended guidelines for fiber.

throughout the day. A pure bran cereal at breakfast is fine as long as you also get additional fiber from other sources. See Table 6.3 to compare the fiber content of selected foods.

Let's examine two sample daily meal plans for breakfast, lunch and dinner that equal 25 to 30 grams of fiber per day. This will give you a good idea of the combinations of foods that meet the recommended guidelines for fiber. See Table 6.4.

As the sample menus indicate, your fiber needs can be met in many different ways. The following suggestions should help you meet those needs. Eat a total of *at least* five fruits and vegetables per day. You can choose a variety of breads, but include some whole-grain types. Include beans, and occasionally, nuts (in small quantities) for excellent high-fiber sources. Read the fiber content on cereal boxes to include some high-fiber choices (from 5 to 14 grams of fiber per serving). Sometimes, mixing a high fiber cereal with a lower fiber cereal enables you to get the fiber you need with the taste you prefer.

## BENEFITS OF WHOLE GRAINS VS. REFINED GRAINS

In addition to fiber, whole-grain products also have other benefits. They contain more protein and minerals than their refined counterparts, and have at least twice as much vitamin B6, vitamin E, magnesium and zinc. The additional nutrients are found in the bran and germ, the parts removed during refining. Figure 6.2 shows the components of a kernel of wheat.

Most breads and cereals are enriched, which means some of the nutrients lost in the refining process are restored, including iron, thiamin, riboflavin and niacin. Other minerals lost, but not replaced, are magnesium, manganese, chromium, zinc, folate, vitamin B6 and copper. Researchers are discovering that a substantial number of Americans may not consume enough of these nutrients, since they eat so few whole-grain foods.

### DON'T BE FOOLED BY "WHEAT BREAD" LABELS

Manufacturers seem to have caught on that Americans want to eat more whole-grain bread but prefer the soft, fluffy texture of white bread. So they label some breads "wheat bread" and add caramel color to make it look like whole wheat bread. In fact, the

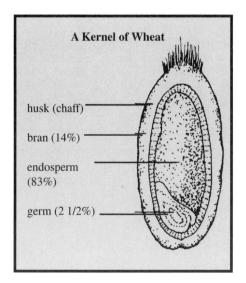

**A Kernel of Wheat**

husk (chaff)

bran (14%)

endosperm (83%)

germ (2 1/2%)

Figure 6.2 A kernel of wheat. The husk or chaff is inedible to humans and is usually fed to livestock. The remaining wheat kernel has three main parts: the endosperm, the germ and the bran. The endosperm is the soft, inside part of the kernel, which contains starch and protein, and is the only part of the kernel used to make refined white flour. The germ has high nutritive value since it contains the concentrated food, including vitamins and minerals, to support new life after the wheat seed is planted. The bran forms a protective coating around the kernel, and is also rich in nutrients and fiber. (Corn, oat and rice grains have similar structures.)

bread may be made primarily with refined flour, with only a small proportion of whole wheat flour added. Therefore, the texture is soft like white bread. It is fine to eat this bread occasionally, but be aware that the fiber and trace minerals of true whole wheat bread are not present.

If you want to buy whole-grain wheat bread, look at the list of ingredients and buy those that list "whole wheat flour" as the first ingredient. If "wheat flour" is listed first, this usually means *refined* wheat flour, or "white flour."

## OTHER GRAIN PRODUCTS

Bread is just one source of whole grain foods. There are many other nutritious grain products that can bring interesting tastes and textures to your table. Try to incorporate more of these into your diet. These include barley, which is excellent in soups, salads or casseroles; oats and oat bran, which come in a variety of forms; brown rice and wild rice; and the many different types of wheat grain products, the most common being cracked wheat, bulgur and wheat germ. The following list describes a wide variety of grain products.

## TYPES OF RICE

*Brown Rice* is the whole rice grain. Only the outer husk has been removed from the kernel. It contains more fiber, protein, phosphorus and potassium than white rice. It has a nutty flavor and chewy texture.

*Regular-milled White Rice or Polished Rice* has had its husk, bran, aleurone (a thin layer under the bran) and germ removed during processing. It loses about 20% of its protein, more than half its minerals, and most of its vitamins in this process. Often it is enriched, replacing some of the lost nutrients.

*Parboiled or Converted White Rice* has undergone a special steam-pressure process that pushes some of the nutrients from the outer bran into the starchy center of the grain. This rice has less fiber and protein than brown rice but more nutrients than other forms of white rice.

*Precooked or Instant Rice* has been cooked, rinsed and dried by a special process. It is the least nourishing and the most highly processed. It is also the most expensive white rice.

*Wild Rice* is not true rice, but is the unmilled grain of an aquatic grass. It is relatively expensive, because its supply is limited. Wild rice is very nutritious because it is never refined.

## WHEAT GRAINS

*Bulgur* or cracked whole wheat, has been precooked, dried and cracked into small pieces. It comes in three sizes: small, medium and large. It has a nutty taste and is delicious by itself or mixed with salads, soup or rice. It contains all the nutrients of whole-grain wheat.

*Couscous* is finely cracked wheat grain that has been steamed and dried. It is usually light in color and refined, so it does not contain the fiber and nutrients of a whole-grain product. It can be substituted for rice in most dishes.

*Wheat berries* are whole wheat kernels. They are similar in appearance to rice but the grains are larger. They take a long time to cook (3 hours), but once cooked, they make a crunchy cereal with a naturally sweet taste. Wheat berries can also be used in breads and muffins.

*Wheat Germ* is the embryo or germ of the wheat kernel. It contains essentially all the fat of the kernel and is a good source of B vitamins, vitamin E and iron. Available as tan flakes in vacuum-packed jars, it should be refrigerated after opening to prevent oxidation.

## CORN PRODUCTS

*Hominy* is the endosperm of the corn kernel, without the bran and germ. It is milled into very fine pieces to make hominy grits. Because it does not include the bran or germ, it is comparable in nutrients to refined wheat.

*Cornmeal* is a granular product of corn which may be made either with or without the germ and most of the bran. Refined cornmeal and hominy grits may be enriched, improving the nutritional quality.

## OTHER GRAINS

*Barley* can be purchased in two forms. Processed or "pearled" barley, which has had the hull and bran removed, but not the germ, is the more common variety available in grocery stores. Higher in protein than other grains, it is used primarily in soups. Unpearled barley, found mainly in health food stores, is a richer source of dietary fiber.

*Buckwheat* is actually not a grain but is used as one. Its seed contains a glutinous substance that can be made into flour so it is commonly considered in the grain family. Fine buckwheat flour is similar to refined white flour, but has somewhat less protein. It is used primarily in making griddle cakes and is valued for its distinctive flavor.

*Rye* is used chiefly as a flour-making grain. Darker in color than wheat flour, it is used to make pumpernickel bread. It is also combined with wheat flour to make rye bread. It is similar in quality and nutrients to wheat flour. When used in breads or crackers, it may either be refined or whole grain.

*Oats* are used chiefly in making oatmeal, including both rolled oats and ground or cut oats (oat bran). In processing, the outer hull is removed, but most of the germ and bran remain. Therefore, it retains the nutrients of a whole-grain product, providing a good source of thiamin and other B vitamins and iron. Oat bran is one of the best sources of soluble fiber.

*Millet* is a small grain that comes from a type of cereal grass. A nutritious whole-grain product, it is a good source of magnesium and copper. Millet can be prepared and eaten like rice or precooked and used in yeast breads, lending a delicate flavor and texture.

## A WORD ABOUT BEANS

Some have called beans or legumes "the perfect food," because they contain an abundance of so many important nutrients—starch, high-quality protein, fiber, vitamins and minerals. They have been an important carbohydrate/protein staple for many civilizations throughout history. An adult's complete daily protein requirement can be met with just two cups of legumes served with a grain product, and two cups of milk or its equivalent.

From a nutrition standpoint, there are definite advantages to changing our protein sources, i.e., incorporating more beans, while eating less meat. This way,

the diet is lower in fat and cholesterol and higher in fiber. Beans are an excellent source of both soluble and insoluble fiber.

When adding beans to your diet, start slowly to help alleviate problems with intestinal gas. Start by sprinkling them on salads, using them in soups, or otherwise eating small servings so your system can get accustomed to them. Split peas and lentils are easier for the body to adjust to than other types of beans. In research studies, it has been found that when eating beans on a daily basis, most people stop having excessive gas after two or three weeks.

## TIPS FOR ADDING MORE
## WHOLE GRAINS AND BEANS

• In recipes calling for all-purpose flour, substitute 1/3 of the flour with whole wheat flour. The taste and texture of baked goods change very little with this amount of substitution. (Exceptions are very light angel food cakes, sponge cakes and some white cakes.)

• In some stir-fry dishes or casseroles, reduce or eliminate the meat and replace it with cooked beans. Black beans, kidney beans or garbanzo beans usually combine well with meat dishes.

• Use more whole wheat varieties of processed foods, such as English muffins, waffles or pasta. With pasta, try mixing whole wheat pasta with regular pasta at first, so the change in texture is not too great.

• Sprinkle bran flakes, wheat germ and/or bran on top of casseroles for crisp toppings. These also can be used as a filler with low-fat ground meats.

• Substitute brown rice for white rice or add wild rice to white rice dishes.

• When shopping for snack foods, look for whole-grain products. There are some excellent low-fat, high-fiber varieties available, including Norwegian crisp breads and some of the 100% rye crackers and whole wheat crackers. Be sure to check the fat content on the labels.

## TIPS FOR ADDING MORE FRUITS AND VEGETABLES

• When hungry for a snack, choose a fresh fruit.

• Make fresh or cooked fruit a regular dessert item, served alone, or with angel food cake or another low-fat accompaniment.

• Add a variety of raw vegetables or fruits to salad greens.

• Have pealed, ready-to-eat, raw vegetables available in the refrigerator for snacks.

• Add fruits to cereal, ice milk, low-fat frozen yogurt, etc.

• Add raisins or shredded vegetables (carrots, zucchini or sweet potatoes) to muffins and spice cakes.

• Use pita bread to make a veggie sandwich. Fill pocket with fresh or sautéed vegetables and add a small scoop of low-calorie or nonfat salad dressing or plain yogurt for flavor.

• Add sautéed onions, mushrooms and/or sweet peppers to meat sandwiches.

# SEVEN

---

# *Putting It All Together —*
# *Meal Planning and Exercise*

## THE FOOD GUIDE PYRAMID

Changing to a healthier diet means altering eating habits that have been formed over many years. It is not difficult to do, but does require motivation and effort, especially in the beginning. The motivation should come from knowing the many long-term health benefits to be gained.

You have already learned many of the components of a healthy diet, which were discussed in the previous four chapters. Now you will learn how to combine all this information and work it into well-balanced meals.

In the past, planning well-balanced meals meant choosing a specified number of servings from the Basic Four Food Groups. The primary consideration was getting enough vitamins, minerals and protein in the diet. Little, if any, consideration was given to the amounts of fat, cholesterol or fiber.

All this has changed with the influx of new information on the impor-

tance of these factors in the diet. Over-consumption of fat, cholesterol and animal protein; and under-consumption of fiber can also be very damaging to a person's health, especially in the long term.

The Food Guide Pyramid, shown in Figure 7.1, is the best place to start in planning healthy meals. The pyramid shape indicates at a glance the foods that should be the mainstay of your diet and those that should be eaten more sparingly. Following the serving suggestions and accompanying guidelines of the Food Guide Pyramid will ensure that you not only get enough of the essential nutrients, but that you also incorporate into your meals all the other aspects of a healthy diet — reducing total fat, especially saturated fat, relying less on animal sources for protein needs and eating adequate amounts of fiber.

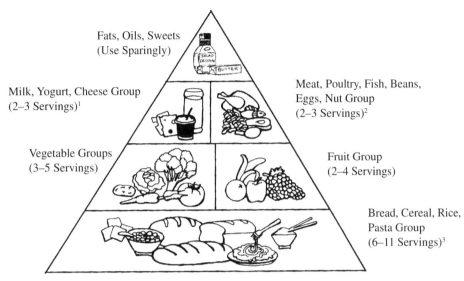

**Food Guide Pyramid**
**A Guide to Daily Food Choices**

Fats, Oils, Sweets
(Use Sparingly)

Milk, Yogurt, Cheese Group
(2–3 Servings)[1]

Meat, Poultry, Fish, Beans,
Eggs, Nut Group
(2–3 Servings)[2]

Vegetable Groups
(3–5 Servings)

Fruit Group
(2–4 Servings)

Bread, Cereal, Rice,
Pasta Group
(6–11 Servings)[3]

Figure 7.1 Adapted from the U.S. Department of Agriculture "Food Guide Pyramid."

[1] One serving equals 1 cup or 1 ounce cheese. Use skim or low-fat dairy products. Adult men and women over 25 years old require 2 servings/day (except for women who are pregnant, nursing or over 50 years.) The recommendation for children up to 9 years is 2–3 servings/day; for children 9 to 12 years, 3–4 servings/day; for ages 12 to 24 and pregnant women, 3 to 4 servings/day; for nursing mothers, 4 servings per day; and for women over 50 years, 3–5 servings/day.

[2] In order to minimize saturated fat and cholesterol, eat more beans and fish and less meat. To limit fat to 20% of total calories, eat *a daily maximum of:*
- 3–4 oz. cooked lean meat, poultry, shrimp, crab or lobster or
- 4–6 oz. cooked fish, clams, scallops and oysters

*plus,* eat *an average of:*
- 1/2 to 3/4 cup beans per day. (Use nuts sparingly.)

Eggs should be limited to no more than 4 per week from all sources, including baked goods and sauces. If you have elevated cholesterol, it is preferable to use egg substitutes or egg whites, which can be consumed in unlimited quantities.

[3] Include at least 3 to 5 servings of whole grain foods.

## MEAL PLANNING

Meal planning is critical to improving your diet. It is best to plan one to two weeks at a time, including three meals a day, plus snacks. That way you can see if you are choosing the right amounts each day from the six food groups. It also makes it easier to plan variety into your menus. Eventually you may only need to plan your evening meals if your breakfasts, lunches and snacks consist of fairly similar types of foods.

It is not necessary to immediately incorporate into your diet all the recommended daily servings from each food group. In some cases, it works best to concentrate on one food group at a time, and to gradually meet the suggested guidelines of the Food Guide Pyramid.

Use snacks to improve your diet. For example, if you're not eating enough fruits, vegetables or whole grain foods, choose these for snacks. Frequent snacking can be part of a healthy diet, if done with the right kinds of foods.

Do not overlook your fluid requirements. You should drink eight 8-ounce glasses of liquids per day, not including beverages high in caffeine. It is especially important to drink enough fluids when you increase your fiber intake because fiber attracts water, and thus more is needed to move it through the colon. Inadequate fluids, with or without increased fiber consumption, can cause constipation or mild dehydration.

## MEETING OUR PROTEIN NEEDS

Consuming sufficient protein is essential for the body's proper functioning. It is needed to build muscles, tendons, ligaments, skin, hair and nails; to produce enzymes, hormones and antibodies; to maintain proper fluid balance; and to monitor a host of other body functions.

The amount of protein needed is based on age and ideal body weight. Growing children and pregnant women need proportionately more protein because they are experiencing increased growth of new body tissue. If they follow the recommendations in the Food Guide Pyramid, including the higher dairy requirements, they will be sure to

receive adequate protein (even though portion sizes of foods will be smaller for small children).

The Recommended Dietary Allowance (RDA) for protein for an average adult male over 14 years of age is 56 grams a day; for an average female over 18 years of age, it is 44 grams a day. This is based on an "average" ideal body weight of 154 for a male, and 120 for a female.

You can calculate your own protein RDA, based on your ideal body weight (IBW), in two simple steps as shown in Figure 7.2.

As you can see from Figure 7.2, the protein RDA for a 5'6" woman is 48 grams

Figure 7.2 The two-step process to determine the Recommended Dietary Allowance for protein.

---

**How to Calculate Your Protein RDA**

Step 1: Determine your ideal body weight. (See Weight Table, p.15.)
Step 2: Multiply your IBW by 0.37 to get your protein RDA in grams per day.

For an example, we will use a 5'6" woman with an ideal body weight of 130 pounds.
Step 1: Ideal body weight = 130 pounds.
Step 2: 130 pounds x 0.37 = 48 grams of protein per day.

---

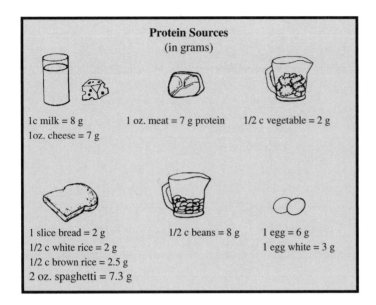

Figure 7.3 The principal sources of protein in the diet.

Protein Sources
(in grams)

1c milk = 8 g
1oz. cheese = 7 g

1 oz. meat = 7 g protein

1/2 c vegetable = 2 g

1 slice bread = 2 g
1/2 c white rice = 2 g
1/2 c brown rice = 2.5 g
2 oz. spaghetti = 7.3 g

1/2 c beans = 8 g

1 egg = 6 g
1 egg white = 3 g

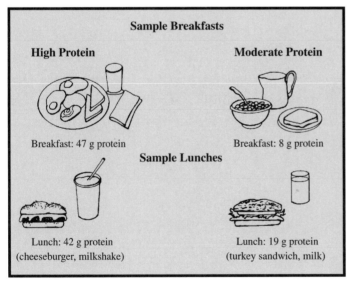

Figure 7.4 Sample breakfasts and lunches showing high and moderate amounts of protein.

Sample Breakfasts

High Protein

Breakfast: 47 g protein

Moderate Protein

Breakfast: 8 g protein

Sample Lunches

Lunch: 42 g protein
(cheeseburger, milkshake)

Lunch: 19 g protein
(turkey sandwich, milk)

per day. This quantity of protein is very easy to meet, and most Americans well exceed the RDA. The National Research Council, concerned with the health hazards associated with too much protein, has suggested a *maximum* daily protein consumption of 0.7 grams/pound, based on your IBW. This is approximately double the RDA.

Let's examine the amount of protein in various types of food (Figure 7.3), in order to have a better understanding of our protein sources. Use this chart to help you find combinations of foods to meet your protein needs.

Meeting protein requirements can be accomplished with a variety of different food combinations. It is not absolutely necessary to have 3 to 6 oz. of meat, poultry or fish each day to do this. The RDA for protein also can be met by eating less meat or fish and more beans and grains.

When relying on beans as a source of protein, however, be sure to complement them with a grain product, such as bread, pasta, rice or wheat in order to have a complete protein.

### MORE THAN ENOUGH PROTEIN

Many Americans go overboard with protein consumption. In fact, the average American diet contains 11 ounces of meat a day, 50 to 75% over the RDA for protein. Let's look at two typical high-protein meals, illustrated in Figure 7.4, to show how easily this can happen. A breakfast of 2 eggs, 3 ounces of ham, a glass of milk and 2 slices of toast contributes 47 grams of protein, enough to meet an entire day's RDA for an average size woman. A lunch of a quarter-pound cheeseburger with a 12-ounce milk shake provides 42 grams of protein—again, almost a full day's recommended amount.

As a healthier alternative, a breakfast of 1 ounce of cereal with 1/2 cup milk, and a piece of toast contributes a more desirable 8 grams of protein. For lunch, a turkey sandwich (lettuce, tomato and 1 ounce of turkey meat), and a glass of milk yields 19 grams of protein. These two meals alone total 27 grams of protein. If you have a dinner of 4 ounces of fish, potatoes, vegetable and salad, this would add an additional 38 grams of protein, or a total of 65 grams for the day. As these examples show, it is very easy to meet and often exceed the RDA for protein.

### IS TOO MUCH PROTEIN HARMFUL?

There are no benefits and there may be harm associated with the overconsumption of protein (greater than 15% of total calories). In fact, the excess protein is wasted, since it is broken down and either converted to glucose to supply energy for the body, or stored as fat.

High consumption of protein, especially animal protein, is associated with higher rates of obesity, heart dis-

ease, cancer and diabetes. Animals fed high-protein diets develop enlargement of their livers and kidneys.

Diets too high in protein are often deficient in fruits, vegetables and whole grain products, resulting in inadequate intakes of certain nutrients. High-protein diets also increase the body's excretion of calcium, which means you need more calcium-rich foods to avoid the effects of calcium deficiency—weak bones and teeth. Care should be taken when making daily meal plans to make sure that protein is adequate, but not excessive.

## SAMPLE DAILY MEAL PLANS

The following pages provide two weeks of sample meal plans. Preparing these menus should help you keep fat intake to approximately 20% of total calories, and should provide you with adequate amounts of protein, fiber and all the essential vitamins and minerals. Portion sizes will vary depending on caloric needs.

The starred items indicate that the recipes are included in the recipe section of the book. If your time is limited during the week, some of the suggested foods, particularly homemade desserts or muffins, can be made in advance, perhaps on the weekends. You may also save time by buying parts of a meal at the supermarket; for example, baked beans (preferably vegetarian), packaged rice mix or muffins. (Be sure to read the label or inquire about the grams of fat in baked goods. Some are very high.)

The suggested meal plans should give you a good idea of the variety of foods you can and should enjoy, knowing you are following a diet for optimal good health. However, don't limit yourself to these meal plans since there are many other delicious recipes in this book that are healthy and low in fat, and with minimal planning, can provide the balance needed in your diet.

## EXERCISE

Exercise is an essential part of a healthy life-style. Regular aerobic exercise not only burns calories, but also complements the health benefits of a prudent diet. Diet and exercise work as a team to keep the body at its physical best.

### BENEFITS OF EXERCISE

The health benefits attributed to exercise are numerous. Exercise improves the cardiovascular system by raising HDL or "good" cholesterol and by lowering triglycerides and blood pressure. Exercise also reduces the risk of developing adult-onset diabetes and increases bone mass which helps prevent osteoporosis (fragile bones). Regular aerobic exercise is essential to weight reduction, enabling dieters to lose weight more readily and to keep the pounds off. It can also relieve anxiety and stress by releasing certain chemicals called endorphins into the brain. Exercise can also help relieve constipation if done in combination with a diet plan of increased fiber and fluids. With all these benefits, how can anyone choose not to exercise?

**Sample Meal Plan**
**WEEK I**

| | Sunday | Monday | Tuesday | Wednesday | Thursday | Friday | Saturday |
|---|---|---|---|---|---|---|---|
| **Breakfast** | orange juice<br>whole grain cereal with milk<br>coffee/tea | orange juice<br>*French Toast with whole wheat bread<br>coffee/tea | banana<br>bagel with light cream cheese<br>coffee/tea | orange juice<br>all-bran cereal with raisins and skim milk<br>coffee/tea | orange juice<br>scrambled egg substitute<br>whole wheat toast<br>coffee/tea | instant oatmeal<br>orange<br>whole wheat toast<br>coffee/tea | whole grain cereal with raisins, sliced banana, milk<br>bagel<br>coffee/tea |
| **Morning Snack** | apple | *Oatbran Muffin<br>coffee/tea | apple | 1 oz. pretzels<br>fruit juice | low-fat, high-fiber crackers<br>carbonated drink | pear | orange |
| **Lunch** | ham sandwich<br>*Minestrone Soup (canned or home made)<br>skim milk | turkey sandwich on whole wheat<br>cranberry-orange relish<br>baked beans | ham sandwich on rye<br>*Black Bean Salad<br>fruit salad<br>strawberry shake | *Tuna Pasta Salad<br>French bread<br>cantaloupe<br>skim milk | turkey sandwich on whole wheat<br>baked beans<br>marinated asparagus | tuna salad (with nonfat mayonnaise) on whole wheat<br>fruit salad<br>Skim milk | turkey sandwich on hard roll<br>*Tropical Fruit Slaw<br>skim milk |
| **Afternoon Snack** | nectarine | apple | *Oatbran Muffin<br>coffee/tea | apple | skim milk<br>banana | apple | banana |
| **Dinner** | roast turkey breast (leftovers for stir-fry Tues.)<br>*Mashed Potatoes w/ nonfat turkey gravy<br>cranberry-orange relish (canned)<br>*Green Beans Amandine<br>rolls | *Pasta with Red Clam Sauce<br>steamed carrots and peas<br>crusty French bread<br>*Spinach Salad with Honey Mustard<br>skim milk | *Stir-fry Chicken and Vegetables (substitute turkey) over rice<br>multi-grain bread<br>*Baked Tomatoes<br>Fig Newtons<br>skim milk | *Bean Stroganoff<br>steamed Brussels sprouts<br>french bread<br>skim milk<br>*Granola Apple Cobbler | *Flank Steak Chile<br>*Bran Muffins (purchased or homemade)<br>skim milk<br>canned fruit (in light syrup) | *Stuffed Baked Potato<br>*Tropical Fruit Slaw (make enough for next day)<br>whole wheat bread or rolls<br>skim milk | *Marinated Salmon<br>*Mashed Potatoes with Chives<br>steamed carrots<br>tossed salad<br>*Chocolate Chip Bundt Cake |
| **Evening Snack** | 2 large low-salt pretzels<br>soft drink | low-fat frozen yogurt | low-salt pretzels<br>apple juice | banana | cereal with skim milk | bagel with jam<br>beverage | *Bran Muffin<br>skim milk |

* Recipes appear in Recipe section of book.

## Sample Meal Plan
### WEEK II

| | Sunday | Monday | Tuesday | Wednesday | Thursday | Friday | Saturday |
|---|---|---|---|---|---|---|---|
| **Breakfast** | cantaloupe *Bran Muffin coffee/tea | orange juice oat bran cereal with milk bagel | orange juice cereal combination: All-Bran and Raisin Bran with milk coffee/tea | cantaloupe oat bran cereal with milk whole wheat toast coffee/tea | grapefruit juice *Oat Bran-Apple Muffin coffee/tea | grapefruit bagel with peanut butter whole wheat toast skim milk | fresh strawberries All-Bran cereal with milk and sliced banana coffee/tea |
| **Morning Snack** | *Bran Muffin skim milk | apple coffee/tea | *Blueberry Muffin | pear | banana | apple coffee/tea | pear coffee/tea |
| **Lunch** | tuna salad (with nonfat mayonnaise) on rye bread baked beans (vegetarian) skim milk | turkey sandwich on whole wheat *Tabouli Salad or applesauce skim milk | ham sandwich on Kaiser roll vegetarian baked beans tossed salad skim milk | *Stuffed Baked Potato fruit salad skim milk | turkey sandwich on whole wheat steamed broccoli applesauce skim milk | *Lentil Soup French bread angelfood cake with ice milk skim milk | *Tuna Stuffed Tomatoes whole wheat bread skim milk |
| **Afternoon Snack** | pear soft drink | *Chocolate Chip Cake coffee/tea | banana | low-fat crackers soft drink | bagel with jam coffee/tea | tangerine | bagel soft drink |
| **Dinner** | *Shrimp Jambalaya *Orange Cornbread tossed salad *Chocolate Chip Bundt Cake (leftover) skim milk | *Beanburgers (mix may be made several days in advance) *Slim Waldorf Salad *Baked Tomatoes fresh strawberries with frozen yogurt skim milk | *Apple-Date Stuffed Tenderloin *Rice-Mushroom Casserole (or use packaged rice mix) green beans cantaloupe skim milk | *Scallops Florentine over Brown Rice dinner rolls sliced tomatoes *Baked Rice Pudding skim milk | *Vegetable Pasta Stir-Fry French bread tossed salad angelfood cake, (purchased) strawberries and vanilla ice milk skim milk | *Chicken n' Dumplings fruit salad whole wheat bread vanilla pudding (made with skim milk) with sliced bananas skim milk | *Light Fried Fish Fillets *Sweet Potato Casserole steamed broccoli *Custard Pie skim milk/water |
| **Evening Snack** | sliced banana with skim milk | pretzels soft drink | frozen yogurt | cold cereal with skim milk | *Baked Rice Pudding | pretzels soft drink | *Custard Pie |

* Recipes appear in Recipe section of book.

Studies have documented the benefits of exercise and the drawbacks of a sedentary life. Researchers at Duke University found that *unfit* people have the same risk of heart disease and stroke as smokers, (2.8 times greater risk) or those 19 years older (3 times greater risk). A study reported in the *Annals of Internal Medicine* found that postmenopausal women who exercised one hour, three times a week, increased their bone mass by 2.6% in one year. On the other hand, sedentary women *lost* an average of 2.4% of bone mass during this same period. Over a number of years, the difference in bone mass between an active and sedentary person could be quite significant.

Long-term exercise can help preserve a youthful mind. Men in their 60s, who have jogged or played racquetball or squash for 20 years or longer, have reaction times that are equal to or better than men in their 20s who are inactive. Reaction time is determined by measuring the length of time it takes to react to a stimulus (such as a buzzing sound) with a response (such as pressing a button).

Exercise has also been shown to help relieve moderate depression. In a study at the University of Wisconsin, it was found that walking and/or running for one hour a day, three times a week, over a 10-week period, worked as well as, or better than, psychotherapy in treating moderate depression.

You're never too old to benefit from exercise. In fact, you can actually increase the size and strength of your muscles even into your 90s. In a study conducted at Tufts-USDA Human Nutrition Research Center on Aging, it was found that a group of men and women who averaged 90 years of age, increased the muscle area of their thighs by 10% through a weight-lifting program. Even more significant, they increased the amount of weight they could lift from an average of 17.6 pounds to 44 pounds.

This increase in strength brought some unexpected benefits. They were able to walk faster, take longer strides or just get around more easily.

## KINDS OF EXERCISE — AEROBIC AND NONAEROBIC

The National Heart, Lung and Blood Institute classifies exercise into three distinct types. The first two types are aerobic which means they benefit the cardiovascular system, reducing the risk of heart disease and stroke. Type I includes the most vigorous exercises (Figure 7.5). Ideally, these exercises should to be done for at least 20 minutes per day, three times a week, for optimal conditioning of the heart and lungs.

Type II exercises are less vigorous, but can condition the heart and lungs if

| **Type I Exercises** | |
| --- | --- |
| Cross-country skiing | |
| Hiking (uphill) | Figure 7.5 Type I Exercises. These condition heart and lungs if done for at least 15 minutes per day, three times a week. |
| Ice hockey | |
| Jogging | |
| Jumping rope | |
| Rowing | |
| Running in place | |
| Stationary cycling | |

| **Type II Exercises** | |
| --- | --- |
| Bicycling | |
| Downhill skiing | |
| Basketball | |
| Calisthenics | Figure 7.6 Type II Exercises. These can condition the heart and lungs if done vigorously for at least 30 minutes per day, three times a week. |
| Field hockey | |
| Handball | |
| Racquetball | |
| Soccer | |
| Squash | |
| Swimming | |
| Tennis (singles) | |
| Walking | |

| **Type III Exercises** | |
| --- | --- |
| Baseball | |
| Bowling | Figure 7.7  Type III Exercises. These do not condition the heart and lungs, but do improve coordination and muscle tone. |
| Football | |
| Golf (on foot or by cart) | |
| Softball | |
| Volleyball | |
| Weight lifting | |

done briskly (Figure 7.6). They should be done vigorously for at least 30 minutes per day, three times a week, to get approximately the same conditioning benefits as Type I exercises. Aerobic exercise done several times a day for shorter periods of time also can benefit the heart and lungs, but to a slightly lesser degree.

Type III exercises are nonaerobic, which means they do not condition the heart and lungs, but they are beneficial in other ways (Figure 7.7). They improve coordination and muscle tone, and can reduce stress.

## STRENGTH-TRAINING EXERCISE

Strength or weight training is a nonaerobic exercise that only recently has been recognized as being vitally important to health and well-being. In fact, many exercise physiologists consider it the most important exercise for those over 65 years old.

In strength-training exercise, you work your muscles to become stronger through repeated resistance motions. This can be done through weight lifting (with free-weights or multifaceted machines), using dumbbells or ankle weights; or by doing push-ups, chin-ups, etc. In a complete program, you work the major muscle groups of the shoulders, back, chest, arms, legs and abdomen.

Strength training is increasingly important at middle age and beyond, because as we age, we lose a significant amount of muscle. From age 20 to 70, a sedentary person loses 30% of muscle mass, and much of the remaining muscle slowly shrinks or wastes away. A weight-training program can restore

10% of muscle mass, and even more remarkably, can triple muscle strength. For older folks, this can mean the difference between being able to take care of oneself, or being institutionalized. It can also mean avoiding a fall and the consequences of a broken bone.

Weight training can begin at any age, and requires only a minor time commitment — just two or three sessions per week, 30 to 40 minutes each time. Unlike running, fast walking or other aerobic exercises, weight training must be taught and requires the use of some props or exercise equipment. Weights of some sort are a necessity, such as barbells, dumbbells, ankle weights and/or homemade weights made from milk cartons filled with water or sand.

In a weight-training session, you work the various muscle groups by doing 8 to 12 repetitions of each exercise, such as arm curls, and then rest briefly. Each set of exercises is repeated two more times. Each time, you should feel thoroughly fatigued by the tenth or twelfth repetition. If not, you should increase the weight to create greater resistance.

Aerobics and strength training work together to make you look and feel your best. The former burns calories and fat, and at the same time benefits the cardio-vascular system, while the latter tones and builds muscle and increases strength.

### GETTING STARTED — DESIGNING AN EXERCISE PROGRAM

Choose an exercise that you enjoy from Type I or II category. If you are doing something you like, the chances are much greater that you will continue it on a long-term basis. If you prefer exercising with others, find a friend or group and set up a regular schedule.

To begin a strength-training program, consult a qualified exercise physiologist at your local YMCA, health club or spa. They should be prepared to advise you on a safe, effective program based on your goals and physical condition. If you do not want to join a health club or spa, an exercise physiologist should be able to design a program you can do at home.

The key is to start all forms of exercise gradually, pacing yourself according to your level of fitness. Before beginning an exercise session, either aerobic, strength training or a combination of both, be sure to include a 10-minute warm-up. This should consist of five minutes of low-intensity aerobics (walking around briskly); followed by 5 minutes of gentle, relaxing stretching exercises. You also need to include a 5-minute cool-down period of walking around, after your exercise session is complete. If you combine aerobics and strength training into one session, the recommended order is warm-up, aerobics, strength training and cool-down.

Remember that your goal is to work up to three to five days per week of aerobic exercise, and two to three days per week of strength training exercise. It is fine to take several months to arrive at that goal.

### ARE YOU EXERCISING VIGOROUSLY ENOUGH?

There is a way to tell if you are exercising vigorously enough to benefit your cardiovascular system. This is determined by taking your pulse immediately after exercising. Your pulse, or heart rate, should be 60 to 70% of your maximum heart rate, which is approximately 220, minus your age. See Table 7.1 to find the average maximum heart rate and heart rate "target zone" for your age. The "target zone" is the rate your heart should beat immediately following exercise in order to provide optimal benefit to your heart and lungs.

As an example, for a 40-year-old, the chart shows that the average maximum heart rate is 180, and the heart rate "target zone" is 108 to 135 beats per minute. If your heart rate immediately following exercise is below the suggested target zone range for your age, exercise a little harder, and if above, exercise with less vigor. After exercising six months or longer, your heart rate can safely go as high as 85% of your maximum heart rate. However, it is not necessary to exercise that hard to stay in good condition.

### SHOULD YOU SEE A DOCTOR BEFORE EXERCISING?

For most people, it is not necessary to see a doctor before beginning an exercise program. The National Institutes of Health recommends seeing your doctor only if one of the following conditions applies to you:

1. Your doctor said you have heart trouble, a heart murmur, or you have had a heart attack.
2. You frequently have pains or pressure—in the left or mid-chest area, left neck, shoulder, or arm—during or right after you exercise.
3. You often feel faint or have spells of severe dizziness.
4. You experience extreme breathlessness after mild exertion.
5. Your doctor said your blood pressure was too high and is not under control; or you don't know if your blood pressure is normal.
6. Your doctor said you have bone or joint problems such as arthritis.
7. You are over age 60 and not accustomed to vigorous exercise.
8. Your father, mother, brother or sister had a heart attack before age 50.

To find your heart rate Target Zone, look for the age category closest to your age and read the line across. For example, if you are 43, the closest age on the chart is 45; your heart rate target zone is 105 to 131 beats per minute.

| Age | Heart Rate Target Zone 60–75% | Average Maximum Heart Rate 100% |
|---|---|---|
| 20 years | 120–150 beats per min. (60–75% of 200 beats) | 200 beats per minute |
| 25 years | 117–146 beats per min. | 195 |
| 30 years | 114–142 beats per min. | 190 |
| 35 years | 111–138 beats per min. | 185 |
| 40 years | 108–135 beats per min. | 180 |
| 45 years | 105–131 beats per min. | 175 |
| 50 years | 102–127 beats per min. | 170 |
| 55 years | 99–123 beats per min. | 165 |
| 60 years | 96–120 beats per min. | 160 |
| 65 years | 93–116 beats per min. | 155 |
| 70 years | 90–113 beats per min. | 150 |

Your maximum heart rate is usually 220 minus your age. However, the above figures are averages and should be used as general guidelines.

To see if you are within your heart rate Target Zone, take your pulse immediately after you stop exercising. Count it for 30 seconds and multiply by two. If your pulse is below your Target Zone, exercise a little harder the next time. If you're above your Target Zone, exercise a little easier. And if it falls within the Target Zone, you're doing fine. Once you're exercising within your Target Zone, you should check your pulse at least once each week during the first 3 months and periodically thereafter.

Source: *The National Heart, Lung and Blood Institute,* National Institutes of Health

9. You have a medical condition not mentioned here which might need special attention in an exercise program. (For example, insulin-dependent diabetes.)

## SPECIAL DIET TIPS FOR ATHLETES

• To replace the fluid lost during exercise, drink two glasses of water for every pound of weight lost while exercising.

• There is no need to drink a "sports drink" to replace electrolytes lost during exercise. Proportionally more water is lost than electrolytes. The next nutritious meal will replace the small amount of electrolytes lost.

• For endurance athletes (exercising vigorously for more than 90 minutes), it is best to take fluid with some calories during performance. Good choices are a 7 to 10% solution of sugar water (the sugar concentration in a soft drink), apple juice or a banana with water.

• Weight lifters should keep protein intake to no more than 15% of total calories, which is the upper limit recommended for the general public. This is equivalent to approximately 0.7 gram of protein per pound of body weight. For a 150-pound man, this would be a *maximum* of 105 grams of protein per day. (150 pounds x 0.7 grams/pound = 105 grams of protein.)

(Excess protein, greater than 15% of total calories, does not build larger muscles nor is it stored in muscle tissue. Rather, it is broken down into its components, including urea, which is excreted from the body; the remainder is converted to carbohydrate or stored as fat. Eating too much protein usually means you are not eating enough carbohydrate, the most important energy source for athletes. Carbohydrate is stored in the muscle as glycogen, which is the fuel the body needs during exercise.)

# EIGHT

# *Vitamin and Mineral Supplements*

## SUPPLEMENTS IN THE DIET

In the past, vitamin supplements were taken primarily to prevent nutritional deficiencies or when there was a special medical need, such as during pregnancy. All that changed, beginning in the late 1980s, after a number of studies touted the benefits of vitamin supplements. Now, 40% of Americans take supplements, not only to meet nutritional needs, but also in hopes of pumping up immunity or reducing the risk for certain diseases, including cancer, heart disease, osteoporosis, cataracts and colds.

What do these recent studies show? First of all, taking vitamin/mineral supplements will never be an adequate substitute for eating fruits, vegetables, whole-grain foods and other nutritious foods. The evidence is overwhelming that eating these foods provides the greatest protection against disease. However, it appears that supplements may enhance the benefits of a healthy diet and life-style, and in some cases, may help compensate for deficiencies in the diets of certain groups of people, such as the elderly.

## ANTIOXIDANTS

There are some very promising studies involving the antioxidant supplements beta carotene, and vitamins E and C. (Selenium, an essential part of an antioxidant enzyme, is also being studied as a possible anticancer agent.) Some of the studies suggest that these antioxidants may play a role in reducing the risks of heart disease, cancer and cataracts. In each of these diseases, oxidation is thought to be one of the major culprits.

These three antioxidants are alike in that they help prevent harmful oxidation from occurring in the body. Each one, though, plays a different role in the body's defense system. Vitamin C is water soluble and works in the watery inner parts of the cell. Vitamin E is the principal fat-soluble vitamin. It lodges within the fat-containing cell membranes and inside LDL cholesterol ("bad" cholesterol) particles, protecting them from attack by free radicals (the unstable molecules which cause oxidation). Beta carotene also resides inside LDL particles and, in addition, works effectively in areas where there are low levels of oxygen, such as the capillaries of muscle tissue. Their protective roles do overlap. Vitamin E is thought to protect beta-carotene molecules from being oxidized, and vitamin C "spares" or protects vitamin E.

The study of antioxidants for the prevention of disease is still in its infancy. Not until around the year 2,000, when clinical trials now underway are completed, will there be sufficient data to possibly make a public policy recommendation advocating the use of antioxidant supplements. At present the data is not conclusive, and researchers are unsure how the antioxidants inter-act with each other, or what dosages are appropriate for various age groups.

As with all scientific research, the information gleaned from various studies is never static. New studies regarding antioxidants may question or reinforce what appears beneficial today. Therefore, without specific recommendations by a reputable authority such as the National Institutes of Health, or the National Cancer Society, you should check with your physician before self-prescribing megadoses of any vitamin or mineral. Together you can determine the best approach based on your medical history, life-style and health concerns.

The following provides a summary of the major human studies relating to antioxidant supplements completed prior to May 1994. (In animal studies to date, antioxidant supplements have not prolonged life, but have improved the quality of life by slowing down the development of certain chronic diseases that are common in humans.)

## ANTIOXIDANTS AND HEART DISEASE

Two studies from Harvard School of Public Health, published in November 1992, show promising results regarding vitamin E supplements reducing the risk for heart disease. One study involved 87,000 nurses, and the other 40,000 male health professionals. In the nurses' study, after eight years, those who consumed at least 100 International Units (IU) of vitamin E were 34% less likely to suffer a heart attack than those who did not take the supplement; with the male health professionals, after four years, those who took from 100 to 249 IU of vitamin E were 37% less likely to suffer heart attacks. There was no greater benefit for males who consumed more than 250 IU of vitamin E. High supplemental intakes of vitamin C did not show a decrease in risk for either group. Beta-carotene intake in the supplemental range showed a decrease in risk in the women's study, but in the men's study only smokers showed a reduced risk of heart disease.

As part of the ongoing Harvard Physicians' Health Study, a subgroup of 333 male physicians with known coronary artery disease were given either a beta-carotene supplement of 80,000 IU every other day or a placebo (inactive pill). After a period of seven years, it was found that those who took the beta-carotene supplement experienced a 54% reduction in the incidence of heart attack, stroke, bypass surgery or coronary death than the control group, who did not take the supplement.

## ANTIOXIDANTS AND CANCER

Antioxidants do not appear to be protective against all forms of cancer as once thought, but certain antioxidants appear to be protective with some cancers. To determine the effectiveness of antioxidants in inhibiting cancer, blood serum levels of beta carotene, vitamin E and vitamin C were measured to see if high levels in the blood corresponded with reduced risks of cancer, or vice versa. The antioxidants present in blood serum came from either foods or supplements.

A number of studies have shown that people with higher levels of beta carotene in their blood consistently have a reduced risk of lung cancer, sometimes as much as one-half the risk. One study, however, published in 1994, showed the opposite effect. It involved male smokers from Finland who took beta-carotene supplements of 33,000 IU per day or a placebo. The men who took the supplements showed an 18% increase in the incidence of lung cancer, compared to those who did not take the supplement. In discussing the results of the study, the authors state that, although the results "may well be due to chance..., it does raise the possibility that these substances (antioxidant supplements) may have harmful as well as beneficial effects."

Higher blood serum levels of beta carotene showed a lower incidence of stomach cancer, a form of cancer uncommon in the United States. With other cancers, there was no definitive link between blood serum levels of beta carotene and the incidence of cancer.

In studies involving vitamin E, only with pancreatic cancer was there a link between low blood serum levels of that vitamin and an increased incidence of cancer. Regarding vitamin C, several studies have shown a reduced risk of stomach cancer with increased levels of vitamin C, but no difference with lung, rectum or colon cancer.

### ANTIOXIDANTS AND CATARACTS

Vitamin C supplements may be more protective against cataracts than cancer. As part of the Nurses' Health Study, conducted by Harvard School of Public Health, it was found that women who took vitamin C supplements (at least 250 mg/day) for at least a decade had a 45% lower risk of developing cataracts. Multivitamins with smaller amounts of vitamin C did not provide protection. Other studies involving vitamin E and beta carotene also showed a lower risk of cataracts with supplements of these antioxidants.

## ASPIRIN AS A SUPPLEMENT

In the Physicians' Health Study conducted by Harvard University, it was found that men over the age of 50 who took a regular aspirin (325 mg) every other day, had a 44% lower risk of heart attack than those who took a placebo. Other studies have shown that a baby aspirin (80 mg) taken every day may be just as effective.

Aspirin may also reduce the risk of colon cancer. In 1992, the *Journal of the National Cancer Institute* reported that, based on a questionnaire completed by over 750,000 participants, those who took one aspirin tablet at least 15 times a month cut their incidence of colon cancer in half. *Taking aspirin at these levels, however, increases the risk of developing a stomach ulcer, or suffering a hemorrhagic stroke, so it only should be taken under a doctor's supervision.*

## SUPPLEMENTS AND THE ELDERLY

It appears that vitamin/mineral supplements may be particularly beneficial to older populations, who are less likely to achieve a balanced diet from foods alone. This may be a result of poor absorption of nutrients, difficulty in chewing, inadequate appetite or the inability to prepare balanced meals.

In a Canadian study published in 1992, a group of 96 senior citizens aged 66 to 86 were given either a multivitamin/mineral supplement plus 44 IU vitamin E and 25,000 IU beta carotene, or a placebo. After one year, those taking the supplements had only one-half as many infections, and the colds or infections they had lasted only half as long. Blood tests revealed enhanced immune response in those taking the supplements, evidenced by increased levels of

T-cells and other lymphocytes that fight infection.

In a Tufts University study involving 1,200 adults over the age of 65, it was found that about 30% of them were at increased risk for heart disease because they had decreased levels of three B vitamins—B6, B12 and folate. Deficiencies in these nutrients result in high levels of homocysteine, a chemical present in the blood that when elevated increases the risk of heart attack by three or four times. The researchers were able to bring down the homocysteine levels to normal concentrations in nearly all those in the study simply by increasing their intake of the three B vitamins. The Tufts research suggests that the recommended intakes of these three B vitamins for older adults should be 400 mcg of folate, which is twice the Recommended Dietary Allowance (200% RDA); 1.9 mg of B6; and 12 mcg of vitamin B12, again twice or 200% the RDA.

## SELECTING VITAMIN/MINERAL SUPPLEMENTS

Given the realities of the American diet—that 54% of women get less than two-thirds the RDA for calcium; 30% of adults over 65 years old are deficient in the B vitamins B6, B12 and folate; and only 18% of Americans eat five or more fruits and vegetables per day—makes a strong case for advocating the use of vitamin/mineral supplements. *However, supplements never should be considered a substitute for eating a low-fat balanced diet, which is the basic prerequisite for achieving optimal health.*

### HOW TO CHOOSE MULTIVITAMIN/MINERAL SUPPLEMENTS

Walking up to the vitamin counter at your local drugstore or supermarket can be a bewildering experience. The amount of nutrients vary from one brand to another; some are promoted as "natural," "stress vitamins," "preservative-free," "generic" and on and on. Which are the better choices?

The following information should be helpful. First of all, natural is no better than synthetic, except perhaps with vitamin E. Natural vitamin E is listed as "d-alphatocopherol," not "dl-alphatocopherol." Generic store brands are generally identical in quality to name brands, since the vast majority of supplements are manufactured by a small group of multinational firms.

Vitamins should meet a 45-minute dissolution test, to ensure that they dissolve while in the small intestine. If they are not dissolved in the digestive tract, they will not be absorbed into the blood. The supplement meets this standard if it states on the label that the product meets the U.S. Pharmacopoeia (USP) standards, or that it "passes a 45-minute laboratory dissolution test." If this information is not on the label, you can call the company that manufactures the vitamins to ask if their product meets this test. Some products are formulated to pass this test, although it is not stated on the label.

Finally, be sure to check the expiration date. Make sure it will not be outdated before you finish the bottle.

The next question is how much of each nutrient is ideal? Nobody really knows for sure the "optimal" intake levels for nutrients. The committee that sets the official Recommended Dietary Allowances (RDAs) is not setting "optimal" levels, but rather recommending intakes of essential nutrients that "meet the known nutrient needs of practically all healthy persons." The RDAs are established primarily to avoid nutrient deficiencies and to ensure that toxicity not result because of overconsumption of certain nutrients. Even though RDAs do not pretend to be "optimal," they do represent the best basis for choosing a supplement.

Therefore, when selecting a vitamin/mineral supplement, ignore all the advertising hype, and look directly at the list of ingredients with the percentage of the RDAs. Choose one that pro- vides a wide variety of vitamins and minerals in amounts equal to or close to 100% of the RDAs. Keep in mind that the foods you eat also contain vitamins and minerals, so it isn't necessary to receive your entire RDAs from a supplement. To avoid toxicity, choose a vitamin/mineral supplement that provides no more than the RDAs of vitamins A and D, or any mineral. Also avoid those that provide more than five times (500%) the RDA for any other nutrient. (If giving children a multivitamin/ mineral supplement, make sure it is appropriate for their age and nutritional requirements by first checking with your pediatrician.)

Regarding vitamin A, supplements that provide more than the RDA of vitamin A listed as "beta carotene" may be taken in quantities greater than 100% RDA. Postmenopausal women are the only exception for exceeding the RDA for vitamin D. It may be beneficial for them to take vitamin D supplements of up to 800 IU (200% RDA) to reduce the risk of fractures from osteoporosis. Vitamin D helps the body absorb calcium, and several studies have shown a reduction in hip, wrist, arm and pelvic fractures with supplements of 400 to 800 IU.

## ANTIOXIDANT SUPPLEMENTS

A typical antioxidant supplement contains 200 to 400 IU of vitamin E, 10,000 to 25,000 IU beta carotene and 250 to 500 mg vitamin C. (Antioxidant vitamins at these dosages are sometimes included in a multivitamin.) In a report published by the National Heart, Lung and Blood Institutes in June 1992, the authors noted that these antioxidant supplements have no known toxic side effects at reasonable dosages. They considered the following to be "high (but safe) doses" for testing the effectiveness of antioxidants: 400 to 800 IU vitamin E, up to 1 gram vitamin C and beta carotene at any "nonyellowing" dose. (Beta carotene has no known toxic side effects, but may cause skin pigment to turn yellow, which is considered harmless.) See Figure 8.1 to compare the U.S. Recommended Dietary Allowances (USRDAs) with the typical supplemental ranges of the three major antioxidants.

It is possible to consume close to the supplemental ranges of beta carotene and vitamin C through foods alone if special care is taken to select the foods highest in those nutrients. However, that is not the case with vitamin E. The best food sources of vitamin E are plant oils, nuts and other high fat foods, all of which should be eaten in limited quanitities. To consume 200 IU of vitamin E, you'd need to eat four cups of almonds or almost 14 cups of peanuts per day. (Refer to Tables 6.1 and 6.2 for the best food sources of beta carotene and vitamin C.)

Consult your physician before taking antioxidant supplements in amounts greater than five times the USRDA. Although highly unlikely, it is possible that such amounts could cause harm in the long term. Your physician can advise you, based on whether he or she feels the potential benefit outweighs the risk.

Figure 8.1 The USRDAs of the three major antioxidants and the typical supplemental ranges.

| Antioxidant | USRDA | Typical Supplemental Range |
|---|---|---|
| Beta carotene | none* | 10,0000 – 50,000 IU |
| Vitamin C | 60 mg | 250 – 1,000 mg |
| Vitamin E | 8 IU (women) 10 IU (men) | 200 – 800 IU |

* The USRDA for vitamin A is 5000 IU, which is often in the form of beta carotene and/or acetate.

## SPECIFIC VITAMIN NEEDS

The need for specific vitamin/mineral supplements varies based on a person's age, sex and dietary habits. Because of these variables, some individuals or age groups are at greater risk for developing certain deficiencies. The following provides a discussion of specific nutrient needs based on age, sex and dietary habits. Looking at your own needs, you can decide if a supplement(s) can help you avoid a possible deficiency.

For older populations, there are several vitamins and minerals commonly found to be deficient. These include calcium, especially for women, the B vitamins (B6, B12 and folate) and vitamin D, particularly for non-milk-drinkers during the cold winter months. Drinking four glasses of milk per day supplies all the dietary calcium and vitamin D needed. Being exposed to sunshine for a short period of time each day also provides the necessary vitamin D, except for those who live in the northern states during the winter months.

In supplement form, approximately 100% of the RDA for the B vitamins should be adequate, even though the Tufts University study showed that the B12 and folate needs of the elderly exceeded the RDA. Foods should be able to make up the difference. A vitamin D supplement at 100% of the RDA is sufficient except for postmenopausal women at high risk for osteoporosis, who may want to take up to 800 IU (200% RDA).

The recommended calcium intake for postmenopausal women at high risk for developing osteoporosis is 1500 mg per day. This includes women who are thin, have a family history of the disease, are sedentary or are not taking estrogen-replacement therapy. For postmenopausal women at low risk, the recommended amount is 1,000 mg per day. The average intake of calcium from foods for women over 50 years old is 475 mg per day. (An 8-ounce glass of milk or cup of yogurt supplies 300 mg calcium.) Therefore, supplements may need to supply from 600 to 1000 mg calcium per day. It may take several pills a day to reach that level. Figure 8.2 lists the recommended calcium intakes for men and women based on age and risk of osteoporosis.

Young women have different vitamin needs. Women who are of child-bearing age should be sure to get the RDA of folic acid for pregnant women (400 mcg) prior to conception, in order to reduce the risk of "neural tube" birth defects. To avoid osteoporosis, they also may need calcium supplements if they do not have several daily servings of calcium-rich foods including dairy products, canned fish with bones, tofu or green leafy vegetables. The calcium RDA for men and women up to age 25 is 1,200 mg a day and 800 mg for men over 25. Premenopausal women over age 25 who are at low risk for osteoporosis should consume 800 mg calcium per day, while those at high risk should have 1,000 mg.

| Sex | Age | Calcium Requirements (low-risk osteoporosis) | Calcium Requirements (high-risk osteoporosis) |
|---|---|---|---|
| Males | 11–24 | 1200 mg | NA* |
| | 25–50 | 800 mg | NA |
| | 50+ | 800 mg | NA |
| Females | 11–24 | 1200 mg | 1200 mg |
| | 25–50 | 800 mg | 1000 mg |
| | 50+ | 1000 mg | 1500 mg |

\* Men do not experience the same rate of bone loss after the age of 50 as women, and therefore are not considered at high risk for osteoporosis.

Figure 8.2 Calcium requirements based on age and sex. Women are considered at high risk for osteoporosis if they are thin, have a family history of the disease, are sedentary or are not taking supplemental estrogen after menopause.

Menstruating or pregnant women, who typically have from one-fourth to one-half the stored iron of men, are sometimes deficient in that mineral. Iron supplements should not exceed 100% of the RDA, unless they are taken under a doctor's supervision. Vegetarians who do not consume dairy products should take a supplement that provides the RDA for vitamin B12, or they will develop a deficiency, which can cause anemia and damage to the central nervous system.

There are a several other nutrients that adults may want to take as an individual supplement because they are usually not included in a multivitamin, or if so, at a small percentage of the RDA. These include chromium, selenium and magnesium. The RDAs of these minerals for adults are 50 to 200 mcg for chromium, 55 to 70 mcg for selenium and 280 to 350 mg magnesium. A chromium deficiency may lead to glucose intolerance according to some studies, and selenium may play a role in reducing the risk of cancer. Although magnesium deficiencies are uncommon, this mineral plays an important role in metabolism and the absorption of other minerals.

It appears that vitamin/mineral supplements can do more than prevent deficiency diseases, but exactly how much more is still to be determined. In the meantime, taking supplements in a judicious manner seems a logical choice, if done in conjunction with a balanced, low-fat diet.

# NINE

## Medical Tests for Blood Pressure and Cholesterol: Knowing Your Numbers

### MOTIVATION FOR CHANGE

Blood-pressure and cholesterol tests help determine the risk for heart disease. Cholesterol tests tell us if excessive artery-clogging fat is circulating in the blood. If so, positive steps can be taken to reduce these levels through diet; and if that is not enough, with the addition of drugs.

Blood-pressure measurements indicate whether the heart and blood vessels are being overly stressed while pumping blood throughout the body. If this condition goes unchecked, it can cause enlargement of the heart, weakening of blood vessel walls and can lead to strokes. Changes in diet and life-style can reduce blood pressure.

Many of us do not adopt a healthy life-style unless a medical test indicates we are at risk. These tests can thus serve as the impetus for positive changes. It makes more sense, though, to adopt a healthy life-style regardless of test results, because everyone is at risk to some extent and test results do not tell us everything.

### SCREENING TESTS READILY AVAILABLE

Health care professionals in many communities have provided opportunities to have blood-pressure and cholesterol-screening tests done at little or no cost. The tests are conducted at shopping malls, drug stores, fairgrounds and other popular locations. If you have an abnormal screening test, or if you think the results are questionable, it would be wise to have the test repeated at your doctor's office. There is no excuse for being unaware of these two very important numbers. It can improve your chances for a longer and healthier life.

### CHOLESTEROL TESTING

#### WHO SHOULD BE TESTED?

All adults over the age of 20 should have their cholesterol checked, according to guidelines of the National Cholesterol Education Program. Children should be tested if there is a family history of heart disease or if one of the parents has high cholesterol. Still, some pediatricians are in favor of screening all school-age children, since some parents do not know their cholesterol levels.

## WHAT ARE DESIRABLE CHOLESTEROL VALUES?*

A cholesterol-screening test measures total blood cholesterol. It can be done as a finger-prick test, or a vial of blood can be drawn from a vein in your arm. In either case, no fasting is required. Figure 9.1 summarizes the risk classifications based on total cholesterol levels. Values of less than 200 milligrams per deciliter (mg/dl) are "desirable" or "low risk." Those between 200 and 239 are "borderline/high risk," and those 240 and above are considered "high risk." This puts over 50% of adult Americans above the desirable level and 25% in the high-risk category. If your cholesterol level is below 200, you do not need further testing. You should still follow a prudent diet (less than 30% of calories from fat) to keep it low, and be tested again within five years.

## CHOLESTEROL VALUES OVER 200 (MG/DL)

If your cholesterol level is over 200, you should have the test repeated at your doctor's office. The average of the two results is used to make decisions regarding treatment. If the difference in the two values is greater than 30, it is recommended that the test be repeated.

Figure 9.1 Risk of heart disease based on total blood cholesterol.

| Risk of Heart Disease Based on Total Cholesterol | |
|---|---|
| **Total Cholesterol (mg/dl)** | **Classification** |
| Less than 200 | Desirable (Low risk) |
| 200 – 239 | Borderline/High risk |
| 240 and above | High risk |

## LIPOPROTEIN ANALYSIS

Once your correct value is established, a lipoprotein analysis may be recommended. This is a blood test which measures the HDL or "good" cholesterol, LDL or "bad" cholesterol, and triglycerides. This test should be done if your cholesterol level is above 240; or if it is between 200 and 240, *and* you have obvious signs of heart disease or at least two other heart disease risk factors. A 12-hour fast prior to this test is required. (See Figure 9.2 for the list of risk factors.)

*The recommendations regarding cholesterol levels are based on the guidelines of the National Cholesterol Education Program's, "Report of the Expert Panel on Detection, Evaluation, and Treatment oif High Cholesterol in Adults," October 1987.

**Risk Factors for Heart Disease**
**(in addition to high cholesterol)**

Male gender
Family history of premature heart disease (before age 55)
Cigarette smoking
High blood pressure
Low HDL cholesterol(less than 35 mg/dl)
Diabetes mellitus
Circulatory disorders
Extreme obesity (more than 30% over ideal body weight)

Figure 9.2 Risk factors for heart disease.

(In February 1992, an expert panel of the National Heart, Lung and Blood Institute, recommended that *all* adults have their HDL cholesterol measured as part of standard cholesterol testing. It will probably be just a matter of time before it becomes part of routine cholesterol testing.)

A lipoprotein analysis gives a more precise picture of your blood lipids (fats) than total blood cholesterol. By breaking down blood lipids into various components, this test enables your doctor to see the type and degree of cholesterol problem you have. He can then recommend the best treatment for your particular case. You may be at high risk if your LDL cholesterol is too high or your HDL cholesterol is too low.

## Desirable LDL Values

The higher your LDL value, the greater your risk for heart disease. There are three classifications of risk based on LDL cholesterol, just as for total cholesterol, as shown in Figure 9.3. The "desirable" level is less than 130; "borderline/high risk" is from 130 to 159; and "high risk" is 160 and above.

Decisions regarding dietary or drug treatment will depend not only on the LDL cholesterol level, but also on other risk factors. Those who have definite signs of heart disease *or* two or more other risk factors (Figure 9.2), should reduce LDL cholesterol levels to less than 130. For those who do not have these risk factors, an LDL cholesterol of less than 160 is the goal.

Keep in mind that these goals are *minimal,* and are used to justify the use of drugs if the appropriate LDL level cannot be achieved by diet alone. If even lower levels (below 130) can be achieved, risk is further reduced. Research has shown that the lower the LDL level, the greater the chance to stabilize or reverse atherosclerosis.

Diet modification is the first step in treating high LDL cholesterol. As a start,

| Risk of Heart Disease Based on LDL Cholesterol | |
| --- | --- |
| **LDL Cholesterol (mg/dl)** | **Classification Based On LDL Cholesterol** |
| Less than 130 | Desirable (Low risk) |
| 130 to 159 | Borderline/high risk |
| 160 and Above | High risk |

Figure 9.3 Classification of heart disease risk based on LDL cholesterol.

the American Heart Association recommends that calories from fat should account for less than 30% of total calories, with no more than 10% from saturated fat. This may be sufficient to bring cholesterol levels to the desirable range. However, if LDL levels are still elevated after several months, more substantial reductions in total fat and saturated fat should be attempted. It may be necessary to reduce total fat to 10% or 20% of total calories and saturated fat to less than 7% of calories to achieve adequate reductions in blood cholesterol levels through diet alone. Chapter 3 explains how to implement a diet of 20% or 10% of calories from fat. Diet therapy should be maintained for at least six months before drugs are considered, unless total cholesterol levels are extremely high (over 300) and other risk factors are present.

### HDL CHOLESTEROL—A SEPARATE RISK FACTOR

The higher the HDL cholesterol, the lower the risk for heart disease. The function of HDL is to pick up excess cholesterol from the bloodstream, vessel walls and tissues, and carry it back to the liver, where it is converted to bile acids and excreted from the body.

Average HDL levels for men are 40 to 50, and for women are 50 to 60. Higher levels have been shown to be protective against heart disease. Levels below 35 are considered a signal of high risk for heart disease. Figure 9.4 lists the risk classifications that correspond with HDL levels. (In a preliminary report that appeared in *Circulation* in November 1993, it was noted that a not-yet-published study conducted by the University of Minnesota found that having low HDL—below 35 for men and below 45 for women—did not increase the risk of heart disease if total cholesterol was less than 200. The study involved 13,500

| Risk of Heart Disease Based on HDL Cholesterol | |
| --- | --- |
| **HDL Cholesterol (mg/dl)** | **Classification Based On HDL Cholesterol** |
| Above 40 | Desirable |
| 35 to 40 | Borderline/high risk |
| Less than 35 | High risk |

Figure 9.4 Risk of heart disease based on HDL cholesterol.

men and women over a five-year period.)

It is more difficult to raise HDL than lower overall cholesterol. Diet changes do not have much effect. The best ways to increase HDL levels, other than drugs, are to maintain ideal body weight and to participate in regular aerobic exercise, 20 to 30 minutes per day, three to five times per week.

## TRIGLYCERIDES

Triglycerides make up 95% of the lipids (fats) circulating in the body. They travel in the bloodstream in lipoprotein packages, i.e., they are surrounded by protein, just like cholesterol. Triglycerides below 250 (mg/dl) are considered acceptable, although below 150 is desirable. (If cholesterol levels are normal, there is no greater risk for heart disease as long as triglyceride levels are less than 250.) Levels from 250 to 500 are considered moderately elevated, and those above 500 are high.

The role of triglycerides in heart disease is less understood than HDL and LDL cholesterol. Often, an elevated triglyceride level is accompanied by an increase in total cholesterol and LDL cholesterol, and/or a decrease in HDL cholesterol. When two or more of these factors act together, there is an increased risk for heart disease. Most researchers feel, however, that moderately elevated triglycerides alone is not a cause for concern. As a result, most doctors do not advocate treating moderate elevations if HDL and LDL cholesterol levels are in the desirable range.

William Castelli, renowned director of the Framingham Heart Study, advocates a more aggressive approach. He recommends treatment (first diet for six months, then drugs if needed) if triglycerides are above 150 while HDL is below 40. His research has shown a definite risk factor when even slightly low HDL is combined with triglycerides over 150.

If triglyceride levels are greater than 500, they present a risk not only for heart disease but also for pancreatitis or inflammation of the pancreas. Levels this high call for aggressive diet and drug treatment. Less than one person in 1,000 has this condition.

Some of the dietary and life-style factors that lower triglycerides also have a positive effect on LDL and HDL cholesterol. Reducing saturated fats and losing weight (if overweight) lowers triglycerides as well as LDL cholesterol. Regular, vigorous exercise increases HDL values, while decreasing triglycerides.

There are certain dietary factors that sometimes raise triglycerides but do not appear to increase the risk for heart disease. These include a high-carbohydrate diet and moderate intakes of alcohol.

Neither of these adversely affects cholesterol values. Refer to Figure 9.5 for a summary of the dietary and life-style factors that reduce the risk for heart disease.

## CHOLESTEROL RATIOS

The cholesterol ratio is sometimes used to predict the likelihood of developing heart disease. It is determined by dividing total cholesterol by HDL cholesterol. For example, if your total cholesterol is 180 and your HDL is 50, your cholesterol ratio would be 180/50 or 3.6.

The ideal ratio, which indicates a very low risk for heart disease, is under 3.5. The ratio which represents an average risk of heart disease for men is 5.0; while for women, it is 4.5. The lower the ratio, the lower the risk. Although the ratio is helpful in predicting the likelihood of CHD, dietary and/or drug treatment is based primarily on the HDL and LDL values.

Figure 9.5 A summary of the dietary and life-style recommendations to reduce the risk for heart disease.

**Dietary/Life-Style Methods
to Reduce Risks of Heart Disease**

**Ways To Lower LDL Cholesterol**
Reduce fat intake, especially saturated fat and cholesterol
Lose weight, if overweight
Reduce stress
Eat foods high in soluble fiber

**Ways to Raise HDL Cholesterol**
Lose weight, if overweight
Do regular aerobic exercise
Stop smoking

**Ways to Lower Triglycerides**
Reduce fat intake, especially saturated fat
Lose weight, if overweight
Do regular aerobic exercise
Reduce alcohol consumption
Eat fewer concentrated sweets

**Ways to Lower Blood Pressure**
Lose weight, if overweight
Reduce sodium intake
Reduce alcohol consumption
Do regular aerobic exercise

## CHOLESTEROL LEVELS FOR CHILDREN

We also need to be concerned with the cholesterol levels of children, since heart disease does not begin in middle-aged adults. Rather, the earliest signs of the disease are evident in young children and teens in the form of fatty streaks that line the aorta and coronary arteries. Studies of U.S. soldiers, who died in Korea and Vietnam, showed that many had plaque and a few even had severe blockage of the coronary arteries at a very young age.

Research has shown that cholesterol levels "track" well from childhood into adulthood. In other words, a given measurement tends to keep the same rank as the child gets older. *A child with high cholesterol has an 80% chance of having an elevated level as a young adult.*

## DESIRABLE LEVELS

The National Institutes of Health make the following recommendations regarding children's cholesterol. If the cholesterol level is below 170, which corresponds with the 75th percentile, it is in the "desirable" range for children. These children should still be encouraged to follow a prudent low-fat diet consisting of less than 30% of total calories from fat, of which no more than 10% should be saturated fat. (See Chapter 3 to see what constitutes a diet of 20% or 30% of calories from fat.)

Children whose cholesterol levels are between 170 and 185 (the 75th and 90th percentile, respectively) should closely follow a low-fat diet of 20% or 30% of calories from fat. The goal is to reduce their level to below 170. They should be retested in a year.

Children who have cholesterol levels from 185 to 200 (90th to 95th percentile) may need to restrict fat intake further than 30% of total calories. Restricting it to about 20 to 25% of total calories is sometimes necessary to bring cholesterol to the "desirable" level. Cholesterol levels of 200 in children correspond to values of 260 in an adult.

If cholesterol levels are above 200 (95th percentile), children may have a hereditary form of high cholesterol. These children should closely follow the dietary regimen mentioned previously. Most children respond very well to diet alone. However, if diet produces insufficient response after at least six months, the guidelines (by the National Institutes of Health) suggest that these children "should be considered for treatment" with a cholesterol-lowering drug. Thus far, their use appears to be safe with children. Tests have shown that they have no effect on growth and development. Your pediatrician will make a recommendation on this, taking other risk factors into account.

## PARENTAL APPROACH IS IMPORTANT

Parents should be careful to use a positive approach in dealing with children whose cholesterol levels are too high. The children should not be made to feel that they have some type of disease or that foods are a form of medicine. The emphasis should be on encouraging all the aspects of a healthy life-style and healthy diet. These include regular exercise, maintaining ideal body weight and no smoking. In the long run, this is more important than significantly reducing a moderately elevated cholesterol level.

Overzealous parents can do more harm than good. Some parents may feel that if restricting fat produces good results, that reducing it further will be better. This is not necessarily the case. Restricting fat too much (to less than 20% of total calories) can be harmful to growing children, who need the nutrients and caloric density of at least this much fat.

### THE GRADUAL RISE IN CHOLESTEROL LEVELS

Cholesterol levels do not rise during childhood as they tend to do during adult years. In fact, they usually drop slightly following adolescence. In general, not until people reach their 20s does cholesterol begin its upward climb. (See Figures 9.6 and 9.7.)

The increases with age can be greatly reduced if a low-fat diet is adopted and followed from childhood throughout adulthood. The longer a low-fat diet is observed, the greater the reduction in mortality rates from heart disease.

## DRUGS TO TREAT HIGH-CHOLESTEROL LEVELS

There are a number of drugs on the market to treat high cholesterol. These drugs are recommended *only* when a low-fat diet fails to lower cholesterol adequately. Table 9.1 lists the cholesterol-lowering drugs, with a

Figure 9.6 How cholesterol levels for white males at the 10th, 50th and 90th percentiles change throughout a lifetime (ages 5 to 70+).

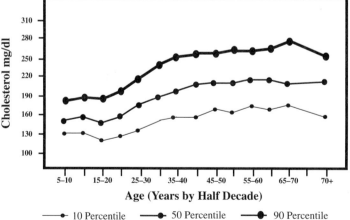

**Cholesterol Levels (mg/dl) Change with Age**
**Percentiles for White Males**

Source: Adapted from the Lipid Research Clinics Population Studies Data Book.

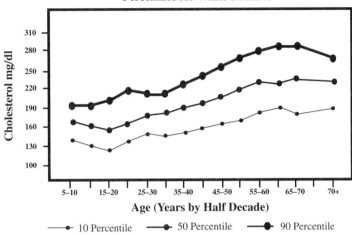

**Cholesterol Levels (mg/dl) Change with Age Percentiles for White Females**

Figure 9.7 How cholesterol levels for white females at the 10th, 50th and 90th percentiles change throughout a lifetime (ages 5 to 70+).

Source: Adapted from the Lipid Research Clinics Population Studies Data Book.

breakdown of their average costs, effectiveness in decreasing LDL or increasing HDL cholesterol, side effects and special precautions.

## BLOOD PRESSURE MEASUREMENTS

High blood pressure is the greatest risk factor for heart disease—even more significant than high cholesterol. It is a major cause of heart failure, kidney failure and stroke. You need to know if your level is high, so you can do whatever is necessary to lower it and reduce the associated health risks. Everyone should have yearly blood pressure checks.

There are still many people who are unaware that they have high blood pressure, but the number is dwindling. Before 1970, only about one-quarter of the estimated 60 million Americans with high blood pressure knew it and only a quarter of these were adequately treated. By 1984, one-half of the hypertensive population were aware of their condition and two-thirds of these received some form of antihypertensive therapy.

### WHAT LEVELS CONSTITUTE HYPERTENSION?

For adults, a diagnosis of hypertension is made if the systolic blood pressure (top number) is greater than 140 millimeters of mercury (mm Hg) and/or the diastolic blood pressure (bottom number) is greater than 90 (mm Hg).

An optimal blood pressure reading is below 120/80, and when blood pressure climbs above this level, risk gradually increases. At levels of 140/90 and above, there is a 50% increase in mortality related to heart disease. Therefore, even

## Major Cholesterol-Lowering Drugs

| Drugs | Average Cost/mo | Well-Tolerated? | Decrease in LDL* Cholesterol | Effect on HDL* Cholesterol | Side Effects | Special Precautions |
|---|---|---|---|---|---|---|
| Cholestyramine Questran Cholybar Colestipol Colestid | $75–95 | varies | 15–30% | slight increase | Upper and lower gastrointestinal (GI) disturbances (constipation, excess gas, stomach acidity). | May alter absorption of other drugs. May increase blood triglyceride levels. |
| Nicotinic acid, Nicobid, Niacin, Time-release niacin | $4–8 | varies | 15–30% | increase | Flushing, itching, upper GI disturbances (stomach acidity or nausea). Flushing is decreased by pretreatment with aspirin or Advil. | Monitor for increased blood uric acid levels, hyperglycemia and liver abnormalities. Not for use in patients with peptic ulcer, liver disease or gouty arthritis. |
| Lovastatin Mevacor Simvastatin Zocor | $120–175 | yes | 25–45% | increase | Generally well-tolerated. Most common side effects include GI disturbances and muscle pain (less than 5% of patients). | Patients should be monitored for changes in liver function. Increased risk of muscle inflammation, if used with niacin or gemfibrozil. |
| Gemfibrozil Lopid | $65–95 | yes | 5–15% | increase | Infrequent side effects, most common being GI disturbances. | Not for use in patients with gallbladder disease. Increases the effect of blood-thinning drugs. May increase LDL cholesterol in those with high triglyceride levels. |
| Probucol Lorelco | $105–120 | yes | 10–15% | decrease | Generally well-tolerated. Uncommon side effects include diarrhea, gas, nausea or abdominal pain (less than 5% of patients). | Lowers HDL cholesterol. Not recommended for patients with abnormal EKG. |

*LDL is the "bad" cholesterol, while HDL is the "good" cholesterol
Adapted from: National Cholesterol Education Program, *Report of the Expert Panel on Detection, Evaluation and Treatment of High Blood Cholesterol in Adults*, 1989.

Table 9.1 Cholesterol-lowering drugs.

modest elevations carry substantial risks. On the other hand, reductions of any amount lower the health risks related to hypertension.

One elevated reading does not necessarily mean you need to be treated for high blood pressure. Instead, a diagnosis is based on the average of *at least* two readings taken on *at least* two different occasions.

Some individuals have a condition called *labile hypertension* in which blood pressure levels climb when they are under stress. They can experience wide fluctuations in their blood pressure, from day to day and even hour to hour. When this is the case, a physician may suggest that they record their blood pressure several times throughout the day, (with a portable blood pressure machine) over a two-to-four-week period; or they may be advised to use a 24-hour recording device to determine blood pressure during normal activities. (A doctor's office can be a stressful environment for some.) Treatment for labile hypertension is based on the average of the home-recorded blood pressures.

### HYPERTENSION IN CHILDREN AND ADOLESCENTS

Children and adolescents can also have hypertension. The National Heart, Lung and Blood Institute considers the following levels to be too high for the various age groups: 116/76 (mm Hg) (3 to 5 years old); 122/ 78 (6 to 9 years old); 126/82 (10 to 12 years old); 136/86 (13 to 15 years old; and 142/92 (16 to 18 years old). Your pediatrician can advise you on treatment if your child's level is higher than those listed above.

## RECOMMENDED TREATMENT FOR HIGH BLOOD PRESSURE

### DIET AND BEHAVIOR MODIFICATION

A low-salt diet (from 1,500 to 2,400 milligrams of sodium per day) is highly recommended for anyone whose blood pressure is above 120/80, regardless of whether drugs are required. Another equally important factor in controlling blood pressure is to lose weight if overweight. (Losing as few as five pounds enables some individuals to bring blood pressure levels into the desirable range, and thereby reduce the risk of heart disease and perhaps avoid the use of drugs.)

Other factors that have been shown to be effective in reducing blood pressure levels in some individuals are regular aerobic exercise, limiting alcohol consumption to no more than one drink per day (see p. 56 to see what constitutes a "drink") and eating more potassium-rich foods. If you are taking medication for hypertension, check with your doctor first before increasing your potassium intake, because certain medications cause the kidneys to retain potassium.

### DIASTOLIC PRESSURE IS TOO HIGH

For those whose diastolic blood pressure (bottom number) is moderately elevated (from 90 to 100), the diet and behavior modification mentioned previously is sometimes all that is needed to bring the level below 90. Those whose diastolic pressure is above 100 almost always require some type of medication.

Generally, drugs are recommended for anyone whose average diastolic pressure remains above 90. The drugs available to treat hypertension include diuretics, beta blockers, angiotensin converting enzyme (ACE) inhibitors, and calcium entry blockers.

The drug of choice depends on the severity of the disease, degree of elevation and individual side effects. Diuretics are usually the first-choice drug for those with moderately elevated blood pressure because they have been proven effective and the side effects are minimal. Beta blockers are most effective for those who have elevated blood pressure affected by stress. For some, a combination of drugs works best. If you take blood pressure medication and are experiencing unpleasant side effects, discuss this with your doctor. He or she may suggest a different drug or combination of drugs that will work better for you.

### SYSTOLIC PRESSURE IS TOO HIGH

Treatment of high systolic blood pressure in the absence of high diastolic pressure is still debatable. Although studies have shown an increased risk for heart disease with high systolic pressure, it has not yet been proven that drugs reduce mortality or help in disease prevention.

Still, the overall recommendation is to use conservative drug treatment with a goal of 10% reduction in systolic blood pressure. If drugs produce bothersome side effects, they are usually discontinued.

The thresholds for initiating drug treatment are based on age. The following guidelines suggest who should receive treatment: those under 35 years old who have systolic blood pressure greater than 140; those 35 to 59 years old whose systolic pressure is greater than 150; and those over 65 years old who have systolic pressure over 160.

# TEN

## *Weight Control*

### WEIGHT LOSS AND HEALTH

Sixty-two percent of American adults consider themselves overweight, according to a poll conducted by Weight Watchers, Inc. Actually, 25 to 30% are truly overweight. That is still a high percentage—and the numbers are increasing.

Why are so many overweight? National food surveys tell us it is not because we consume an inordinately high number of calories. Our ancestors from the early 1900s consumed more calories than we do today and yet fewer of them were overweight. The reason for this is that we get less exercise, and have a higher percentage of fat in our diet; 40% vs. 25 to 30% for our ancestors.

Calories from fat turn into body fat much more efficiently than calories from carbohydrate or protein.

For those who are overweight, the health benefits of sensible weight loss are numerous. For every 2 pounds of weight lost, cholesterol levels drop an average of three points. Those with "high normal" blood pressures (diastolic pressure between 80 and 89) who lose just 9 pounds of weight have only half the risk of developing "high" blood pressure (diastolic pressure over 90). Maintaining a desirable weight also reduces the risks of several types of cancers, heart disease, stroke and adult-onset diabetes.

### FACTORS THAT INFLUENCE BODY WEIGHT

#### FAT FROM FOODS

The higher the percentage of fat in the diet, the greater the likelihood of being overweight. There are two reasons for this. The first is that fat calories are converted to body fat more readily than carbohydrate or protein calories. Excess

fat from foods is converted to body fat using only 3% of its calories, whereas excess carbohydrate uses 23% of its calories in the process of conversion to body fat. This means fewer of the excess calories from carbohydrate will be converted to and stored as fat. Of course, neither dietary fat nor carbohydrate will be converted to body fat unless *excess* calories, over and above what the body needs to maintain itself, are consumed.

The second reason that higher fat intake means greater weight gain is that it takes more calories to satisfy your appetite or "fill you up" when there is a higher percentage of fat. This is because fat is much more dense than carbohydrate or protein. It contains 9 calories per gram, whereas carbohydrate and protein both contain 4 calories per gram.

To emphasize this point, let's compare the calories in similar quantities of food when 20% of calories come from fat vs. 40% of calories from fat. The difference in calories is significant. For example, a plateful of food, with 20% of the calories from fat, has 650 calories; the exact same quantity of food, with 40% of the calories from fat, contains 1,050 calories. It is easier to feel satisfied with fewer calories when you can eat a greater volume or quantity of food.

Another example, shown in Figure 10.1, is to compare one cup of fresh strawberries, which has negligible fat, with a strawberry snack pie, where 37% of its calories come from fat. The cup of strawberries has only 45 calories, compared with 340 calories in the snack pie. They have a similar amount of bulk or volume, but the pie has over seven times as many calories. (The concentrated sugar in the snack pie is also a significant contributor to calories.)

On the other hand, you will probably feel hungry again *sooner* after eating the strawberries than the snack pie because fat provides a longer-lasting feeling of satiety (satisfaction and fullness) than carbohydrate or protein because it is digested more slowly. Still, you'll be consuming fewer calories in the long run when eating foods lower in fat, even if you feel the need to snack on low-fat foods between meals.

## EXERCISE

Exercise is the second factor that affects body weight, since calories are burned during exercise. The more vigorous the exercise, the more calories that

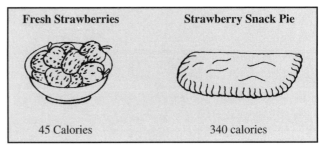

Figure 10.1 A strawberry snack pie, with 37% of its calories from fat, has over seven times as many calories as one cup of fresh strawberries, which has only a trace of fat. Both have approximately the same volume.

**Fresh Strawberries**

**Strawberry Snack Pie**

45 Calories

340 calories

are burned in a given period of time. Refer to Figure 10.2 for a comparison of the approximate number of calories burned in various forms of exercise.

Exercise is an aid to weight control in more ways than just burning calories. It enhances the breakdown and loss of body fat, while helping preserve lean muscle tissue. Furthermore, when dieting, the basal metabolic rate slows down, which means the body burns fewer calories while at rest. Exercise while dieting is credited with helping the body return to a normal metabolic rate after dieting has stopped. This is very important in weight maintenance.

Exercise also helps dieters psychologically. Regular exercise encourages an overall feeling of well-being and fitness. This positive feeling helps dieters continue toward dietary goals.

## HEREDITY

The third and final factor affecting weight is heredity. Recent studies conducted in the late 1980s and early 1990s, show that heredity plays a greater role in weight control than once thought. A Quebec study reported in 1990 that genes determine how the body handles excess calories. Some people's bodies handle the excess calories very inefficiently, converting them to muscle protein rather than body fat. Since it takes nine times as much energy to turn food into muscle as it does to store it as fat, those who turn excess calories into muscle tissue burn up many of their excess calories in the process.

In the Quebec study, 12 pairs of identical twins were hospitalized for 120

| Number of Calories Burned during Exercise | |
|---|---|
| **Activity** | **Calories per 30 minutes** |
| Domestic work | 90 |
| Walking, 2 1/2 mph | 105 |
| Bicycling, 5 1/2 mph | 105 |
| Gardening | 110 |
| Golf, lawn mowing (power mower) | 125 |
| Bowling | 135 |
| Walking, 3 3/4 mph | 150 |
| Swimming, 1/4 mph | 150 |
| Square dancing, volleyball | 175 |
| Roller skating | 175 |
| Wood chopping, hand sawing | 200 |
| Tennis | 210 |
| Cross-country skiing, 10 mph | 300 |
| Squash, handball | 300 |
| Jogging, 7 mph (9-minute miles) | 300 |
| Bicycling, 13 mph | 330 |
| Running, 10 mph (6-minute miles) | 450 |

Figure 10.2 Approximate number of calories burned by a 150-pound person while performing various activities for 30 minutes.

days so their diets and physical activity could be closely monitored. For the first 30 days, they were fed the equivalent of their usual diet, which maintained their weight during that period. For the next 90 days, each pair of twins was fed 1,000 extra calories over their maintenance diet. They were not allowed to do strenuous exercise, but were required to do a specified amount of walking.

The results were surprising to everyone concerned. Within each pair of twins, the weight gain was nearly the same. But there was a great variation from one pair of twins to another. The weight gain of the pairs varied from 9 pounds to 29 pounds.

What this study showed was that some people, because of their genetic makeup, have a greater tendency to put on weight. Of course, all who ate excess calories over the three-month period did gain weight, but some gained three times as much as others. One can deduce from this study that the reverse is also true — it is easier for some people to lose weight or maintain weight than others. Weight control is within everyone's reach, but some will always have to work harder at it than others.

## OUR BODY'S REACTION TO DIETING

Whenever anyone is dieting, i.e. when calorie intake is restricted to less than what it takes to maintain weight, the body reacts as if it is being starved. To protect itself, the body slows down its metabolism to conserve limited food. What this means is that the body burns fewer calories than usual while at rest. This makes it more difficult, but not impossible, to lose weight.

Weight loss should be gradual, not exceeding 1 to 2 pounds per week. The slower the weight is taken off, the more likely it will stay off. When weight loss is no more than 2 pounds per week, approximately 60 to 80% of the weight is lost as fat, and just 20 to 40% as lean body mass. In quick-loss starvation diets, a much greater proportion is lost as lean body mass and fluids. To protect against excess muscle loss, women are encouraged to consume at least 1,200 calories per day; and men, a minimum of 1,500 calories per day.

After dieting for a period of time, many dieters complain of reaching a plateau, where they cannot seem to lose more weight. When weight is lost, 10 to 20 pounds for example, less food is needed to maintain the lower weight. It takes fewer calories to maintain 140 pounds than 160 pounds. If additional weight loss is desired, either food intake needs to be restricted further or exercise increased.

Once the desired weight is reached by a gradual method of weight loss in combination with regular exercise, the metabolic rate increases to a rate normal for the new weight. The new metabolic rate is generally within 10% of the original metabolic rate. Still, former dieters must eat less than they did previously to maintain the lower weight.

## WHAT IT TAKES TO GAIN/LOSE WEIGHT

To gain a pound of weight, you must consume an excess of approximately 3,500 calories. That means 3,500 calories over and above what you need to maintain your weight. One piece of pecan pie (495 calories) will not do it.

The reverse is true if you are trying to lose weight. If your goal is to lose a pound a week, you must eliminate about 3,500 calories over a week's time, either through exercise or calorie reduction. This averages out to 500 fewer calories per day. You can either eat 500 fewer calories, exercise enough to burn 500 calories, or a combination of both, which is preferable. For weight loss of 1 to 2 pounds per week, you will need to eliminate 500 to 1,000 calories per day.

# TYPES OF DIETS

## MEDICALLY SUPERVISED LIQUID DIETS

These diets are characterized by extreme calorie restriction; usually no more than 420 to 800 calories per day. For the first two to three months, nutritional needs are met by a liquid formula only, which contains protein, vitamins and minerals. After the liquid diet phase, solid food is gradually reintroduced. The expected weight loss while on liquid diets is 3 to 5 pounds per week. The more popular medically supervised liquid diets are Optifast, Medifast and Health Management Resources (HMR).

All of these programs are fairly expensive, ranging from about $1,000 to $3,500, and they last anywhere from 6 to 18 months. All are available only through hospitals and clinics, and most require that participants be at least 50 pounds or 20% over their ideal body weight. The dropout rate is high—usually about 40 to 50%.

There are a number of serious drawbacks to rapid weight loss diets. The most obvious is that dieters who lose weight this quickly will most likely not *keep* the weight off. Based on studies of liquid diet programs at university medical centers, it is estimated that no more than 10% keep the weight off a year or two after completing the program. What makes subsequent weight gain nearly inevitable is that fat cells cannot shrink fast enough, nor metabolism readjust adequately when weight loss is this rapid. The body tries to make up for the deficiencies it experienced by putting weight back on with only a minimal amount of calories—perhaps only 1,200 to 1,500 calories a day. This makes it extremely difficult to keep pounds off when solid foods are reintroduced.

Another drawback is that proportionately more lean muscle mass and less fat is lost with liquid diets. *The body is capable of losing no more than 1 to 2 pounds of fat per week.* Any pounds lost over and above this are muscle and water. Consequently, not much more, and sometimes even less fat is lost with this type of diet than with a conventional low-calorie diet.

Unpleasant side effects usually occur as the body responds to starvation diets. First, to conserve calories, the body temperature drops, causing a "chilly" feeling. Second, the body cuts back its blood supply to the tiny vessels near the skin's surface, which creates rough, dry skin. Third, exercise becomes difficult as the result of being in a weakened state. It is often met by dizziness or cramps.

The medical rationale for these diet programs is that these patients have not been able to lose weight using more conventional methods and that their obesity is increasing their risks for heart disease, high blood pressure, stroke and diabetes. Even though it does not work for many, i.e. not many succeed in *keeping* the pounds off, it does work for some. Starvation or liquid diets should be diets of last resort.

### OVER-THE-COUNTER LIQUID DIETS

Some self-prescribed liquid diet products are available at the grocery stores and drug stores and require no professional supervision. Slender by Carnation encourages you to use only their product, with no supplements of real food. If you drink four servings per day, as recommended, you will consume 880 calories. It claims to contain 100% of the RDAs for protein, vitamins and minerals.

Another product, Ultra Slim Fast, comes in powdered form to be mixed with 8 ounces of milk, water or fruit juice. The instructions recommend three servings per day—at breakfast, lunch and an afternoon snack—plus a regular meal at dinner. The three servings of liquid formula contain 660 calories plus 12 grams of fiber.

These diets are characterized by a yo-yo form of weight loss, i.e., rapid weight loss followed by quick weight gain when off the liquid diet. (See "Medically Supervised Liquid Diets," above.) This tendency is slightly lessened if there is at least one regular meal per day. A major concern with unsupervised liquid diets is that dietary deficiencies can occur, and without proper medical supervision, the heart and gallbladder can be adversely affected. In addition, yo-yo dieting has been found to be less healthy than maintaining a slightly higher steady weight.

## REAL FOOD DIETS WITH REQUIRED SPECIAL PRODUCTS

Two popular diet programs that require special products are Jenny Craig and Nutri/System. Both stress nutrition education and behavior modification, and encourage regular aerobic exercise. Their weight loss goal is 1 to 2 pounds per week. They require the use of pre-packaged meals during the weight loss period. The use of these foods is essentially their way of choosing low-fat foods and monitoring calorie intake for you.

These diets are beneficial for those who do not want to count calories or make their own food choices. On the other hand, it would be very difficult for those who must eat out frequently. In the beginning of a diet program, pre-packaged meals may be helpful in educating dieters on food selection and recommended portion sizes.

There are two main disadvantages to using this type of diet plan. One is that their foods are more expensive than buying similar types at the grocery store. The cost of the pre-packaged meals is $60 to $70 per week, not including the fresh produce and skim milk you buy on your own. Another disadvantage is that eventually, when your weight-loss goal is reached, you will be required to select your own foods, and this may be difficult if you have not had to do it all along.

Both programs continue for one year after the weight loss goal is reached to help with the maintenance diet. Educating clients on how to make healthy food choices on their own is the goal during this phase.

## REAL FOOD DIETS WITHOUT SPECIAL PRODUCTS

The strengths of these programs lie in their educational efforts to teach dieters how to make the right food choices on their own without the use of special products. If good eating habits are learned and implemented by the dieter during the period of weight loss, it should be easier to adjust to a maintenance diet once the goal has been reached. Three diet programs that offer this approach are Diet Workshop, Weight Loss Clinic and Weight Watchers.

Diet Workshop and Weight Watchers educate their clients on food selection, exercise, etc. through weekly group meetings headed by trained "graduates" of their programs. Weight Loss Clinic encourages short (5 to 10 minutes) one-on-one meetings with staff members, as often as the client desires, Monday through Friday. Staff members may be nurses, dietitians or company-trained counselors.

Weight loss recommendations from these programs are similar. Diet Workshop recommends a weight loss of 1 1/2 to 2 pounds/week; Weight Watchers, 1 to 2 pounds/week; and Weight Loss Clinic, 2 to 3 pounds/week. Maintenance phases vary from 4 weeks to 6 months. Both Diet Workshop and Weight Watchers offer free lifetime memberships for those who maintain their losses.

The costs of Diet Workshop and Weight Watchers are similar. Both have modest initial membership fees plus weekly charges until maintenance. Weight Loss Clinic is a more expensive program. Prices vary slightly in different locations, so check the prices in your area.

## TIPS ON CHOOSING THE BEST DIET PLAN FOR YOU

All diet programs have advantages and disadvantages, and some people have more success with one type than another. This is because there are many different reasons why people are overweight. Included at the end of this chapter is a specific weight-loss plan, based on the weight-loss principles outlined in this chapter.

No matter what method you choose to lose weight, there is only one way to *keep* the weight off. It requires a *lifelong commitment* to making wise, low-fat food choices on a regular basis and incorporating an exercise program into your life-style.

The following is a list of points to consider in choosing a diet plan:

1. Can you follow your own diet plan or one outlined in a book, without joining a specific weight-loss program? Many are able to do so successfully by reducing fat and exercising regularly, but some need the regimentation of a program or the encouragement and support of a group or weight-loss counselor.

2. Can you live with the diet plan indefinitely? Some programs are set up in the very beginning so that you can continue with them indefinitely. Obviously, you cannot live with a liquid diet or pre-packaged meals forever; but perhaps the maintenance phase of some of these diet programs could be continued indefinitely.

3. Do you need special assistance to aid in proper food selection and portion control (prepackaged meals and snacks); or, with proper education, can you make the right choices on your own?

4. Is the program individualized to take into account different rates of metabolism and caloric needs?

5. Does the program put you in touch with health professionals, such as physicians, dietitians or nurses? If not, ask your physician if the program is reputable. Some programs have been developed by health professionals and have well trained staffs who are knowledgeable about nutrition, behavior modification and the importance of exercise.

6. Is the recommended rate of weight loss the generally accept-

able 1 to 2 pounds per week?

7. What percentage of the program's clients reach their goal weight and maintain it for at least one year? Generally, these numbers are not well documented, but it is still worth asking.

8. Will the maintenance plan fit your needs? Is it long enough and is the educational component adequate?

9. Can you afford the program? There is a wide variation in costs of different types of programs. The more expensive are not necessarily better.

## A SUGGESTED WEIGHT-LOSS PLAN

The following is a suggested weight-loss plan, which incorporates all the aspects of healthy low-fat eating discussed in the previous chapters. This is not a 4-week or 12-week plan, but a plan that should be satisfying for the rest of your life, with only slight modifications made after your weight-loss goal is reached. Diets and deprivation do not work. They only encourage the yo-yo effect of rapid weight loss, followed by weight gain, and on and on. What is needed is a fundamental change in lifestyle and eating habits.

The two primary elements of this weight-loss plan are eating very low-fat foods (which in most cases enables you to eat until you are satisfied without consuming excessive amounts of calories) and a regular exercise program (consisting of a combination of aerobic and strength-training exercises). It is important to take a multivitamin/mineral supplement with any weight-loss program, to ensure that you are getting adequate amounts of all the essential nutrients.

### PLAN A BALANCED LOW-FAT DIET

When you decide you want to lose weight, focus on more than just improving your appearance. Remind yourself that your objectives are also to feel better, have more energy and live a longer, healthier life. The latter objectives should help motivate you to make healthy food choices. If you are starving yourself, eating the wrong kinds of foods or depriving yourself of necessary nutrients, you will not feel better. You may be able to lose weight in those ways, but you will cause harm to your body in the long run.

The Food Guide Pyramid should serve as the focal point for planning a balanced diet. When formulating your meal plan for the day, include at least the minimum number of servings from each of the five major food groups. The minimum number of daily servings is given in Figure 10.3. To see what constitutes a single serving, refer to Figure 10.4.

The number of servings may seem large to you. However, when you eat a meal, such as a spaghetti dinner, the amount of pasta you eat may actually count as two or three servings. Most people eat at least 1 cup of pasta at a meal, which would be two servings.

| Minimum Servings of Food per Day | |
|---|---|
| Bread group | 6 servings |
| Vegetable group | 3 servings |
| Fruit group | 2 servings |
| Milk group | 2–3 servings |
| Meat group | 2 servings |

Figure 10.3  The minimum number of servings per day from the five major food groups, based on the Food Guide Pyramid.

Figure 10.4  The amount of food which constitutes a single serving from each of the five major food groups of the Food Guide Pyramid.

| What Constitutes One Serving? | |
|---|---|
| **Breads, cereals, rice and pasta**<br>1 slice of bread<br>1/2 cup cooked rice or pasta<br>1/2 cup cooked cereal<br>1 ounce ready-to-eat cereal | **Milk, yogurt, and cheese**<br>1 cup milk or yogurt<br>1 1/2 to 2 ounces cheese |
| **Vegetables**<br>1/2 cup chopped raw or cooked vegetables<br>1 cup leafy raw vegetables | **Meat, poultry, fish, dry beans, eggs, and nuts (protein group)**<br>2 1/2 to 3 ounces cooked lean meat, poultry or fish |
| **Fruits**<br>1 fruit or a melon wedge<br>3/4 cup juice<br>1/2 cup canned fruit<br>1/4 cup dried fruit | Count 1/2 cup cooked beans or 1 egg as 1/3 serving |

## LIMIT FAT GRAMS

*Women should limit fat to 30 grams per day; men should limit fat to 40 grams per day.* The procedure that works best is to split approximately half your daily fat-gram allowance between breakfast and lunch, and use the remaining half for dinner. A pocket-sized Fat Gram Counter book is essential when you start out, since it is impossible to guess how much fat is in foods. It can be purchased at most bookstores for a cost of $3 to $8.

Nearly all foods are "allowed," but if you consistently choose low-fat foods, you will have more variety in the foods you can eat before reaching your daily fat allowance. For example, if you start the day with a sausage biscuit at McDonald's, you will be consuming 28 grams of fat. Consequently, a woman will have only 2 grams of fat remaining for the rest of the day, and a man will have just 12 grams remaining. On the other hand, if you eat a melon wedge and a bagel with jelly, you will consume only 2 grams of fat. That leaves a woman with up to 28 fat grams, and a man up to 38 grams of fat to consume in the remaining two meals of the day. Once you reach your limit for the day, you need not starve yourself, but simply choose only nonfat foods the rest of the day. This would include an assortment of fruits, vegetables, rice, nonfat crackers and breads.

Snacks should be fat free, or very low fat. There are many choices available—nearly all fruits and vegetables, pretzels with or without salsa, melba rounds and bagels (with small amounts of jelly or jam, or a nonfat variety of margarine or cream cheese).

What about fat-free cookies, coffee cakes and desserts? These foods are fine to eat occasionally, but one of the pitfalls in dieting is that there are certain foods that are very difficult to eat in moderation—our craving for them is too strong. This includes most concentrated sweets, and salty, high-fat snack foods, such as potato chips. Unless you have a high degree of self-control, limit the fat-free sweets to special occasions.

Be sure to drink the recommended amount of fluids while on a weight-loss regimen—at least eight glasses of liquids per day, not including caffeinated beverages. Drinks high in sugar should be limited or avoided. Sometimes, people "feed" their thirst, that is, they eat because the misinterpret their body's thirst signal for a hunger signal. When you think you are hungry, drink a glass of water and see if that satisfies you. If it does not, then eat a healthy snack, such as a fruit.

To sum up the food segment of this weight-loss plan, there are two factors involved: a balanced diet and a daily fat gram allowance. In order to take both these factors into account, it works best to write down a weekly meal plan, including snacks. If you know you are going out to dinner on a particular night, and that you will exceed your fat gram allowance that day, limit your fat grams more severely on the previous two days. Think of the weekly meal plan as just 15 to 20 minutes of time spent each week creating great-tasting, nutritious menus.

In addition to writing down a weekly menu, you should also keep a diary of the foods you actually eat each day, including all snacks. At the end of each week, compare the plan with what you actually ate. In this way, you can determine how well you followed your plan, and discover the pitfalls, if any, you want to avoid in the future. Once you are successfully losing 1 to 2 pounds a week, you can discontinue the diary.

## 15-DAY MEAL PLAN

The following pages provide 15-day sample meal plans which limit fat to less than 30 grams per day. The meal plans are similar to the two-week meal plan in Chapter 7, where fat is limited to approximately 20% of calories. However, since the goal of this meal plan is to lose weight, some changes were made to bring the fat and calorie content down further. These menus were designed to be a guide for you to create your own delectable meals. Do not let them stifle

## 15-Day Meal Plan[1]

| | Day 1 | Day 2 | Day 3 | Day 4 | Day 5 | Day 6 | Day 7 | Day 8 |
|---|---|---|---|---|---|---|---|---|
| **Breakfast** | orange juice whole grain cereal w/ skim milk (2g) coffee/tea | melon wedge whole wheat toast w/ jelly (2 slices; 2g) coffee/tea | 1/2 grapefruit bagel w/ nonfat cream cheese (2g) coffee/tea | orange juice cooked cereal w/ raisins and skim milk (2g) coffee/tea | orange juice scrambled egg substitute (2 eggs; 1g) whole wheat toast w/ jelly (1 slice;1g) coffee/tea | instant oatmeal w/ sugar, cinnamon, milk (2g) orange coffee/tea | whole grain cereal w/ 1/2 banana, skim milk (2g) toast w/ jelly (1 slice; 1g) coffee/tea | honeydew wedge *Bran Muffin— plain (low-fat; 2g) coffee/tea |
| **Morning Snack** | apple | Graham crackers (2 squares; 2g) | plum | pretzels (1oz.; 1g) | low-fat crackers (Melba Rounds) (1/2oz.; 1g) non-caloric beverage | apple | orange | *Bran Muffin— low-fat (2g) |
| **Lunch** | ham sandwich[2] (3–6g) minestrone soup (1 cup; 2g) skim milk | turkey sand-wich[2] on whole wheat (3–6g) fresh fruit salad (1 cup) beverage | tuna pasta salad (5g) French bread—plain (1 slice; 1g) skim milk | ham sandwich[2] on rye (3–6g) cantaloupe wedge non-caloric beverage | *Black Bean Salad (4g) whole wheat bread plain (1 slice; 1g) pineapple slice skim milk | tuna salad w/ nonfat yogurt or mayonnaise on whole wheat (3–5g) steamed broccoli or raw carrots skim milk | turkey sand-wich[2] on hard roll (3–6g) *Tropical Fruit Slaw (1g) skim milk | tuna salad w/ non-fat yogurt or mayonnaise on rye (3–5g) baked beans-vegetarian (1/2 cup; 1g) skim milk |
| **Afternoon Snack** | baby-cut carrots | apple | large hard pretzel coffee/tea | apple | non-caloric beverage | Graham crackers (2 squares; 2g) | banana | pear |
| **Dinner** | roast turkey breast (3oz.; 2g) *Mashed Potatoes w/ Nonfat Turkey Gravy Cranberry-orange relish (1/4 cup) steamed broccoli w/ Butter Buds roll-plain (1g) skim milk | *Pasta w/ Red Clam Sauce (8g) steamed carrots or peas w/ Butter Buds French bread-plain (1 slice) *Spinach Salad w/ nonfat dressing skim milk | *Stir-Fry Chicken and vegetables (substitute turkey) (5g) whole grain bread–plain (1 slice; 1g) *Baked Tomatoes skim milk | fast food restaurant dinner grilled chicken breast sand-wich[2] (no mayo; 6g) carrot (1 large) tossed salad w/ low-fat dressing (2g) 1% milk | *Round Steak Chile (6g) *Bran Muffin–low-fat (2g) steamed mixed vegetables w/ Butter Buds tossed salad w/ low-fat dressing (2g) skim milk | *Stuffed Baked Potato (3g) *Tropical Fruit Slaw (make enough for next day; 1g) multi-grain bread (1 slice; 1g) skim milk | *Marinated Salmon (6oz.; 9g) *Mashed Potatoes w/ Chives (2g) steamed carrots w/ Butter Buds tossed salad w/ nonfat dressing *Chocolate Chip Bundt Cake (2.5g) | *Shrimp Jambalaya (4g) whole grain bread—plain (1 slice; 1g) tossed salad w/ non-fat dressing *Chocolate Chip Bundt Cake (2.5g) skim milk |
| **Evening Snack** | large hard pretzel non-caloric beverage | peach | pretzels (1oz.; 1g) non-caloric beverage | popcorn (air-popped) | baby-cut carrots non-caloric beverage | pretzels w/ salsa (1oz.; 1g) non-caloric beverage | skim milk non-caloric beverage | non-caloric beverage |
| **Fat Grams Daily Totals** | 12–15 grams | 15–18 grams | 15–17 grams | 16–19 grams | 19–20 grams | 11–14 grams | 21–24 grams | 16–18 grams |

1. Meal plans contain 1,250 to 1,450 calories per day.
2. Sandwich condiments and spreads should be nonfat or low-fat and limited to 11/2 teaspoons; meat fillings should be limited to 1 to 2 oz.
*Recipes appear in book.

## 15-Day Meal Plan[1]

| | Day 9 | Day 10 | Day 11 | Day 12 | Day 13 | Day 14 | Day 15 |
|---|---|---|---|---|---|---|---|
| **Breakfast** | orange juice oatbran cereal w/ raisins and skim milk (3g) coffee/tea | orange juice cereal combination All-Bran and Raisin Bran w/ skim milk (2g) coffee/tea | fresh strawberries (1 cup) oatbran cereal w/ sugar, cinnamon and skim milk coffee/tea | grapefruit half *Oat Bran-Apple Muffin (3g) coffee/tea | cantaloupe wedge whole wheat toast w/ jelly (2 slices; 2g) skim milk | Corn Flakes Cereal w/ 1/2 banana (sliced), skim milk (1g) coffee/tea | orange juice scrambled egg substitute (1 egg; 1g) whole wheat bread w/ non-fat creamcheese (1 slice; 1g) coffee/tea |
| **Morning Snack** | apple | fresh strawberries (1 cup) | pear | grapefruit half | popcorn (air-popped) | banana (1/2) | low-fat crackers—Melba Rounds or Wasa Crispbread (1oz.; 1–2g) |
| **Lunch** | *Curry Chicken Salad (6g) whole grain bread—plain (1 slice; 1g) skim milk | ham sandwich on Kaiser roll[2] (3–6g) vegetables—steamed or raw skim milk | fast-food restaurant: regular hamburger (9g) side salad w/ low-fat dressing (2g) soft drink | *Minestrone Soup (2 cups; 1g) whole wheat bread—plain (1 slice; 1g) skim milk | *Lentil Soup (11/2 cups; 1g) whole wheat bread—plain (1 slice; 1g) angelfood cake (1/12 cake) skim milk | *Tuna Stuffed Tomatoes (2g) whole wheat bread w/ non-fat cream cheese (1 slice; 1g) skim milk | *Black Bean Salad (4g) whole wheat bread—plain (1 slice; 1g) fresh strawberries (1 cup) non-caloric beverage |
| **Afternoon Snack** | non-caloric beverage | baby-cut carrots | carrots or celery | applesauce—unsweetened (1/2 cup) | tangerine | apple | baby-cut carrots |
| **Dinner** | *Beanburger (1) (7g) *Slim Waldorf Salad (1g) *Baked Tomatoes fresh strawberries skim milk | *Apple-Date Stuffed Tenderloin (4oz.; 6g) *Rice-Mushroom Casserole (2g) green beans—steamed w/ Butter Buds cantaloupe wedge skim milk | *Scalloped Florentine over Brown Rice (5g) French bread—plain (1 slice) tossed salad w/ low-fat dressing (2g) sliced tomatoes *Baked Rice Pudding (3/4 cup; 1g) skim milk | *Lentil Burrito (1; 5g) French bread—plain (1 slice) *Steamed Carrots w/ Onions (2g) tossed salad w/ low-fat dressing (2g) angel food cake w/ fresh strawberries skim milk | *Chicken and Dumplings (1 serving; 10g) fresh fruit salad (1 cup) whole wheat bread (1 slice; 1g) skim milk | *Light Fried Fish Fillets (4–5oz.; 7g) *Sweet Potato Casserole (3g) steamed broccoli w/ Butter Buds tossed salad w/ low-fat dressing (2g) skim milk | *Pork Medallions w/ Mushroom Sauce (6g) *Rice-Mushroom Casserole (1 cup; 2g) mixed vegetables—steamed w/ Butter Buds tossed salad w/ low-fat dressing (2g) skim milk |
| **Evening Snack** | non-caloric beverage | fresh strawberries (1 cup) | peach | baby-cut carrots | non-caloric beverage | baby-cut carrots | low-fat frozen yogurt (1/2 cup; 2g) |
| **Fat Grams Daily Totals** | 18–19 grams | 14–17 grams | 22–23 grams | 14–15 grams | 15–16 grams | 16–17 grams | 20–21 grams |

1. Meal plans contain 1,250 to 1,450 calories per day.
2. Sandwich condiments and spreads should be nonfat or low-fat and limited to 11/2 teaspoons; meat fillings should be limited to 1 to 2 oz.
*Recipes appear in book.

your imagination — there are many more delicious recipes in this book.

Men can use the same meal plans and simply increase quantities of food, adjusting the fat grams based on serving size. The recipes from this book are marked with an asterisk (*). You probably will be surprised at the variety and quantity of food you can eat while dramatically limiting your fat intake. The menus consist of 1,250 to 1,450 calories per day. The approximate fat grams are listed beside each food, and totals are given for each day.

When using these meal plans, there are some specific guidelines you need to follow to keep the calories under 1,450 and fat grams in the range specified. Portion sizes are given for some foods, especially those with a significant amount of calories or fat. When preparing recipes from this book, consider the serving size to be the same as that specified in the recipes.

Condiments used on sandwiches or other foods should be low-fat or nonfat. If using low-fat mayonnaise on a sandwich, limit the amount to a light scraping or 1 1/2 teaspoons. Meat filling in sandwiches should be limited to 1 to 2 ounces. (The average deli sandwich contains 5 ounces of meat filling.) One thin slice of low-fat cheese may be substituted for light mayonnaise or 1 ounce of meat. Add raw or sautéed vegetables as desired. A range of 3 to 6 grams of fat is given for sandwiches to allow for these variations.

The fat grams listed for breads or bagels do not include added fat in the form of butter, margarine, etc. If you use these on your bread, be sure to add on the appropriate number of fat grams. It would be preferable, though, to eat breads or bagels plain or with a nonfat topping.

When cooking foods in a skillet, use non-stick pans, and if necessary, only a light coating of vegetable cooking spray to keep foods from sticking. This would apply when preparing scrambled eggs, or sautéing vegetables or stir-fry dishes.

On days that you do not have time to prepare a meal, you can substitute a frozen dinner or a hearty canned soup for the meal on the menu. Choose one with less than 20% of calories from fat, that is, one that has no more than 2 grams of fat for each 100 calories. For example, if the frozen dinner or soup contains 300 calories, it should have no more than 6 grams of fat; for 400 calories, no more than 8 grams of fat. Supplement the meal with skim milk, plain bread, fruits and/or vegetables, if desired.

## THE EXERCISE FACTOR

Exercise is a critical component in weight loss and weight maintenance. A regular exercise program gives you a feeling of control which affects the way you eat, making you less likely to binge. Exercise also increases muscle mass, which raises your metabolic rate. This means that you will burn more calories while at rest, because muscle requires more calories to sustain itself than body fat.

The best exercise program for weight loss and weight maintenance combines aerobic and strength-training exercise. In strength training, you work all the large muscle groups to become stronger through repeated motions such as weight lifting. The ideal program includes five days per week of aerobic exercise 20 to 60 minutes per day, depending on the intensity of the exercise; and two to three sessions per week of strength training. A complete strength-training session takes from 30 to 40 minutes. However, whatever amount you can work into your schedule will be beneficial. (See pages 91–98 for additional information on aerobic and strength training exercises.)

## PITFALLS TO ACHIEVING SUCCESS

People overeat for many different reasons—loneliness, depression, stress or habit. In some cases, it is very difficult to overcome these obstacles without getting to the root of the problem, which may require counseling.

Another factor which makes weight loss challenging is a slow basal metabolic rate. Some people must work harder at weight loss because of this. Increasing the amount and intensity of exercise, both aerobic and strength training, is the best method to increase the metabolic rate while burning calories. Remember, the greater muscle mass you create through exercise, the more calories you will burn while at rest. In addition, you may need to be more watchful of food portions or fat grams consumed each day.

Another major pitfall to successful weight loss is having high-fat foods around the house. Sometimes people feel that because their children like potato chips and other high-fat foods, they need to stock their cupboards with them. You'll be doing yourself and your children a favor by not having these foods around. There are much healthier alternatives for children's snacks than chips, foods that do not tend to put on unwanted extra pounds.

Watching fat grams when eating away from home can be a real challenge, especially if eating out constitutes a large proportion of your meals. In trying to please the palate, chefs generally use more fat in foods than necessary. For example, the marinara sauce you make at home may contain 3 grams of fat per serving, while the same type of sauce at your favorite Italian restaurant may have 19 grams of fat.

Do not become discouraged. There are a number of lower-fat food choices that will enable you to stay roughly within the fat-gram allowance when eating out. The best selections will be discussed in the next chapter. Another alternative, if you do not have a luncheon or dinner meeting to attend, is to bring a bag lunch from home.

# ELEVEN

## Helpful Hints for Special Situations

### EATING IN RESTAURANTS

If you are a typical American, you eat out at least one meal in three, and by the year 2,000, half of your food expenditures will go to the restaurant industry. For those who dine out frequently, it is imperative to make healthy food choices when you do. Otherwise, the tendency is to eat too much fat, cholesterol and sodium, and not enough calcium, fiber, fruits and vegetables. Gone are the days when you could justify abandoning your diet for the special occasions when you would eat out. For most people, eating out is no longer reserved just for special occasions.

Contrary to popular thinking, you can combine good taste with healthy food choices when eating out. Today there is a greater selection of low-fat menu items than ever before because of the increased demand for it by American consumers. In some cases, lower-fat choices are marked with the American Heart Association symbol to designate that they are "heart healthy." This makes the selection process easier, but you must be careful not to add excess fat in the form of salad dressings, butter, sour cream or bacon bits. This could bring the meal well over the guidelines of the American Heart Association.

If you are unsure about how the food is prepared, do not be afraid to ask. You can also request that it be prepared a certain way, or that the sauce be on the side. Most restaurants are happy to oblige you if it is possible, since they want to have happy customers who will return. Also, inquire if substitutions are permissible, such as a vegetable or fruit, instead of hash browns or French fries. (Refer to the chart of Menu Terminology, Figure 11.1, to become familiar with the composition of sauces, various methods of food preparation, etc.)

If you are at a buffet where most of the fare is laden with mayonnaise and high-fat sauces, don't be discouraged. Take small portions of these foods, or omit them entirely, and fill up on breads and fruits, which are almost always

**Menu Terminology**

**Au gratin** — a thick, creamy cheese sauce usually mixed with sliced potatoes or other vegetables and baked in an oven until a light brown crust is formed.

**Bearnaise Sauce** — a creamy sauce for beef or fish made with egg yolks, butter, vinegar, white wine and spices.

**Bechamel Sauce** — a white sauce made of cream, butter, flour, etc.

**Blackened** — a method of cooking meat, fish or poultry which was popularized as a form of Cajun (highly spiced) cooking. The food to be blackened is usually first dipped in oil, then covered by hot Cajun spices, and pan-fried at a very high temperature, thus "blackening" the fish or meat on the outside, while preserving the interior juices.

**Bordelaise Sauce** — a brown sauce flavored with red wine and shallots.

**Bouillabaisse** — a chowder made with several kinds of fish and shellfish, vegetables, seasonings, etc.

**Braised** — meat or poultry cooked slowly in a covered utensil in a small amount of liquid or in steam.

**Creamed** — as in creamed potatoes or creamed peas. Generally, a sauce made with flour, butter and cream or whole milk, that accompanies a vegetable.

**Fricasseed** — a method of cooking meat whereby it is cut into small pieces, stewed or fried, and served in a sauce of its own gravy.

**Hollandaise Sauce —** a creamy sauce, usually for fish or vegetables, made of butter, egg yolks, lemon juice, etc.

**Poached** — to cook in a boiling or simmering liquid. Fish or eggs are the foods most often cooked this way.

**Ratatouille** — a French appetizer or side dish containing eggplant, tomatoes, onions, green pepper and seasonings. It may be served hot or cold.

**Sautéed** — fried quickly, usually in a small amount of fat, although in some cases, greater amounts of fat are used.

**Scalloped** — to bake in a casserole with a milk or cream sauce and usually with bread crumbs.

Figure 11.1 Definitions of terms that commonly appear on restaurant menus.

available. When traveling by air, you can contact the airlines at least 24 hours in advance to order a low-fat, low-cholesterol or vegetarian meal.

## Best Choices When Eating Out

The following suggestions should make it easier to choose healthy meals when eating out. The suggestions are far from complete, but should serve as a helpful guide.

### Breakfast

- Egg whites or egg substitutes (no yolks), scrambled or in omelet form without cheese
- Bread, toast, English muffins, bagels preferably with nonfat cream cheese, jellies or jams; or a thin scraping of light cream cheese or margarine
- Waffles or pancakes with syrup (preferably no butter, and little or no margarine)
- Cereal, cooked or cold, with 1% or skim milk
- Fruits and fruit juices
- Low-fat cottage cheese

## LUNCH

- Soups — broth-based or bean, including lentil, minestrone, split pea (avoid creamed soups)

- Sandwiches — plain turkey, chicken or tuna (without heavy mayonnaise); with mustard or thin scraping of mayonnaise. Add vegetables as desired.

- Salads — Choose from an assortment of greens and add plain or marinated vegetables when at a salad bar. Top with vinegar, lemon juice or a low-calorie salad dressing. Avoid or limit salads mixed with mayonnaise, including chicken salad, potato salad and macaroni salad. If salad comes with meal, ask for salad dressing on the side. (Limit or avoid bacon, egg and cheese.)

- Small hamburger (no mayonnaise, cheese or special sauce)

- Fresh fruit salad

- Baked potato, topped with low-fat cottage cheese, plain yogurt, baked beans or nonfat sour cream.

- Vegetarian chili, chicken fajita, bean burrito (Limit cheese and sour cream.)

## DINNER—APPETIZERS

- Shrimp or crab meat with seafood cocktail sauce

- Steamed shellfish including clams and mussels, served plain, with seafood cocktail sauce, or in broth (no butter or cheese sauces)

- Vegetables, fresh or marinated (Preferably in vinegar with no oil — if oil is used, let most of the oil drip off.)

- Fresh fruit

## DINNER—ENTREES

- Fish, shellfish, chicken, or turkey prepared with *little or no fat* — baked, grilled, blackened*, poached, steamed, roasted or stir-fried.

- Lean beef, pork tenderloin or lean ham. (Ideally, portions should be limited to 4 ounces.) Best beef choices include stir-fry dishes, shish kabobs, round steak and filet mignon, prepared with little or no added fat

- Create your own vegetarian entree by combining several side dishes of grains and vegetables

- If you order a large portion of meat (7 ounces or more), split it with a companion, or take half of it home to eat later. Order an extra side dish of fruit, vegetables, rice, etc., prepared with little or no fat

- Entrees made with wine or tomato sauces are better than those made with cream sauces

## DINNER—SIDE DISHES

- Fresh garden salads with low-fat dressings on the side. (Limit mayonnaise-based salads, including cole slaw, most pasta salads and potato salad.)

*Blackened foods should be ordered only occasionally, because this cooking method encourages the formation of HAs, a carcinogen formed when meats and fish are charred at very high temperatures.

• Baked potato topped with low-fat cottage cheese or plain low-fat yogurt and chives. (Limit butter or sour cream to a teaspoon.)

• Bring your own Butter Buds, or a similar powdered nonfat butter product, to use on a baked potato or steamed vegetables.

• Vegetables, with little or no fat. (Omit those with cheese or cream sauces.)

• Whole wheat and rye breads are preferable, but all plain breads are fine.

(Avoid croissants and pre-buttered rolls or garlic bread.)

### DINNER—DESSERTS

• Fresh fruit

• Sherbet, fruit ices, gelatin, sorbet, meringue shells with fruit, or angel food cake.

• The fillings in fruit pies are generally low in fat, but pie crusts are very high in fat. Cut down on fat by not eating the pie crust.

## ETHNIC RESTAURANTS

Since America is the great "melting pot," we are blessed with a wide variety of ethnic restaurants. Many of the foods available to us are as authentic as that of the home country. These restaurants provide us with an endless choice of foods, many with names we cannot even pronounce. The following provides a sampling of some of the best and worst food choices (from a health standpoint) available at these restaurants.

These suggestions, of course, make up only a small portion of all the foods that are available. When dining out, if in doubt, be sure and ask how the food is prepared, the ingredients in a particular sauce, and/or approximately how much fat (butter, margarine or cooking oil) is used in the preparation. *Bon appetit!*

## CHINESE AND INDOCHINESE

Authentic Chinese foods are characterized by large amounts of vegetables and grains, primarily rice, and limited portions of animal protein—a good start toward healthful eating. Chinese foods offered in most American restaurants, though, have far more fat and meat than do traditional dishes.

The worst offenders are those that combine meat with peanuts or cashews; and the deep-fried foods, including bat-

ter-dipped meats or seafood, egg rolls and fried won tons. These should be avoided when trying to limit fat, as well as the crispy chow mein noodles and fried rice.

The best dishes are those with lots of vegetables and smaller amounts of meat or seafood. They can be prepared by boiling or steaming, or sautéed or stir-fried in *small* amounts of oil. White sauces generally have less fat than brown sauces. To minimize fat, cholesterol and sodium, ask for extra rice, and eat proportionally more white rice and vegetables and less sauce.

If you wish to limit sodium, ask for dishes prepared without monosodium glutamate (MSG) or soy sauce. Plain steamed vegetables are available at some restaurants. You may want to add a sweet-sour sauce or a very small amount of soy sauce at the table for flavor. For an alternative flavor, you could request that your dish be prepared using fresh minced ginger and garlic. Soups are best avoided when limiting sodium.

Thai and Vietnamese cooking are generally low in fat, while full of interesting flavors.

## ITALIAN

Pasta is the cornerstone of many Italian dishes. High in complex carbohydrates, it comes in all shapes and sizes and can be used with a variety of sauces. The type of sauce used will determine whether the pasta dish is high or low in fat. Those low in fat include pasta with red clam sauce; pasta with a marinara sauce (tomato-based), plain or with shrimp, unbreaded chicken pieces, or vegetables. Pasta with white clam sauce is another good choice, but be sure to request that the chef go light with the olive oil.

Chicken Marsala is cooked in a wine-based sauce, and is generally lower in fat. If the sauce appears oily, leave most of the sauce on the plate. Other lower-fat options include simply prepared, unbreaded chicken, shellfish and fish dishes, and thick-crusted pizzas with a limited amount of cheese, covered with a variety of vegetables, Canadian bacon or shrimp.

Some of the highest-fat Italian foods to avoid are pizzas with pepperoni or sausage, lasagna and breaded veal and chicken dishes topped with cheese. High-fat sauces are those that contain large amounts of ground beef or sausage, lots of cheese, or butter and cream. The combination butter, cream and cheese sauces over pasta, such as Fettucine Alfredo, are the highest in fat, with much of it saturated fat.

## FRENCH

French restaurants can pose a real challenge because of their rich, high-fat sauces. Still, there are entrees that can be enjoyed without a guilty conscience, including those with a wine sauce, such as coq au vin (chicken with wine), or bouillabaisse, a fish chowder. Other good choices are steamed mussels; fish en papillote (fish baked in paper to preserve natural juices and seasonings); and ratatouille, a mixture of eggplant, tomatoes and other vegetables. The French also have many simple vegetable dishes and some fat-free desserts—sorbets and pears in wine.

Foods to avoid are French onion soup, because of its high sodium and high fat (from the cheese), quiche Lorraine, duck a l'orange, and those that contain hollandaise, béarnaise, or béchamel sauces.

## GREEK

Some good choices at Greek restaurants are plaki (fish cooked with tomatoes, onions and garlic), meat and vegetable shish kabobs, tabouli (parsley-wheat salad), rice pilaf and couscous (steamed, finely cracked wheat). To reduce the fat and sodium in Greek salads, omit or limit the olives and feta cheese, and request that the dressing be served on the side.

Most foods made with lamb or phyllo dough are high in fat, so it is best to avoid them, as well as all deep-fried foods. Eggplant is low in fat but when made into babaganoosh, an appetizer, it too is very high in fat.

## JAPANESE

A variety of Japanese dishes are prepared with a minimal amount of fat. To begin with, one of the staples of Japanese cooking is steamed rice. Low-fat accompaniments for the rice include steamed fish, sushi (raw fish), and yakimono (broiled) fish and chicken. Other good choices are chicken or fish teriyaki, and tofu (soybean curd) dishes.

Request that foods be broiled without fat.

Dishes that should be bypassed are tempura and other deep-fried foods, such as tonkatsu (deep-fried pork), katsudon (deep-fried pork, onion and poached egg), and torikatsu (deep-fried chicken). To limit sodium, ask that salt, MSG and/or soy sauce be omitted or used sparingly.

## MEXICAN AND SOUTHWESTERN

These highly spiced meals are often a good source of fiber because whole grains and beans are important components of Mexican dishes. Choose corn over flour tortillas (made with lard), and make sure that they are baked, not fried. Poultry or shellfish and vegetables, cooked with little or no extra fat (request that they prepare it this way), provide good fillers for the tortillas. Baked tortillas without high-fat meat or cheese fill-

ings would also be healthy choices.

Other wholesome meals include rice and beans, either plain or with onions, tomatoes and spices; bean, chicken or seafood burritos; and enchiladas.

Refried beans are usually cooked in a small amount of lard, so do not eat large quantities of them. Rice is preferable. Be mindful that sour cream, cheese and avocado, which often accompany Mexican dishes, are very high in fat.

## INDIAN AND THE FAR EAST

Because of their preference for yogurt-based sauces and dals (legume dishes), these restaurants usually have many healthy, highly spiced varieties to choose from. In addition to the dals, other good choices are biryanis and pilafs (rice-based dishes), vegetable curries and tandoori chicken or fish. Baked breads are good, but avoid fried breads.

Sometimes ghee (clarified butter) and large amounts of oil are used in the preparation of entrees. You can request that the restaurant prepare your entree without ghee and only a minimal amount of oil. Also, stay away from curries made with coconut milk, and lamb dishes, since they are both high in saturated fat.

## VEGETARIAN

Although vegetarian dishes do not have meat, this does not necessarily mean that they are low in fat. Some vegetarian entrees are prepared with a large quantity of oil, high-fat dairy products, eggs and/or nuts. Still, vegetarian restaurants usually feature a variety of whole-grain products, vegetables, and bean dishes—all very good. It would be best to request that they limit or omit butter, margarine, sour cream, cheese, cooking oil and/or eggs. Also request

that only a sprinkling of nuts and seeds be used.

These suggestions are not all-inclusive, but hopefully will be helpful to you the next time you eat in an ethnic or vegetarian restaurant. As you can see, there are still many interesting entrees to choose from when following a healthy low-fat diet. If, on rare occasion, you eat a high-fat meal, be sure to pay especially close attention to eating low-fat meals several days after to compensate.

## FAST-FOOD RESTAURANTS

Fast-food restaurants are here to stay. Children love them; they make eating out affordable for the whole family; and since they are quick and predictable, they are often the perfect answer to eating while traveling. Even though these restaurants have a notorious reputation for serving unhealthy foods, high in fat and sodium, that need not be the case if you choose foods carefully. Eating a

modest amount of fat is possible if you know what to order, what "special" sauces to eliminate, etc. Restricting sodium is more difficult to do.

In response to the consumer's desire for healthier, lower-fat foods, new choices have been added to fast-food menus. Some of the newcomers to the scene are grilled (not deep-fried) chicken breast sandwiches and a variety of salads. If you omit the mayonnaise, these chicken sandwiches generally contain from 6 to 8 grams of fat. With the mayonnaise, the total fat is roughly doubled. If you want to use a condiment, use catsup or mustard instead, which have no fat. Another choice offered by most fast food franchises is a small burger, most of which contain just 10 grams of fat.

Many fast-food restaurants have taken the guesswork out of their food composition. They now provide consumers with a printout of the nutrient contents of all their foods, including quantities of fat, cholesterol, sodium, etc. When this information is not provided, the best way to cut down on fat at fast-food establishments is to avoid the major fat culprits—deep-fried foods, cheese, mayonnaise and most special sauces. Figure 11.2 shows how much fat can be eliminated from a fast-food item just by removing a major fat contributor. (Also refer to Appendix, page 387, for more complete nutrient information on fast foods.)

### Adjusting the Fat Downward

| Kentucky Fried Chicken Original Recipe | | Hardees' Chicken Filet Sandwich | |
|---|---|---|---|
| Drum & Thigh | | | |
| As Prepared | 28g Fat | As Prepared | 14g Fat |
| – Skin | – 18g Fat | – Mayonnaise | – 7g Fat |
| Lower Fat Version | 10g Fat | Lower Fat Version | 7g Fat |
| **McDonald's Filet-o-Fish** | | **Wendy's Baked Potato with Cheese** | |
| As Prepared | 18g Fat | As Prepared | 24g Fat |
| – Tartar Sauce | – 9g Fat | – Cheese | – 23g Fat |
| Lower Fat Version | 9g Fat | Lower Fat Version | 1g Fat |

Figure 11.2 These examples show how you can drastically reduce the fat in fast foods by simply removing one of the high-fat components. Low-fat condiments, such as low-calorie salad dressings or catsup, can be used to add flavor in place of the cheese or high-fat sauces.

# PICNICS AND OUTDOOR GRILLING

Outdoor grilling has become a popular American pastime, suitable for a most elegant meal or a simple outdoor picnic. It makes cooking an adventure in which the whole family, and even guests, can participate. In addition, it opens up a whole new world of interesting flavors through the use of marinades, sauces, etc.

When cooking outdoors, be mindful of more than just creating outstanding entrees enhanced by a charcoal or mesquite flavor. Also consider which foods are best for grilling from a health standpoint, and the safest ways to grill foods. Grilled meats and fish will be discussed first, followed by side dishes that accompany an outdoor meal.

## MEATS AND FISH—GRILL WITH CARE

Care should be taken when grilling meat or fish to reduce the carcinogens that can form when fat is burned. These carcinogens, called PAHs (polycyclic aromatic hy-

---

**Safe Grilling Tips**

- Select the leanest cuts of meat.
- Trim all visible fat from meat before grilling. This will help prevent flare-ups from dripping fat.
- Choose fish or chicken over beef and pork, since they are generally lower in fat. (Lean beef and pork are still appropriate on occasion.)
- Avoid eating charred parts of meat.
- If you grill frequently (several times a week), consider precooking (microwaving or parboiling) the meat so it is not on the grill as long. Grill immediately after precooking.
- To keep fat from dripping onto the coals and producing smoke, place aluminum foil on top of grate and place food directly on the foil, turning up the sides slightly to contain the meat juices; or put a metal drip pan beneath the food to be grilled.
- Baste with barbecue sauce or marinate in low-fat salad dressings, or other marinades low in fat
- Serve food from the grill on a clean platter, not one that has raw, possibly contaminated, meat juices on it.
- Grill vegetables with little or no added fat.
- Mesquite produces more PAHs than hardwood because it is a softwood and burns at a higher temperature. Therefore, you may want to limit its use.
- Clean the grill after each use.

---

**Good Choices for Outdoor Grilling**

- Shish kabobs with vegetables. Use lean beef, chicken or fish and serve over a bed of long grain and wild rice.
- Marinated chicken breast, grilled. Serve on a bun with lettuce, tomato and condiments of choice.
- Grilled pork tenderloin. Baste with honey mustard. Serve with a rice casserole and fruit salad.
- Barbecued chicken. Remove skin before grilling, place chicken pieces on aluminum foil, and brush with barbecue sauce.
- Grilled seafood of any type.

---

drocarbons), are formed when fat drips onto a flame or heating element. The PAHs travel upward with the smoke and are deposited on the grilled meat. They are also present in charred foods. Grilled meats are the principle source of PAHs in the diet.

The best way to prevent PAHs from forming is to keep fat from dripping onto the heat source. Below is a list of safe grilling tips, which should reduce the number of PAHs. It is impossible to tell how great a threat they pose, but most experts feel that those who grill frequently, i.e. several times a week, should take care to follow the precautions. If you grill once a week, your risk is probably insignificant.

Care should also be taken when broiling or pan-frying meats to limit the formation of a different carcinogen, HAs (heterocyclic amines). They are formed by the burning of amino acids and other substances in meats. Their numbers can be reduced by cooking more slowly, rather than at very high temperatures.

## SIDE DISHES FOR PICNICS

Some of the customary side dishes and snack foods served at picnics are fairly high in fat—potato chips have 8 grams of fat for 10 medium-size chips; potato salad has from 7 to 13 grams of fat per one-cup serving. Many fruit or vegetable salads with mayonnaise, heavy cream, or sour cream have 10 to 20 grams of fat per serving. If your goal is to keep fat intake to within 35 to 45 grams per day, you need to limit most of these higher fat side dishes, especially if your picnic meal includes a meat dish.

Another concern about side dishes at picnics is that they not be allowed to stand at room temperature or outdoors for too long before being eaten. In hot

---

**Suggested Side Dishes to Accompany Grilled Foods**

- Baked potato with nonfat sour cream or yogurt, chives and/or 1 teaspoon tub margarine (optional)
- Corn on the cob served with Butter Buds (powdered nonfat butter flavor) or margarine (less than 1 teaspoon).
- Rice-Mushroom Casserole*
- New Potato Salad*
- Tropical Fruit Slaw*
- Fresh fruit salad
- Congealed salads with fruits or vegetables (without sour cream or cream cheese)
- Vegetarian baked beans
- Creamy Cucumber Salad*
- Marinated Vegetable Salad*
- Taboule*
- Slim Waldorf Salad*

*Recipes appear in recipe section.

Figure 11.3 Low-fat side dishes to accompany a picnic meal.

weather (85 degrees F and above), food should not sit out over an hour; at room temperature, perishable foods should not be left out over 2 hours. To prevent bacteria from multiplying and causing illness, hot foods should stay at 150 degrees F or higher and cold foods at 45 degrees F or lower. (Refrigerator temperature should be 40 degrees F or lower.) Leftovers should be refrigerated promptly. The foods at greatest risk for bacterial multiplication are meats, gravies, cream sauces, eggs, dairy products, mayonnaise and custards.

When planning your next picnic, you may want to choose your side dishes from the list provided in Figure 11.3. Those marked with an * appear in the recipe section of this book. All have less than 4 grams of fat per serving.

## NUTRITIOUS SNACKS

Snacking accounts for 15 to 20% of American adults' daily calorie intake, so you need to choose your snacks wisely. Creating healthy snacks that are tasty and easy to prepare can be lots of fun. If you have young children, they will love helping you. Just use your imagination in trying different combinations of foods. One example is a banana yogurt shake. Use a food processor to blend a banana with low-fat frozen yogurt, adding both nutrients and flavor to the yogurt. The banana actually makes the shake taste thick and "creamy."

Another choice popular with children is a fresh or canned pear half, filled with a dab of peanut butter. If using canned pears, it is best to buy the pears in light syrup, to avoid too many empty calories from sugar. Lightly sweetened cold cereals, plain or with fruit, also make excellent snacks. Figure 11.4 provides a list of healthy snacks, which require little or no preparation time.

Figure 11.4 A sampling of healthy snacks which require minimal preparation time.

---

**Quick Healthy Snacks**

- Pretzels, preferably low-salt
- Graham crackers
- Frozen yogurt, nonfat or low-fat
- Fresh fruit
- Dried fruit—raisins, prunes, or apricots
- Canned fruit in light syrup, with or without low-fat cottage cheese
- Jello with fruit
- Prepackaged instant hot cereals
- Ice milk, plain or topped with fruit
- Cold cereals served with skim milk (with whole milk for children under two years old.)
- Bagel, plain or raisin, topped with light scraping of margarine, peanut butter, or jelly

---

# FOOD STORAGE AND SAFETY

Each year, approximately 7 million Americans suffer from food borne illnesses, also called food poisoning. Some are not aware of the cause of their affliction, thinking they have the flu or some other ailment. An estimated 85% of these food poisonings are avoidable, if people would just handle foods properly. The following includes some helpful hints from the U.S. Department of Agriculture to reduce the risk of food poisoning.

## BUYING AND STORING FOODS

1. If food is stamped with a "use-by" date, eat it before that date.

2. When you buy refrigerated foods, make sure they are cold to the touch; frozen foods should be rock solid; and canned goods should be free of dents, cracks or bulging lids.

3. The refrigerator should run at 40 degrees F or less, the freezer at 0 degrees F. Generally you should keep your refrigerator as cold as possible without freezing your milk or lettuce.

4. Freeze fresh meat or poultry immediately if you can't use it within a few days. Ground meat and fish should be used in one or two days.

5. Put packages of raw meat, poultry or fish on a plate in the refrigerator so their juices will not drip on other food. Also, when preparing meats or fish, keep raw juices from coming into contact with ready-to-eat foods, since these juices often contain bacteria.

## PREPARING FOODS

1. When cutting raw meats or fish, use either plastic or wooden cutting boards. Thoroughly wash the cutting board in hot soapy water, or preferably in a dishwasher, before using again. In addition, use hot soapy water to wash hands, utensils and work areas that have come into contact with the raw meat or fish.

2. Do not thaw food on the kitchen counter, but rather in the refrigerator or in the microwave.

3. Marinate foods in the refrigerator, rather than the kitchen counter. (You can safely marinate foods on the kitchen counter if the marinating time is 30 minutes or less.) Reserve a portion of the marinade for a dip or basting sauce that hasn't had raw meat in it. Do not

re-use the marinade used on raw meat unless it's been boiled.

4. In order to kill potentially harmful bacteria, cook ground beef, veal and lamb to 160 degrees and ground poultry to 165 degrees F. When cooked to these temperatures, these meats appear gray in color, with no trace of red or pink. Beef, veal and lamb roasts are safe to eat if cooked to 145 degrees or medium-rare, pork roasts to 160 degrees, and poultry to 180 degrees F. (A turkey breast is safely cooked at 170 degrees F.) Use a meat thermometer, inserted into the center of the roast, to make sure the meats are cooked adequately to meet food safety guidelines. Poultry juices should run clear and the flesh should not be pink. Fish should be cooked until it flakes with a fork.

5. Use a clean plate for serving cooked foods. Be especially careful *not* to re-use a plate that had raw meat on it.

6. Cook eggs until the yolk and white are firm, not runny. Scramble eggs to a firm texture. Don't use recipes in which eggs remain raw or only partially cooked. Salmonella, a bacteria that causes food poisoning, can grow inside fresh, unbroken eggs. (Commercial egg substitutes do not carry a risk of salmonella, because they are pasteurized.)

7. When microwaving food, use only microwave-safe containers. Cover foods with a lid or plastic wrap, vented, and do not allow plastic wrap to touch the food. Observe the standing time called for in the recipe, because during this time the food finishes cooking. Insert a temperature probe or meat thermometer in several spots to check that food is done.

8. Rinse all fruits and vegetables prior to eating, even those with an outside shell you do not eat, such as a melon. This will help prevent salmonella and other bacteria from being transferred, when sliced with a knife, from the outside surface to the inside part you eat.

## SERVING FOODS AND HANDLING LEFTOVERS

1. When you serve food, never leave it out over 2 hours. In hot weather (85 degrees F and above), food should never sit out over 1 hour. If these time limits are exceeded, throw the food out. Even reheating it to high temperatures (165 degrees F) will not destroy the disease-causing toxins that may have formed.

2. With poultry or other stuffed meats, remove stuffing and refrigerate it in separate containers.

3. If reheating leftovers, bring sauces, soups and gravy to a boil, and heat other leftovers thoroughly to 165 degrees F.

4. Discard moldy foods, because poisons in molds are often present under the surface of the foods. Exception: Hard cheeses and firm fruits and vegetables with visible mold can be safely used provided a large area around the mold is removed.

5. Never taste food that looks or smells strange to see if you can use it. Just throw it out.

6. Refer to the Cold Storage chart to see how long food can be stored in the refrigerator or freezer at optimum quality.

## Cold Storage

These SHORT but safe time limits will help keep refrigerated food from spoiling or becoming dangerous to eat. These time limits will keep frozen food at top quality.

| Product | Refrigerator (40°F) | Freezer (0°F) |
|---|---|---|
| **Eggs** | | |
| Fresh, in shell | 3 weeks | Don't freeze |
| Raw yolks, whites | 2–4 days | 1 year |
| Hard cooked | 1 week | Don't freeze well |
| Liquid pasteurized eggs or | | |
|     egg substitutes, opened | 3 days | Don't freeze |
|     unopened | 7 days | 1 year |
| | | |
| **Mayonnaise, commercial** | | |
| Refrigerate after opening | 2 months | Don't freeze |
| | | |
| **TV Dinners, Frozen Casseroles** | | |
| Keep frozen until ready to serve | | 3–4 months |
| | | |
| **Deli Products** | | |
| Store-prepared (or homemade) egg, | | |
|     chicken, tuna, ham, macaroni salads | 3–5 days | Don't freeze well |
| Pre-stuffed pork & lamb chops, | | |
|     chicken breasts stuffed with dressing | 1 day | |
| Store-cooked convenience meals | 1–2 days | |
| | | |
| **Soups & Stews** | | |
| Vegetable or meat-added | 3–4 days | 2–3 months |
| | | |
| **Hamburger, Ground & Stew Meats** | | |
| Hamburger & stew meats | 1–2 days | 3–4 months |
| Ground turkey, veal, pork, lamb | | |
|     & mixtures of them | 1–2 days | 3–4 months |

| Cold Storage (cont'd) | | |
| --- | --- | --- |
| **Product** | **Refrigerator (40°F)** | **Freezer (0°F)** |
| **Hot-Dogs & Lunch Meats** | | |
| Hot-dogs, opened package | 1 week | |
|     unopened package | 2 weeks | 1–2 months |
| Lunch meats, opened | 3–5 days | |
|     unopened | 2 weeks | |
| **Fresh Meat** | | |
| Steaks, beef | 3–5 days | 6–12 months |
| Chops, pork | 3–5 days | 4–6 months |
| Chops, lamb | 3–5 days | 6–9 months |
| Roasts, beef | 3–5 days | 6–12 months |
| Roasts, lamb | 3–5 days | 6–9 months |
| Roasts, pork & veal | 3–5 days | 4–6 months |
| Variety meats—tongue, brain, | | |
|     kidneys, liver, heart, chitterlings | 1–2 days | 3–4 months |
| **Meat Leftovers** | | |
| Cooked meat and meat dishes | 3–4 days | 2–3 months |
| Gravy and meat broth | 1–2 days | 2–3 months |
| **Fresh Poultry/Fish** | | |
| Chicken or turkey, whole | 1–2 days | 1 year |
| Chicken or turkey pieces | 1–2 days | 9 months |
| Giblets | 1–2 days | 3–4 months |
| Fish | 1–2 days | 6–12 months |
| **Cooked Poultry, Leftover** | | |
| Fried chicken | 3–4 days | 4 months |
| Cooked poultry dishes | 3–4 days | 4–6 months |
| Pieces, plain | 3–4 days | 4 months |
| Pieces covered with broth, gravy | 1–2 days | 6 months |
| Chicken nuggets, patties | 1–2 days | 1–3 months |

Source: U.S. Department of Agriculture, Food Safety and Inspection Service, Home and Garden Bulletin No. 248.

## COMMON FOOD MISCONCEPTIONS

**Myth:** Children should be discouraged from drinking chocolate-flavored milk because it is a poor source of calcium and contains unhealthy amounts of sugar.

**Fact:** Chocolate milk is actually a good source of calcium for children, especially if they wouldn't otherwise choose milk. Low-fat chocolate milk (1% fat) is a healthier alternative than whole milk. They both have approximately the same number of calories (about 150 for an 8-ounce cup), but whole milk has much more fat. It has 8 grams of fat compared with only 3 grams in 1%-fat chocolate milk. Generally, chocolate milk contains at least 90% of the calcium of white milk.

**Myth:** Snacking is an unhealthy habit.

**Fact:** To the contrary, snacking can be a very healthy practice as long as it is done in moderation with the right foods. Refer to Figure 11.4 for a list of healthy snack choices. Snacking in mid-afternoon may prevent binging at mealtime because of feeling starved.

**Myth:** Cured meats, like other meats, can be frozen in order to preserve them for use at a later time.

**Fact:** Do not freeze cured meats. It adversely affects the taste and texture of the meat, and the seasonings in the meat quicken its rancidity while frozen.

**Myth:** Even moderate amounts of caffeine are harmful to most people and should be avoided.

**Fact:** Moderate use of caffeine, i.e. the equivalent of two to four cups of coffee per day, is not harmful for most people. Studies from the 1970s showing that it increased the risk for heart disease, cancer, fertility problems, ulcers and fibrocystic breast changes have all been discredited. However, it is recommended that you limit consumption if it makes you jittery, or if you have certain health conditions. These include: irregular heartbeats or recent heart attack, peptic ulcer, heartburn, high blood pressure, insomnia, anxiety disorders, or if you are pregnant or nursing. A well-designed study published in 1993 found that drinking one to three cups of coffee a day increased the risk of miscarriage in pregnant women.

**Myth:** You should eat extra protein if you want to build up muscles through weight lifting.

**Fact:** Protein is needed to build muscle, but even serious weight lifters should not exceed the recommended upper limit of protein consumption, which is 15% of total calories. (See p. 88.) The body can use only so much protein, and the excess cannot be stored as muscle. Instead, it is converted to fat and carbohydrate and the by-products are eliminated in the urine. Too much protein can cause health problems including dehydration and kidney damage.

**Myth:** You cannot refreeze an item after it has thawed.

**Fact:** It is perfectly safe to refreeze foods that have been thawed in the refrigerator, but not foods thawed in the microwave or on the kitchen counter. Foods thawed on the kitchen counter may not be safe to eat, because parts of the food may have gotten warm enough for bacteria to begin to grow. Foods thawed in the microwave should be cooked immediately, before bacteria has a chance to develop. *Freezing does not kill bacteria.*

**Myth:** It is unsafe to eat meat, poultry and other foods after they have been in the freezer for more than six months.

**Fact:** As far as safety goes, foods can be kept indefinitely in the freezer provided the temperature is 0 degrees Fahrenheit or colder.

Shorter freezer times are recommended for certain foods to preserve their taste and texture.

**Myth:** Drinking red wine, not white wine, can reduce my risk for heart disease.

**Fact:** In almost all population studies, light drinkers have lower rates of heart disease than nondrinkers. It doesn't matter whether they drink red wine, white wine, beer or hard liquor. Alcohol may be associated with a lower risk of heart disease because of its ability to raise HDL (good) cholesterol, and because it appears to make blood less likely to form clots.

Heavy drinking is associated with higher incidence of cancer, cirrhosis of the liver, high blood pressure, automobile fatalities, and other forms of accidental death. Therefore do not start drinking if you are not presently drinking. If you are a moderate drinker, and would like to derive the maximum health benefits, men should limit themselves to no more than one to two drinks a day and women to no more than one drink a day. (See p. 56 to see what constitutes a "drink.") At that level, you may be able to reduce your risk of heart disease without increasing your risks for cancer and other diseases.

**Myth:** Organic foods are more nutritious than conventionally grown foods.

**Fact:** Organic foods are not more nutritious, that is, they do not contain more vitamins and minerals than conventionally grown foods. "Certified" organic produce, though, has met strict guidelines restricting the use of pesticides and chemical fertilizers. Without the "certified" label, foods sold as organic may contain pesticide residues at the same levels as conventional foods. By the mid-1990s, Congress is scheduled to implement the 1990 Farm Bill which will mandate a single national standard for organically grown produce, which means that all foods sold as "organic" would be certified. In the meantime, by buying "certified" organic you can be relatively sure of purchasing produce without pesticide residues, and in addition, you will be supporting a type of farming that protects the environment.

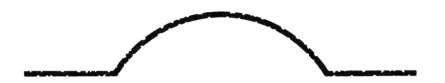

# PART TWO

## The Cookbook

# *Introduction to Recipes*

Important nutrition information is included with each recipe. They have been analyzed, per serving, for: calories, protein, total fat, saturated fat, cholesterol, fiber, sodium, and percentage of calories from fat. The serving sizes given are quite generous — larger than in most low-fat or diet cookbooks.

Optional ingredients are omitted from the nutrition analysis. When the serving size is listed as a range, such as "4 to 6 servings," the figure in the middle, in this case 5 servings, is used for the analysis. When an amount is not specified, such as salt and pepper to taste, the ingredients are not figured into the analysis. If a choice of ingredients is given, i.e., low-fat or nonfat, the first ingredient mentioned is used.

The recipe analysis used Food Processor II software program.* In cases where a recipe ingredient was missing from the program, Bowes and Church's *Food Values of Portions Commonly Used*, 15th Edition, or nutrition information from food labels was used instead.

In certain recipe categories, particularly salads and vegetables, the percentage of calories from fat is often higher than in other food categories. Do not be overly concerned when this is the case, *if* the grams of fat per serving is low. Because the calories from the vegetables themselves are so low, a small amount of added fat has a greater effect on the percentage of calories from fat.

A number of recipes call for "defatted" broth, either chicken or beef. This indicates that the visible fat should be skimmed off the top. The fat can be removed more easily if the broth is first cooled in the refrigerator, but this is not essential.

If you are carefully watching the amount of sodium in your diet, be sure to consider all the foods that will be eaten with the meal. For example, the sodium content of a casserole dish can be higher than for a side dish, since a casserole of meat, starches and vegetables is almost a complete meal in itself. On the other hand, with a side dish, you will probably eat three or four other foods with the meal, which will significantly increase the amount of sodium.

The Preparation Time and Cooking Time have been provided so you

* From ESHA Research, P.O. Box 13028, Salem, Oregon 97309

can tell at a glance approximately how much time is involved in preparing a particular dish. The Preparation Time is the time you spend actively preparing the dish. It includes sautéing time, if you need to be closely observing or frequently stirring a food while it is cooking.

Cooking Time is the time the food takes to cook while you are not actively working on the food, i.e. if the food is baking in the oven or simmering on the stove.

The approximate time it takes from beginning of preparation to when the food is ready for the table is the Preparation Time plus Cooking Time. Marinating time is also included when foods are marinated, and is usually given as a range.

The following is a summary of the recommended consumption levels of certain key nutrients:

**Protein** — the Recommended Dietary Allowance (RDA) for an average adult male over 14-years-old is 56 grams a day; for an average female (not pregnant) over 18, it is 44 grams a day. (To calculate your own RDA for protein (in grams), you multiply your ideal body weight in pounds by 0.37. See p. 88 in text.)

**Fat** — the American Heart Association recommends that fat consumption be limited to less than 30% of total calories. More recent studies have shown that reducing fat to 20 to 25% of total calories is both practical and more effective in reducing the incidence of obesity, cancer and heart disease.

**Cholesterol** — the American Heart Association recommends less than 300 mg per day in the Step-One Diet; and less than 200 mg per day in the Step-Two Diet. (Keep in mind, these are *not target* but *ceiling* recommendations. Lowering intake below the ceiling levels has been shown to be more beneficial in reducing cholesterol values in some individuals.)

**Fiber** — the recommended level is 20 to 30 grams per day.

**Sodium** — the recommended level is less than 2,400 milligrams per day.

# Menus for Entertaining

*Sunday Brunch Buffet*
*Ladies' Summer Luncheon*
*Bridge Club Luncheon*
*Candlelight Dinner*
*Hearty Seafood Supper*
*Traditional Turkey Dinner*
*Dinner at Eight*
*Friday Night Fish Dinner*
*Gourmet Club Dinner Party*
*New Orleans Dinner*
*Labor Day Picnic*
*Summer Picnic at Home*
*Elegant Dinner Party*

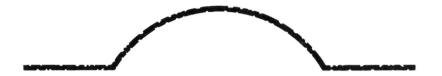

# Sunday Brunch Buffet

◆

### Beverages
*Hot Cranberry Punch, 187, Bloody Mary*

◆

### Buffet
*Crustless Spinach Quiche, 355*
*Baked Apple-Date Delight, 244*
*Mini-Ham Biscuits*
*Fresh Fruit Salad*
*Slim Waldorf Salad, 226*

◆

### Breads
*Lemon Tea Bread, 348*
*Date-Nut Bread, 347*
*Blueberry Muffins, 352*

◆

### Desserts
*Peaches in Wine, 376*
*Frosted Apple Cookies, 378*
*Coffee, Tea*

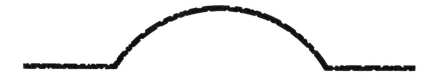

# Ladies' Summer Luncheon

◆

### Beverage
Fruit-Flavored Carbonated Punch

◆

### Entree
Curry Chicken Salad, 211
Spinach Salad with Honey Mustard Dressing, 221
Carrot Bran Muffins, 353

◆

### Dessert
Lemon Custard Delight, 366
Coffee, Tea

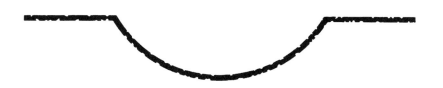

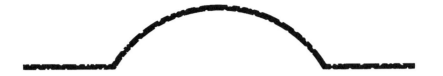

## Bridge Club Luncheon

◆

### Beverage
*Hot Mulled Cider, 187*

◆

### Entree
*Chicken-Seafood Artichoke Casserole, 256*
*Green Bean-Mushroom Salad, 244*
*Bran Muffins, 354*
*Cornbread Muffins*

◆

### Dessert
*Mock Cherry Cheesecake, 365*
*Coffee/Tea*

# Candlelight Dinner

◆

## Appetizers
Oysters Rockefeller, 177
Tabouli, 184, with Melba Rounds

◆

## Entree
Pork Medallions with Mushroom Sauce, 275
Wild Rice Baked Casserole, 332
Baked Apple-Date Delight, 244
Mandarin Salad, 219
Dinner Rolls

◆

## Dessert
Brownie Baked Alaska, 374
Coffee, Espresso

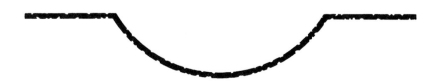

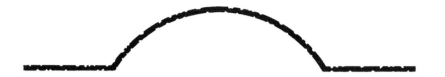

## *Hearty Seafood Supper*

### *Appetizers*
*Tuna Vegetable Dip, 183, with Crackers*
*Spinach Quiche Appetizer, 355*

### *Entree*
*Stuffed Flounder, 287*
*Saffron Rice, 333*
*Steamed Baby Carrots*
*Swiss-Style Garden Salad, 216*
*Dinner Rolls, Date-Nut Bread, 347*

### *Dessert*
*Ice Cream Cake Roll*
*with Blueberry Sauce, 370, 371*
*Coffee, Espresso*

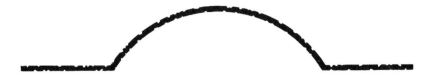

## Traditional Turkey Dinner

◆

### Appetizers
Tangy Shrimp, 174
Artichoke Relish with Pita Chips, 182

◆

### Entree
Baked Turkey Breast
Mashed Potatoes with Nonfat Turkey Gravy, 264
Sweet Potato Casserole, 236
Spinach-Artichoke Casserole, 243
Fresh Cranberry Molded Salad, 228
Dinner Rolls, Banana-Nut Bread, 349

◆

### Dessert
Steamed Date-Nut Pudding with Brandy Sauce, 364, 384
Coffee, Espresso

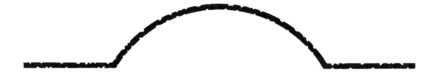

## Dinner At Eight

◆

### Appetizers
*Shrimp Cocktail*
*Hummous, 186, with Pumpernickel Rounds*

◆

### Soup
*Salmon Bisque, 202*

◆

### Entree
*Pork Marengo with "Eggless" Egg Noodles, 279*
*Baked Tomatoes with Spinach, 232*
*Mandarin Salad, 219*
*Dinner Rolls, Bran Mini-Muffins, 354*

◆

### Dessert
*Strawberry Russe, 373*
*Coffee, Espresso*

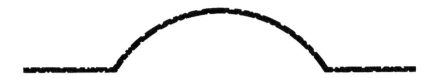

# Friday Night Fish Dinner

◆

### Appetizers
Spinach Quiche Appetizer, 175
Tuna Vegetable Dip, 183, with Melba Rounds

◆

### Entree
Marinated Salmon, 288
Mashed Potatoes with Chives, 234
Green Beans Amandine, 239
Spinach Salad with Honey Mustard Dressing, 221
Dinner Rolls, French Bread

◆

### Dessert
Chocolate Chip Bundt Cake, 359
Coffee, Espresso

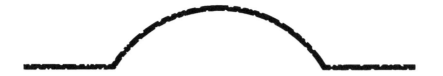

# Gourmet Club Dinner Party

◆

### Appetizers
Crab Canapes, 176
Marinated Vegetables

◆

### Entree
Orange Roughy with Mushroom Sauce, 284
Herbed Red Potatoes, 235
Sesame Broccoli, 240
Fresh Cranberry Molded Salad, 228
Dinner Rolls, Bran Mini-Muffins, 354

◆

### Dessert
Frozen Yogurt Charlotte, 369
Coffee, Tea

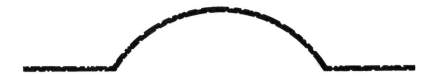

## *New Orleans Dinner*

◆

### *Appetizers*
*Escargots, 180*
*Tuna Canapes ,176*

◆

### *Soup*
*Seafood Gumbo, 192, with Garlic Toast*

◆

### *Entree*
*Shrimp Creole, 300*
*Scrumptious Asparagus, 237*
*Celestial Salad, 220*
*Dinner Rolls, Cornbread Mini-Muffins*

◆

### *Dessert*
*New Orleans Bread Pudding Topped with Hard Sauce, 362, 384*
*Coffee*

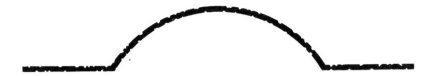

## Labor Day Picnic

◆

### Appetizers
*Fresh Fruit Platter with Yogurt Dip, 179*
*Crabmeat Vegetable Dip with Crackers*

◆

### Entree
*Grilled Breast of Chicken Sandwich, 260–61*
*New Potato Salad, 225*
*Marinated Vegetable Salad, 223*
*Carolyn's Baked Beans, 311*
*Banana-Nut Bread, 349*

◆

### Dessert
*Strawberry Shortcake, 368*
*Lemon-Glazed Spice Bars, 381*
*Coffee, Iced Tea*

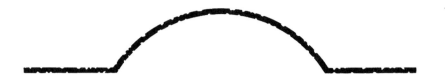

# Summer Picnic At Home

◆

### Appetizers
Stuffed Cherry Tomatoes, 181
Artichoke Relish, 182, with Party Rye

◆

### Entree
Barbecued Shredded Turkey Breast, 261
Served on Hard Rolls
"Sour Cream" Potato Salad, 226
Black Bean Salad, 217
Slim Waldorf Salad, 226
Tomatoes with Chopped Herbs, 233

◆

### Dessert
Carrot Cake with Cream Cheese Frosting, 363
Low-Fat Lemon Bars, 382
Coffee/Tea

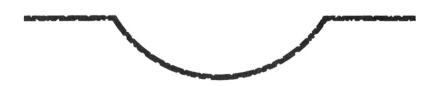

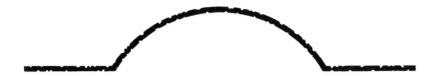

## *Elegant Dinner Party*

◆

### *Appetizers*
*Artichoke Canapés, 181*
*Marinated Mushrooms*

◆

### *Soup*
*Stracciatella, 204–5*

◆

### *Entree*
*Apple-Date Stuffed Tenderloin, 274*
*Rice-Mushroom Casserole, 334*
*Snow-Capped Broccoli, 240*
*Tossed Garden Salad with Lemon-Tahini Dressing, 228*
*Dinner Rolls, Carrot Bran Mini-Muffins, 353*

◆

### *Dessert*
*Guilt-Free Tiramisu, 383*
*Coffee, Espresso*

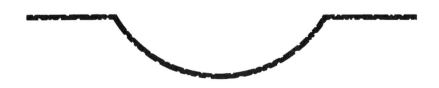

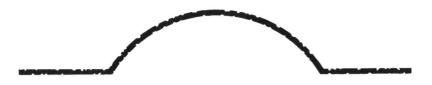

# Appetizers & Beverages

Marinated Chicken Kabobs • Marinated Shrimp with Snow Peas • Tangy Shrimp • Spinach Quiche Appetizer • Tuna (or Crab) Canapés • Oysters Rockefeller • Salmon Teriyaki Appetizer • Fresh Fruit Platter with Yogurt Dip • Escargots • Artichoke Canapés • Stuffed Cherry Tomatoes • Artichoke Relish • Tuna Vegetable Dip • Tabouli • Bean Dip • Hummous • Toasted Pita Chips • Hot Cranberry Punch • Hot Mulled Cider • Banana Yogurt Shake • Christmas Wassail • Light Holiday Eggnog • Hot Chocolate Mix

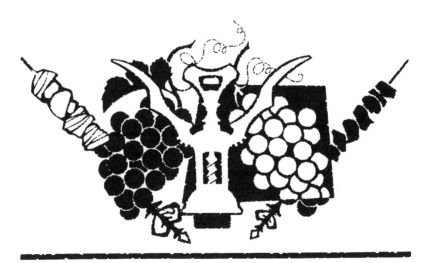

# *Marinated Chicken Kabobs*

4 boneless chicken breasts
1/4 cup reduced-sodium soy
    sauce
1/4 cup prepared barbecue
    sauce
2 tablespoons lemon juice
1/4 teaspoon ground ginger
1/4 teaspoon garlic powder
2 large green peppers, cut into
    1-inch pieces
2 large red peppers, cut into 1-
    inch pieces
18 6-inch wooden skewers
Vegetable cooking spray

### Yield: 12 to 16 kabobs

*For 1 kabob:*
Calories...... 68
Protein (g)... 11
Fat (g)....... 1.7
Sat. Fat (g).. 0.4
Choles. (mg).. 27
Fiber (g)..... 0.4
Sodium (mg)... NA
%Cal-Fat...... 22%

Cut chicken breasts into 1-inch pieces; place in a medium-size bowl or plastic container.

Combine next five ingredients in a small bowl. Stir briskly with a wire whisk. Pour over chicken. Cover and refrigerate at least 2 hours, stirring occasionally to marinate evenly. Do not marinate longer than 8 hours.

Meanwhile, cut red and green peppers into 1-inch pieces.

Remove chicken from marinade, reserving marinade. Place chicken and peppers on skewers in this order: red pepper, green pepper, two pieces of chicken, green pepper and red pepper.

Spray grill with cooking spray. Place kabobs on grill approximately 6 inches from medium-hot coals. Spoon 2 to 4 tablespoons marinade over top. Grill for 15 to 20 minutes or until done, turning as needed; or, kabobs may be broiled in an oven, 6 inches from broiler, for approximately same length of time.

*This appetizer is ideal for a cocktail party with heavy hors d'oeuvres. The red and green peppers make it very colorful.*

Preparation time: 30 minutes

Cooking time: 20 minutes

# Marinated Shrimp with Snow Peas

Blend together oil, vinegar, mustard, parsley, ginger, garlic, dill, salt, pepper and sugar. Mix well and pour over shrimp. Refrigerate at least four hours and up to two days, stirring occasionally.

Cut off tops of snow peas. If peas are fresh, parboil for 30 seconds and plunge immediately into cold water to retain their bright color. Drain. If peas are frozen, thaw and drain. Halve the peas lengthwise and wrap half around each shrimp. Secure with toothpicks and arrange on the lettuce. Garnish with parsley and lemon slices, twisted.

Preparation time: 1 hour

Marinating time: 4 hours–2 days

*1/4 cup olive oil*
*3 tablespoons wine vinegar*
*2 tablespoons Dijon mustard*
*1 tablespoon finely chopped parsley*
*1 teaspoon finely chopped ginger*
*1 clove garlic, minced*
*1 tablespoon chopped fresh dill*
*Pinch salt, pepper, sugar*
*2 pounds large fresh shrimp, cooked and cleaned*
*1/2 pound fresh snow peas, or 10 ounces frozen*
*Curly leaf lettuce or Romaine*
*Parsley and thin lemon slices for garnish*

**Yield: About 30–40 appetizers**

**For 2 appetizers:**
Calories...... 99
Protein (g)... 16
Fat (g)....... 2
Sat. Fat (g).. 0.7
Choles. (mg).. 88
Fiber (g)..... 1.2
Sodium (mg)... 157
%Cal-Fat...... 18%

# Tangy Shrimp

2 tablespoons olive oil
2 cloves garlic, minced
1 tablespoon Dijon mustard
6 tablespoons lemon juice
2 tablespoons red wine vinegar
1 tablespoon chopped fresh dill
Dash of cayenne pepper
1 medium red onion, thinly
   sliced
1 green pepper, cut into 1/4-
   inch strips
2 tablespoons chopped pimiento
1 tablespoon chopped parsley
1 1/2 to 2 pounds cooked
   medium shrimp (60 to 70
   shrimp)

**Yield: 60 to 70 shrimp,
enough for 8 to 12 people**

**For 6 shrimp:**
Calories...... 97
Protein (g)... 16
Fat (g)....... 2
Sat. Fat (g).. 0.6
Choles. (mg).. 147
Fiber (g)..... 0.6
Sodium (mg)... 187
%Cal-Fat...... 19%

In a medium-size bowl, combine oil, garlic, mustard, lemon juice, vinegar, dill and cayenne. Mix well. Add onion slices, green pepper, pimiento, parsley and shrimp, tossing until well coated. Refrigerate, covered, for 1 to 4 hours.

Place shrimp mixture in a serving bowl. Serve with toothpicks.

Preparation time: 25 minutes

Marinating time: 1–4 hours

# Spinach Quiche Appetizer

Preheat oven to 350 degrees.

Combine egg substitutes, milk, salt, pepper and nutmeg in large mixing bowl. Beat slightly. Set aside.

Heat olive oil in medium-size saucepan. Add onion and sauté until onion becomes translucent. Mix thawed and drained spinach with onion mixture. Add to egg mixture.

Toss grated cheese with flour.

Spray 10 x 15-inch jelly roll pan with vegetable cooking spray. Sprinkle cheese evenly over bottom of pan. Pour egg mixture over top.

Bake at 350 degrees for 35 to 40 minutes. Cool slightly and cut into 1 1/4-inch squares.

*The dark green color of this appetizer is especially attractive on a light-colored serving dish. Garnish with fresh sprigs of parsley, or with holly around the Christmas holidays.*

Preparation time: 25 minutes

Cooking time: 40 minutes

8 egg substitutes (2 cups)
1 12-ounce can evaporated skim milk
1/2 teaspoon salt
1/8 teaspoon cayenne pepper
1/2 teaspoon ground nutmeg
2 teaspoons olive oil
1/4 cup chopped onion
2 10-ounce packages frozen chopped spinach, thawed and drained (squeezed dry)
1 cup (4 ounces) shredded Swiss or Cheddar cheese
2 tablespoons flour

**Yield: 96 appetizers**

**For 4 appetizers:**
Calories...... 59
Protein (g)... 6
Fat (g)....... 2.5
Sat. Fat (g).. 1.1
Choles. (mg).. 5
Fiber (g)..... 0.7
Sodium (mg)... 129
%Cal-Fat...... 37%

# Tuna (or Crab) Canapés

1 6 1/2-ounce can tuna in
    spring water, drained and
    flaked
1/2 cup nonfat mayonnaise
1 tablespoon finely chopped
    pimiento
2 tablespoons finely chopped
    green onion,including tops
1/2 cup Parmesan cheese,
    divided
24 small pumpernickel bread
    rounds, or 6 pumpernickel
    slices, quartered

**Yield: 24 appetizers**

**For 1 appetizer:**
Calories...... 43
Protein (g)... 4
Fat (g)....... 0.8
Sat. Fat (g).. 0.4
Choles. (mg).. 3
Fiber (g)..... 0.5
Sodium (mg)... 151
%Cal-Fat...... 16%

In a medium-size mixing bowl, combine tuna, mayonnaise, pimiento, green onion and 3/8 cup (6 tablespoons) Parmesan cheese. Mix thoroughly.

Spread on bread rounds or bread slices, quartered. Sprinkle with remaining 2 tablespoons Parmesan cheese. Place on a baking sheet and broil 5 inches from heat for 4 to 5 minutes, or until slightly browned. Serve hot.

*To make Crab Canapés, substitute 8 ounces backfin crabmeat for the tuna. Be sure to carefully check and remove any shell fragments that may be present in crabmeat. Follow remaining recipe instructions as indicated above.*

Preparation time: 25 minutes

Cooking time: 5 minutes

# Oysters Rockefeller

Wash spinach and remove tough stems. Grind spinach, onions, parsley and lettuce in a food processor.

Place spinach mixture in a large mixing bowl. Add breadcrumbs, Anisette, Worcestershire sauce, Tabasco and salt (if desired). Stir to mix. Return to food processor and puree. Set aside and refrigerate until ready to assemble. (The spinach paste may be made a day ahead.)

Cook oysters: Bring them to a boil in their own liquid. As soon as the liquid comes to a boil, remove from heat. Let oysters stand in hot liquid until ready to assemble.

Preheat broiler to medium setting. Melt margarine in microwave. Rinse oysters.

To assemble: Place small pumpernickel slices on cookie sheet. Top with oyster. Place rounded teaspoon of spinach mixture over each oyster and drizzle with margarine. Sprinkle with Parmesan cheese. Place under broiler 10 to 20 minutes, or until tops begin to brown slightly.

Preparation time: 30–35 minutes

Cooking time: 10–20 minutes

*10 ounces fresh spinach*
*2 green onions, including tops*
*3 sprigs of parsley*
*1/4 head iceberg lettuce*
*1/2 cup dry breadcrumbs*
*2 tablespoons Anisette liqueur
   (licorice-flavored)*
*1 tablespoon Worcestershire
   sauce*
*Dash Tabasco sauce*
*Salt to taste*
*1 tablespoon tub margarine,
   melted*
*3 dozen oysters, packed in own
   liquid*
*36 slices Party Pumpernickel
   (1 8-ounce loaf)*
*6 tablespoons Parmesan cheese*

### Yield: 36 appetizers

For 1 appetizer:
Calories...... 47
Protein (g)... 3
Fat (g)....... 1.2
Sat. Fat (g).. 0.4
Choles. (mg).. 11
Fiber (g)..... 1.3
Sodium (mg)... 94
%Cal-Fat...... 25%

# Salmon Teriyaki Appetizer

1 3-pound salmon fillet
1/4 cup reduced-sodium
  soy sauce
1/2 cup Chablis wine
1/2 teaspoon paprika
3 teaspoons sugar
3 lemons and parsley for
  garnish

**Yield: Approximately 72
1-inch pieces**

**For 2 appetizers:**
Calories...... 66
Protein (g)... 8
Fat (g)....... 3.3
Sat. Fat (g).. 0.6
Choles. (mg).. 23
Fiber (g).....0
Sodium (mg)... NA
%Cal-Fat...... 46%

Prepare marinade by combining soy sauce, wine, paprika, and sugar. Place fish in a shallow container and pour marinade over. Marinate for 30 minutes at room temperature, or 1 to 2 hours in refrigerator.

Meanwhile, set oven control to broil.

Spray broiler rack with vegetable cooking spray. Remove salmon from marinade and place on rack. Spoon 3 tablespoons of marinade over top of fish. Broil approximately 6 inches from heat, skin side down for 10 to 15 minutes, or until fish flakes easily with a fork.

Place salmon fillet on an oval platter, skin side down. Cut into 1-inch squares, leaving skin intact. Garnish with lemon halves with serrated tops and parsley. Serve with toothpicks or cocktail forks.

Preparation time: 15 minutes

Cooking time: 15 minutes

Marinating time: 30 minutes–2 hours

# Fresh Fruit Platter with Yogurt Dip

Cut up fruit into bite-size pieces. Save honeydew shells and pineapple tops (with leaves) for garnish. Cover and refrigerate fruit until ready to assemble tray.

Make yogurt dip by adding brown sugar and cinnamon to yogurt. Mix thoroughly. Set aside until ready to serve.

To serve, line 16 x 20-inch tray with Romaine leaves. Arrange fruit and yogurt dip on tray. Yogurt may be served in hollowed-out honeydew shell with serrated top, or small bowl. Serve with toothpicks.

For garnish on tray: Serrate top edge of melon shell(s). Place shell in center of tray or place one at each end of tray. Place pineapple top(s) with leaves inside melon shell(s).

*Vary quantity of fruit depending on number of guests and other foods served. A 16 x 20-inch tray filled with fruit will be adequate for 20 to 35 guests. Have additional fruit to replenish tray if serving more guests.*

Preparation time: 45 minutes

1 honeydew melon (shell halves reserved for garnish)
1 or 2 fresh pineapples with tops
2 other fruits in season (strawberries, cantaloupe, grapes, watermelon or kiwi fruit)
1 head Romaine lettuce

Yogurt dip:
2 cups nonfat or low-fat plain yogurt
1/4 cup brown sugar, firmly packed
1/4 teaspoon cinnamon

**For 1/2 cup fruit and 2 tablespoons dip:**
Calories...... 64
Protein (g)... 2
Fat (g)....... 0.2
Sat. Fat (g).. 0
Choles. (mg).. <1
Fiber (g)..... 1.3
Sodium (mg)... 27
%Cal-Fat...... 5%

# Escargots (Snails)

1 can (18 count) extra-large snails
1 tablespoon tub margarine
1 1/2 tablespoons flour
1 cup clear chicken broth
1 tablespoon powdered butter flavoring
1 teaspoon minced garlic
2 teaspoons chopped green onion tops
18 snail shells, real or artificial
2 tablespoons grated Parmesan cheese
2 tablespoons fresh minced parsley
1/2 loaf French baguette, sliced thin (optional)

**Yield: 18 appetizers**

**Per 2 appetizers:**
Calories...... 39
Protein (g)... 2
Fat (g)....... 1.3
Sat. Fat (g).. NA
Choles. (mg).. NA
Fiber (g)..... 0
Sodium (mg)... 85
%Cal-Fat...... 29%

Preheat oven to 500 degrees. Drain liquid from can of snails. Rinse and set aside.

In a medium-size skillet, heat margarine over moderate heat. Add flour, stirring with a fork until well blended. Add chicken broth and cook, stirring constantly, until mixture comes to a boil and thickens.

Stir in powdered butter flavoring, garlic and green onion tops. Simmer for 3 minutes, uncovered, over medium-low heat. Place one snail in each snail shell.

Place in snail pan or shallow muffin tins, open side up. Spoon Parmesan cheese over top of each opening.

Bake, uncovered, in a 500-degree oven for 5 minutes, or until cheese is lightly browned and liquid is bubbly.

Remove from oven and cool 5 minutes. Sprinkle minced parsley over top of each opening. Serve immediately. Use cocktail forks to remove snails. If desired, serve on thin slice of French baguette (long narrow French bread).

Preparation time: 20 minutes

Cooking time: 5 minutes

# Artichoke Canapés

Drain artichoke hearts and chop coarsely in food processor. Transfer to medium-size mixing bowl. Drain chopped chilies. Add to artichokes. Add mayonnaise and 1/4 cup Parmesan cheese. Mix thoroughly.

Spread artichoke mixture on bread rounds or bread slices, quartered. Place on baking sheet. Sprinkle with remaining 2 tablespoons Parmesan cheese.

Broil 5 inches from heat for 3 to 5 minutes, or until slightly browned. (Carefully watch canapés while broiling because 30 seconds too long can result in burned edges of bread.) Serve hot.

Preparation time: 15–20 minutes

Cooking time: 5 minutes

*1 14-ounce can artichoke hearts, packed in water*
*1 4.5-ounce can green chilies, chopped (mild)*
*1/2 cup nonfat mayonnaise*
*3/8 cup Parmesan cheese, divided*
*30 small pumpernickel bread rounds, or 8 slices pumpernickel bread, quartered*

### Yield: 30 appetizers

**Per 2 appetizers:**
Calories..... 64
Protein (g).. 3
Fat (g)...... 1
Sat. Fat (g). 0.4
Choles. (mg). 2
Fiber (g).... 2.7
Sodium (mg).. 216
%Cal-Fat..... 14%

# Stuffed Cherry Tomatoes

Cut tops off cherry tomatoes and scoop out pulp. Fill cavity with hummous, using either a teaspoon or a pastry tube. Sprinkle top with fresh, finely chopped parsley. Chill until ready to serve.

Preparation time: 40 minutes

*24 cherry tomatoes*
*3/4 cup hummous (Recipe, page 186)*
*3 sprigs parsley, finely chopped*

### Yield: 24 individual appetizers

**For 2 appetizers:**
Calories...... 27
Protein (g)... 1
Fat (g)....... 0.7
Sat. Fat (g).. 0.1
Choles. (mg).. 0
Fiber (g)..... 1
Sodium (mg)... 38
%Cal-Fat...... 25%

# Artichoke Relish

2 14-ounce cans artichoke
  hearts, drained and chopped
1 4-ounce jar diced pimiento,
  drained
4 green onions, thinly sliced
4 tablespoons freshly grated
  Parmesan cheese
2 cloves of garlic, minced
4 tablespoons lemon juice
2 tablespoons olive oil
1 teaspoon dried whole thyme
1/4 teaspoon pepper
2 tablespoons chopped fresh
  parsley

**Yield: 3 cups of relish
enough for 10 to 14 persons**

**For 2 tablespoons:**
Calories...... 32
Protein (g)... 2
Fat (g)....... 1.6
Sat. Fat (g).. 0.4
Choles. (mg).. <1
Fiber (g)..... 2.7
Sodium (mg)... 34
%Cal-Fat...... 40%

Drain artichoke hearts and chop coarsely in food processor. In medium-size bowl, combine artichokes with remaining ingredients, except parsley. Mix well.

Cover and refrigerate 4 hours or overnight. Sprinkle relish with parsley before serving. Serve with Toasted Pita Chips (Recipe, page 186) or Melba rounds.

*Leftover relish tastes great on a slice of bread, or as part of a sandwich. It can also be served as a side dish for lunch.*

Preparation time: 25 minutes

Marinating time: 4–12 hours

# Tuna Vegetable Dip

Drain can of tuna fish. Place in medium-size bowl, breaking up chunks of tuna. Add remaining ingredients, except bread, and mix well. Chill at least 2 hours before serving.

Serve in hollowed out loaf of bread, or in serving bowl with low-fat crackers.

To serve in bread loaf, slice off top 1/3 of loaf. Hollow out lower 2/3 by pulling out pieces of bread until shell of loaf remains. Fill with dip. Serve with bread removed from loaf, torn into bite-size pieces.

*To make Crabmeat Vegetable Dip, substitute 8 ounces backfin crabmeat for the tuna. Be sure to carefully look through the crabmeat to remove any shell fragments that may be present.*

Preparation time: 25 minutes

*1 9 1/4-ounce can tuna fish packed in water, drained*
*1/2 cup light mayonnaise*
*1/2 cup nonfat mayonnaise*
*1 cup nonfat "sour cream"*
*1 small onion, chopped*
*1 1.4-ounce package Knorr vegetable soup mix*
*1 8-ounce can water chestnuts (chopped)*
*5 ounces chopped spinach (1/2 10-ounce package frozen chopped spinach)*
*1 loaf unsliced round or oval bread, or low-fat crackers*

*Yield: 2 1/2 cups dip*

*For 2 tablespoons:*
Calories...... 56
Protein (g)... 5
Fat (g)....... 1.3
Sat. Fat (g).. 0.3
Choles. (mg).. 5.4
Fiber (g)..... 0.5
Sodium (mg)... 243
%Cal-Fat...... 21%

# *Tabouli*

1 cup fine or medium-grade
  bulgur
Water
1 cup chopped fresh parsley
  (about 1/2 bunch)
1 tablespoon minced fresh dill
  or 1 teaspoon dill weed
1/2 cup chopped green onions,
  including tops
2 medium tomatoes, diced
1 medium cucumber, peeled,
  deseeded, chopped
1/2 cup no-oil Italian dressing
Juice of 1/2 lemon
Freshly ground pepper to taste
Romaine lettuce leaves
Garnish: black olives, tomato
  wedges, parsley sprigs

**Yield: 3 1/2 cups**

**Per 2 tablespoons:**
Calories...... 23
Protein (g)... 1
Fat (g)....... 0.1
Sat. Fat (g).. 0
Choles. (mg).. 0
Fiber (g)..... 1.4
Sodium (mg)... 34
%Cal-Fat...... 2%

Place bulgur in large mixing bowl. Add water to cover and let stand about 1 hour or until bulgur has doubled in size and most of the liquid is absorbed. Drain well and squeeze dry.

Add parsley, dill, green onions, tomatoes and cucumber. Toss gently.

Add Italian dressing, lemon juice and pepper and toss until well mixed. Refrigerate.

Serve with small pita wedges or melba rounds.

*Tabouli, which can also be served as a salad, makes a delicious, low-calorie topping for crackers.*

Preparation time: 30 minutes (plus 1 hour to soak bulgur)

# Bean Dip

Combine first six ingredients in a saucepan and cook until onions are tender.

Place can of black-eyed peas and reserved liquid in a food processor and process to a slightly lumpy paste. Transfer to a medium-size bowl and add ingredients from saucepan. Mix until well blended. Serve hot or cold with bread rounds, melba rounds or toasted pita chips. (Recipe, page 186.)

*This dip also makes a delicious warm burrito filling. To prepare, heat bean dip in saucepan and spoon onto warmed flour tortilla and roll up. Or, if using a microwave, spoon filling onto tortilla and microwave on medium for 1 1/2 minutes.*

Preparation time: 20 minutes

Cooking time: 10 minutes

*1 4-ounce can chopped green chilies, drained*
*1/2 cup tomato sauce*
*4 green onions, chopped*
*1/2 teaspoon ground cumin*
*1/2 teaspoon Tabasco sauce*
*1 clove garlic, minced*
*1 16-ounce can black-eyed peas, drained, (Reserve 2 tablespoons liquid)*

### Yield: 1 1/2 cups

**For 2 tablespoons:**
Calories...... 33
Protein (g)... 2
Fat (g)....... 0.3
Sat. Fat (g).. 0.1
Choles. (mg).. 0
Fiber (g)..... 2
Sodium (mg)... 152
%Cal-Fat...... 7%

# Hummous

2 cups cooked garbanzo beans
(one 16-ounce can, or 3/4
cup raw garbanzos, cooked)
3 tablespoons garbanzo cooking
liquid or juice from can
3 tablespoons sesame seeds or
tahini (sesame seed oil)
2 tablespoons lemon juice
2 cloves garlic, minced
1/2 teaspoon cumin
1/4 teaspoon salt (optional)
Pinch pepper

Yield: 2 cups

For 2 tablespoons:
Calories...... 44
Protein (g)... 2
Fat (g)....... 1.4
Sat. Fat (g).. 0.2
Choles. (mg).. 0
Fiber (g)..... 1.5
Sodium (mg)... 72
%Cal-Fat...... 27%

Drain garbanzo beans, reserving 3 tablespoons liquid. Combine all ingredients, including the reserved liquid, in a food processor. Process continuously for 1 to 2 minutes, until light and fluffy.

*Excellent as a spread on pita bread or low-fat crackers. Fat content is much lower than a cheese spread.*

Preparation time: 15 minutes

# Toasted Pita Chips

6 slices pita bread, whole wheat
or plain
Mrs. Dash original blend
Garlic seasoned salt, or garlic
powder

Yield: 144 pita chips

For 12 pita chips:
Calories...... 82
Protein (g)... 3
Fat (g)....... 0.4
Sat. Fat (g).. 0.1
Choles. (mg).. 0
Fiber (g)..... 0.5
Sodium (mg)... 169
%Cal-Fat...... 5%

Preheat oven to 275 degrees.

Cut each slice of pita bread into 12 pie-shaped wedges using sharp knife. Split wedges, exposing rough inner side of bread. Arrange on several large cookie sheets in a single layer, rough side up. Sprinkle with Mrs. Dash and garlic salt. (For low-sodium chips, use garlic powder.)

Bake at 275 degrees for 30 to 40 minutes, or until crisp and slightly browned. Cool completely. Store in an airtight container.

Preparation time: 10–15 minutes

Cooking time: 30–40 minutes

# Hot Cranberry Punch

In 30-cup percolator coffee maker, place fruit juices, water and brown sugar. In percolator basket, place cloves, cinnamon sticks and salt. Turn on coffee maker, perk and serve.

*A delicious and quick hot drink to serve during the winter months, especially appropriate around the Christmas holidays.*

Preparation time: 15 minutes

Cooking time: 35 minutes (to perk)

9 cups cranberry juice cocktail
9 cups unsweetened pineapple juice
4 1/2 cups water
1 cup brown sugar
4 1/2 teaspoons whole cloves
4 cinnamon sticks, broken
1/4 teaspoon salt

**Yield: 22 8-ounce cups hot punch**

**For an 8-ounce cup:**
Calories...... 153
Protein (g)... <1
Fat (g)....... 0
Sat. Fat (g).. 0
Choles. (mg).. 0
Fiber (g)..... 0.6
Sodium (mg)... 32
%Cal-Fat...... 1%

# Hot Mulled Cider

Combine all ingredients in a large sauce pan. Bring to a boil and simmer, covered, 1 hour. Remove cloves and cinnamon sticks. Serve in coffee mugs.

Preparation time: 10 minutes

Cooking time: 1 hour

1 quart apple cider
2 cups cranberry juice
5 whole cloves
4 sticks cinnamon

**Yield: 6 1-cup servings**

**Per serving:**
Calories...... 118
Protein (g)... <1
Fat (g)....... 0.2
Sat. Fat (g).. 0.1
Choles. (mg).. 0
Fiber (g)..... 0.4
Sodium (mg)... 6
%Cal-Fat...... 2%

# Banana Yogurt Shake

2 cups low-fat vanilla frozen
   yogurt
1 banana

**Yield: 2 8-ounce shakes**

**Per serving:**
Calories...... 292
Protein (g)... 9
Fat (g)....... 5.6
Sat. Fat (g).. 0.1
Choles. (mg).. 13
Fiber (g)..... 0.9
Sodium (mg)... 106
%Cal-Fat...... 17%

Place frozen yogurt and banana in food processor. Process until smooth.

*This makes a great low-fat after-school snack that children love. The banana provides important nutrients and lends a "creamy" texture to the shake. Other flavors of yogurt may be substituted.*

Preparation time: 5 minutes

# Christmas Wassail

2 quarts apple cider
4 cups orange juice
Juice of 2 lemons
3/4 cup honey
4 sticks cinnamon
2 tablespoons whole cloves
2 tablespoons whole allspice
1 teaspoon grated nutmeg

**Yield: 12 8-ounce servings**

**Per serving:**
Calories...... 272
Protein (g)... 1
Fat (g)....... 0.5
Sat. Fat (g).. 0.1
Choles. (mg).. 0
Fiber (g)..... 0.6
Sodium (mg)... 9.7
%Cal-Fat...... 2%

Combine all ingredients in large sauce pan. Heat to boiling and simmer for 10 minutes. Strain out spices.

Serve in a punch bowl decorated with holly or other Christmas greens, or pour from a pitcher.

Preparation time: 15 minutes

Cooking time: 20 minutes

# Light Holiday Eggnog

In large mixing bowl, combine canola oil, egg substitutes and sugar. Beat with wire whisk for 2 to 3 minutes. Add softened ice milk or fat-free ice cream and nutmeg. Stir with wire whisk until smooth.

This eggnog may be served immediately, with or without alcohol; or it may be refrigerated and served later. It will keep several days in the refrigerator. If you prefer a less thick eggnog, thin it by adding skim milk.

Preparation time: 10 minutes (if ice cream is already softened)

*1 teaspoon canola oil*
*4 egg substitutes (1 cup)*
*1/4 cup granulated sugar*
*2 pints ice milk or fat-free ice cream, softened*
*1 teaspoon ground nutmeg, or to taste*
*Rum or brandy to taste (optional)*

*Yield: 6 servings*

*For a 4-ounce serving (using ice milk):*
Calories...... 198
Protein (g)... 9
Fat (g)....... 6
Sat. Fat (g).. 2.7
Choles. (mg).. 13
Fiber (g)..... 0
Sodium (mg)... 144
%Cal-Fat...... 27%

(With fat-free ice cream: 1 g fat/serving)

# Hot Chocolate Mix

*1 25.6-ounce box instant dry
 milk
1/4 cup Hershey's cocoa powder
1 6-ounce box 10x powdered
 sugar
1 16-ounce container chocolate-
 flavored Nestle's Quik*

**Yield: 30 cups hot chocolate**

**For an 8-ounce cup:**
Calories...... 162
Protein (g)... 9
Fat (g)....... 0.8
Sat. Fat (g).. 0.5
Choles. (mg).. 4
Fiber (g)..... 0.2
Sodium (mg)... 171
%Cal-Fat...... 4%

Mix all ingredients together in a large mixing bowl. Pour into jars or containers to store.

To make hot chocolate, place 1/4 cup hot chocolate mix into coffee mug. Pour boiling water over. Stir until all lumps disappear.

Preparation time: 10 minutes

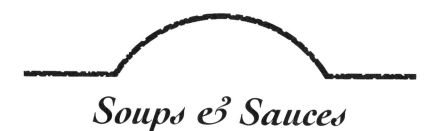

# Soups & Sauces

Seafood Gumbo • Bouillabaisse (Fish Stew) • Chicken Vegetable Soup • New England Clam Chowder • Oyster Stew • Lentil Soup • Minestrone Soup • Southwestern-Style Bean Soup • Louisiana-Style Red Bean Soup • Split Pea Soup • Salmon Bisque • Cream of Broccoli Soup • Cream of Carrot Soup • Stracciatella (Italian Wedding Soup) • Gazpacho Soup • Cabbage Vegetable Soup • Tuna Fish Sauce • Bordelaise Sauce • White Sauce • Tartar Sauce

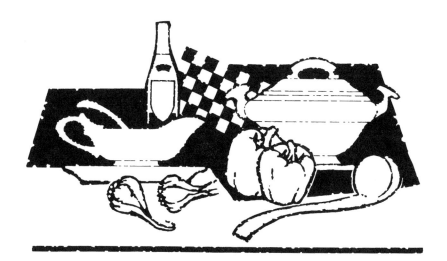

# Seafood Gumbo

2 tablespoons tub margarine
2 tablespoons flour
1/2 cup chopped green onions or
  leeks
1 green pepper, chopped
1/2 cup chopped celery
3 cloves garlic, minced
2 cups okra (fresh or frozen),
  sliced crosswise
2 14 1/2-ounce cans clear
  chicken broth, defatted or from
  own stock, (divided)
1 cup water
1/4 cup flour
1 10-ounce can tomato puree
1/2 pound lump crabmeat
2 tablespoons Worcestershire
  sauce
2 tablespoons brown sugar
1/4 teaspoon thyme
1/2 teaspoon paprika
1/4 teaspoon cayenne, or to taste
2 bay leaves
1 1/2 pounds raw shrimp, peeled
  and deveined
1 pint oysters with juice
6 to 8 cups prepared rice, white
  or brown
Salt and freshly ground pepper
  to taste

**Yield: 8 servings**

**Per serving:**
Calories...... 545
Protein (g)... 39
Fat (g)....... 7.5
Sat. Fat (g).. 1.7
Choles. (mg).. 192
Fiber (g)..... 3.3
Sodium (mg)... 754
%Cal-Fat...... 13%

Heat margarine in large soup kettle. Add 2 tablespoons flour and stir constantly until roux (flour and oil mixture) turns dark brown. Add green onions, green pepper, celery and garlic. Sauté 5 minutes. Add okra and sauté an additional 5 minutes. Stir frequently to avoid sticking or burning.

With a wire whisk, mix 1/4 cup flour into 1/2 cup chicken broth. Add to kettle along with remaining chicken broth and water. Add tomato puree and mix well.

Add crabmeat, Worcestershire sauce, brown sugar, thyme paprika, cayenne and bay leaves. Simmer 1 hour, covered.

Add shrimp and oysters with juice. Simmer until edges of oysters begin to curl, about 10 minutes.

Serve over rice in large soup bowls.

Preparation time: 30 minutes
Cooking time: 70 minutes

# Bouillabaisse (Fish Stew)

In large soup kettle, heat olive oil. Add onion, garlic, leek and mushrooms and sauté for five minutes, or until onion is translucent.

Add chopped tomatoes, clam juice, white wine, basil, bay leaf, saffron, parsley, salt and pepper. Bring to a boil and simmer 20 minutes.

Add lobster, shrimp, scallops, mussels and red snapper and simmer an additional 15 minutes. Remove bay leaf. Serve immediately in large soup bowls.

Serve with Garlic Crustinos (Recipe, page 350), or French bread.

*Traditionally, bouillabaisse, a fish stew, is made with whatever fish is available. Therefore other fish or shellfish, in similar quantities, may be substituted for those given in this recipe.*

Preparation time: 30 minutes
Cooking time: 15 minutes

1 tablespoon olive oil
1 medium onion, chopped
2 cloves garlic, minced
1 leek, chopped finely
4 ounces fresh mushrooms, sliced
1 28-ounce can whole tomatoes, chopped
1/2 cup bottled clam juice
1 1/2 cups dry white wine
1 tablespoon fresh basil, or 1 teaspoon dried
1 bay leaf
Pinch saffron (optional)
2 tablespoons chopped fresh parsley
Salt and pepper to taste (optional)
1 small lobster tail, cut into pieces
1/2 pound raw shrimp, shelled and deveined
1/2 pound scallops
1/2 pound mussels, well scrubbed and debearded
1 pound red snapper, cod, or whitefish, cut into bite-size pieces

## Yield: 6 large servings

**Per serving:**
Calories...... 307
Protein (g)... 40
Fat (g)....... 5.3
Sat. Fat (g).. 0.8
Choles. (mg).. 140
Fiber (g)..... 2.3
Sodium (mg)... 611
%Cal-Fat...... 13%

# Chicken Vegetable Soup

4 chicken breasts, including
    bones, skin removed
10 cups water, divided
5 large carrots, sliced
3 large stalks celery, chopped
4 small onions, thinly sliced
    and cut in half
3 tomatoes, fresh or canned,
    chopped coarsely
3 chicken bouillon cubes
1 15-ounce can corn, including
    liquid
1 10-ounce package frozen
    chopped spinach, thawed and
    drained (optional)
16 ounces ancini di pepe or orzo
    pasta
Freshly grated Parmesan
    cheese

**Yield: 16 cups soup
mixture, 8 cups pasta, or
16 1 1/2 cup-servings soup**

**Per serving:**
Calories..... 192
Protein (g).. 11
Fat (g)...... 1.6
Sat. Fat (g). 0.4
Choles. (mg). 19
Fiber (g).... 2.6
Sodium (mg).. 249
%Cal-Fat..... 7%

Remove skin from chicken breasts and place in a 4 1/2-quart soup kettle with 5 cups water. Bring to a boil, reduce heat and simmer 1 to 3 hours. (The longer it cooks, the more flavor in the broth.) Remove breasts from broth, and when cool enough to handle, separate chicken from bones, shredding chicken. Set aside.

Defat broth. This can be done by pouring into tall, narrow container and skimming fat from top.

Pour defatted broth back into soup kettle, adding remaining 5 cups water. Add shredded chicken, carrots, celery, onions, tomatoes and bouillon cubes. Bring to a boil, reduce heat and simmer 1 hour, or until vegetables are cooked. Add corn, including liquid, and thawed spinach. Bring to a boil and cook an additional 5 to 10 minutes.

Meanwhile, cook pasta according to package directions. Drain and set aside.

To serve, place 1/2 cup pasta in individual soup bowl. With a ladle, scoop about 1 cup soup mixture over top. Sprinkle with Parmesan cheese.

*This is a hearty, wonderfully flavorful soup chock-full of vegetables. If serving as a main dish at a dinner meal, it will provide about 8 large servings.*

Preparation time: 35 minutes
Cooking time: 2 1/2 – 4 1/2 hours

# New England Clam Chowder

Drain clams, reserving liquid.

In heavy soup kettle, melt margarine. Add onion and sauté until it becomes translucent. Add clams, 1/2 cup liquid from clams, water and potatoes. Bring to a boil, reduce heat and simmer for 20 to 30 minutes, or until potatoes are soft.

Mix flour with 1/2 cup skim milk until smooth. Add flour mixture, remaining 1 1/2 cups skim milk, evaporated milk, salt and pepper to soup kettle. Heat just to a boil, stirring occasionally. Serve immediately.

Preparation time: 25 minutes
Cooking time: 30 minutes

*3 6 1/2-ounce cans chopped clams, reserving liquid*
*1 tablespoon tub margarine*
*1/2 cup chopped onion*
*1/2 cup liquid from clams*
*1 1/2 cups water*
*4 cups diced potatoes*
*2 cups skim milk, divided*
*1/4 cup flour*
*1 cup canned evaporated skim milk*
*1 teaspoon salt*
*1/4 teaspoon pepper*

**Yield: 10 1-cup servings, or 4 large main course servings**

**Per 1-cup serving:**
Calories...... 116
Protein (g)... 12
Fat (g)....... 2
Sat. Fat (g).. 0.4
Choles. (mg).. 21
Fiber (g)..... 1
Sodium (mg)... 373
%Cal-Fat...... 15%

# Oyster Stew

3 medium potatoes, peeled and diced
1/4 cup finely chopped onion
2 teaspoons tub margarine
1 pint shucked oysters, with liquid
1 12-ounce can evaporated skim milk
1 teaspoon seasoned salt
Dash of cayenne pepper, or to taste
1 teaspoon Worcestershire sauce
1/4 cup plus 1 tablespoon flour
2 1/2 cups skim milk
Salt to taste
2 tablespoons fresh chopped parsley
Oyster crackers (optional)

### Yield: 6 10-ounce servings

### Per Serving:
Calories...... 186
Protein (g)... 15
Fat (g)....... 3.7
Sat. Fat (g).. 0.9
Choles. (mg).. 49
Fiber (g)..... 1
Sodium (mg)... 446
%Cal-Fat...... 18%

Place diced potatoes in large saucepan with just enough water to cover top of potatoes. Bring to a boil and simmer 15 minutes or until potatoes are tender.

Meanwhile, in medium saucepan, sauté onion in margarine until onion becomes translucent. Add oysters and liquid. Bring to a boil and simmer 10 minutes or until the edges of oysters curl.

As soon as potatoes are tender, drain water. Add oyster mixture, evaporated milk, seasoned salt, cayenne pepper and Worcestershire sauce. Set aside.

In small bowl, mix flour with skim milk until all lumps disappear. Add to potato mixture. Salt to taste. Heat stew, stirring frequently, until it comes to a boil and thickens slightly. Sprinkle with chopped parsley. Serve immediately. Serve with oyster crackers, if desired.

Preparation time: 20 minutes
Cooking time: 20–25 minutes

# Lentil Soup

Rinse lentils; drain and place in soup kettle. Add water, garlic, carrots, celery and onion. Cover and simmer 1 1/2 hours.

Add remaining ingredients and simmer, covered, 30 minutes longer. If soup is too thick, add additional water. Sprinkle with Parmesan cheese, if desired.

*Leftover soup tastes great over pasta or freezes well.*

Preparation time: 25 minutes
Cooking time: 2 hours

*2 cups dry lentils*
*7 cups water*
*1 1/2 teaspoons minced garlic*
*4 medium carrots, chopped*
*3 stalks celery, chopped*
*1 medium onion, chopped*
*16 ounces tomato sauce*
*1 fresh tomato chopped*
*2 tablespoons white wine
    vinegar*
*1 tablespoon reduced-sodium
    soy sauce*
*1 1/2 tablespoons brown sugar*
*1 1/2 teaspoons dried basil*
*1/4 teaspoon black pepper*
*Juice of 1/2 lemon*
*Parmesan cheese (optional)*

### Yield: 8 to 10 servings

**Per serving:**
Calories...... 198
Protein (g)... 14
Fat (g)....... 0.7
Sat. Fat (g).. 0.1
Choles. (mg).. 0
Fiber (g)..... 7.8
Sodium (mg)... 402
%Cal-Fat...... 3%

# Minestrone Soup

1 20-ounce package dried 15-bean mixture
11 cups water
1 large onion, chopped
3 carrots, chopped
2 cloves of garlic, minced
1 28-ounce can tomatoes, chopped
3 chicken bouillon cubes
2 teaspoons basil
1 tablespoon olive oil (optional)
Pepper to taste
Juice of 1/2 lemon
8 ounces dumpling pasta, or "eggless" egg noodles

**Yield: 16 one-cup servings, or 8 2-cup servings**

**Per 1-cup serving:**
Calories...... 122
Protein (g)... 6
Fat (g)....... 0.7
Sat. Fat (g).. 0.3
Choles. (mg).. 0
Fiber (g)..... 5
Sodium (mg)... 296
%Cal-Fat...... 5%

Soak minestrone bean mix overnight or at least 2 to 3 hours in enough water to cover beans. Drain.

In a large kettle, put beans, 11 cups water and remaining ingredients except pasta. Cook over medium heat for 3 hours or until beans are tender.

Shortly before serving, add pasta to soup and boil 10 to 15 minutes longer, until pasta is ready. If soup gets too thick, add more water as needed.

Serve immediately. If desired, sprinkle with Parmesan cheese.

*Soaking beans is not essential, but is recommended. If soaking is omitted, increase cooking time slightly.*

Preparation time: 20 minutes
Cooking time: 3 hours, 15 minutes

# Southwestern-Style Bean Soup

Remove visible fat from top of chicken broth. Combine all ingredients in a 4-quart heavy saucepan. Bring to a boil. Reduce heat, cover and simmer for 45 minutes or longer.

Serve with corn bread, or heavy whole-grain bread.

Preparation time: 20 minutes
Cooking time: 45 minutes

*1 15 1/2-ounce can navy beans or Northern beans, rinsed and drained*
*1 15 1/2-ounce can kidney beans, rinsed and drained*
*1 15 1/2-ounce can pinto beans, rinsed and drained*
*1 15-ounce can clear chicken broth, defatted*
*1 cup water*
*3 fresh tomatoes, chopped coarsely*
*1 10-ounce pkg. frozen whole kernel corn, thawed*
*2 medium carrots, sliced*
*1 large onion, chopped*
*1 8-ounce can tomato sauce*
*1/4 teaspoon minced garlic*
*1/4 teaspoon Tabasco sauce*
*1 to 2 teaspoons chili powder*

### Yield: 4 to 6 servings

### Per serving:
Calories...... 437
Protein (g)... 25
Fat (g)....... 2.9
Sat. Fat (g).. 0.6
Choles. (mg).. 0
Fiber (g)..... 12
Sodium (mg)... 850
%Cal-Fat...... 6%

# Louisiana-Style Red Bean Soup

2 teaspoons olive oil
1 large onion, chopped
1 large green pepper, chopped
  finely
2 cloves garlic, minced
1 large stalk celery, chopped
2 15-ounce cans red kidney
  beans, drained and rinsed
1 14-ounce can clear chicken
  broth, defatted
1 16-ounce can "no salt added"
  tomatoes, chopped
2 cups water
1/2 cup long grain rice,
  uncooked
1/2 teaspoon thyme
1/4 teaspoon cumin
1 teaspoon paprika
1 tablespoon red wine vinegar
Tabasco sauce to taste (1/4 to
  1/2 teaspoon)
Salt to taste

**Yield: 4 to 6 servings**

**Per serving:**
Calories...... 280
Protein (g)... 14
Fat (g)....... 3.3
Sat. Fat (g).. 0.5
Choles. (mg).. 0
Fiber (g)..... 4
Sodium (mg)... 672
%Cal-Fat...... 11%

Heat olive oil in heavy soup kettle and sauté onion, green pepper, garlic and celery, until vegetables are tender, but not brown.

Add remaining ingredients. Bring to a boil, and simmer 30 minutes or until rice is tender.

*Delicious with toasted French bread and a green salad.*

Preparation time: 20 minutes
Cooking time: 30 minutes

# Split Pea Soup

Rinse peas under cold water to remove any foreign particles. Remove visible fat from top of chicken broth.

Place all the ingredients except the pepper and fresh thyme in a large soup kettle. Bring to a boil and simmer, covered, for 2 1/2 to 3 hours. Serve hot.

Sprinkle freshly ground black pepper over individual bowls of soup, and garnish with sprigs of fresh thyme, if desired.

Preparation time: 15 minutes
Cooking time: 3–4 hours

1 pound dried split green peas
4 cups water
2 14 1/2-ounce cans clear chicken broth, defatted
1 clove garlic, crushed
3/4 cup diced carrot
1/2 cup diced celery
3/4 cup diced onion
1 1/2 ounces chopped low-fat boiled ham (2 sandwich slices)
1/2 teaspoon dried thyme
1 bay leaf
Freshly ground black pepper (optional)
Garnish with fresh thyme (optional)

*Yield: 6 to 8 servings*

*Per serving:*
Calories...... 263
Protein (g)... 20
Fat (g)....... 1.9
Sat. Fat (g).. 0.4
Choles. (mg).. 4
Fiber (g)..... 10
Sodium (mg)... 510
%Cal-Fat......6%

# Salmon Bisque

2 14 1/2-ounce cans clear
  chicken broth, defatted
8 ounces fresh salmon
1/2 cup chopped celery
2 tablespoons chives, finely
  chopped
1 6-ounce can tomato paste
3/8 cup sherry (6 tablespoons)
2 12-ounce cans evaporated
  skim milk
1/4 cup plus 2 tablespoons flour
1/4 teaspoon pepper
1 teaspoon seasoned salt
  (optional)

*Yield: 8 to 9 1-cup servings*

*Per serving:*
Calories...... 177
Protein (g)... 14
Fat (g)....... 2.5
Sat. Fat (g).. 0.5
Choles. (mg).. 16
Fiber (g)..... 1
Sodium (mg)... 544
%Cal-Fat...... 13%

Skim fat from top of chicken broth. Pour broth into 4-quart saucepan. Add salmon, celery and chives. Bring to a boil, reduce heat and simmer, covered, for 10 minutes. Carefully remove salmon from broth with a spatula. Set aside.

Add tomato paste and sherry to saucepan, mixing well with a wire whisk. Bring to a boil and simmer an additional 20 minutes.

Meanwhile, remove skin from salmon and mash into small pieces with a fork.

In medium-size bowl, stir flour and evaporated milk with a wire whisk until all lumps disappear. Add milk mixture, salmon, pepper and seasoned salt to saucepan. Heat just until bisque comes to a boil and thickens.* Remove from heat and serve.

*Do not boil more than a few minutes after adding the milk mixture to avoid curdling.*

Preparation time: 20 minutes
Cooking time: 25 minutes

# Cream of Broccoli Soup

Thinly slice 2 cups of broccoli flowerets. Set aside. Coarsely chop remaining broccoli (including stems), onions, celery and carrot.

Place chicken broth in 4-quart heavy saucepan. Add chopped vegetables (except for 2 cups flowerets), minced garlic and water. Bring to a boil and simmer until vegetables are tender (about 30 minutes).

Puree broth mixture in food processor until smooth. Return to saucepan.

In a medium-size mixing bowl, add flour to evaporated skim milk, mixing with wire whisk until smooth. Add to pureed mixture. Add flowerets, thyme and pepper. Bring to a boil over medium heat, stirring frequently. Simmer until flowerets are tender.

Pour into soup bowls. Sprinkle with scallions or Parmesan cheese, if desired.

Preparation time: 25 minutes
Cooking time: 40 minutes

1 bunch broccoli, divided
2 medium onions, chopped
1 cup chopped celery
1 carrot, chopped
2 14 1/2-ounce cans clear
  chicken broth, defatted
1/2 teaspoon minced garlic
1 cup water
1/2 cup flour
2 12-ounce cans evaporated
  skim milk
1/2 teaspoon thyme
1/4 teaspoon black pepper
Chopped scallions (optional)
Parmesan cheese (optional)

**Yield: 8 servings**

**Per serving:**
Calories...... 186
Protein (g)... 16
Fat (g)....... 1.6
Sat. Fat (g).. 0.4
Choles. (mg).. 3
Fiber (g)..... 3
Sodium (mg)... 492
%Cal-Fat...... 7%

# Cream of Carrot Soup

2 pounds carrots, peeled and
   thinly sliced
1 1/2 cups chopped onion
1 cup sliced celery
1 14 1/2-ounce can clear
   chicken broth, defatted
1 1/2 cups water
2 teaspoons tub margarine
1 teaspoon freshly grated
   ginger root
1 5-ounce can evaporated skim
   milk
1 tablespoon sherry
Garnish with sprigs of fresh
   rosemary (optional)

### Yield: 4 to 6 servings

**Per serving:**
Calories...... 150
Protein (g)... 6
Fat (g)....... 2
Sat. Fat (g).. 0.5
Choles. (mg).. <1
Fiber (g)..... 7
Sodium (mg)... 398
%Cal-Fat...... 13%

Combine sliced carrots, onion, celery, chicken broth and water in large saucepan. Bring to a boil. Cover and simmer 20 minutes, or until carrots are tender. Let cool slightly. Drain vegetables, reserving liquid.

Meanwhile, in small frypan, sauté ginger root in margarine for 3 minutes. Add to drained carrot mixture.

In a food processor or blender, puree drained carrots until smooth, gradually adding all the reserved liquid during the processing. Return to soup kettle. Whisk in evaporated milk. Heat slowly until soup almost comes to a boil. Just before serving, stir in sherry.

Garnish with sprigs of fresh rosemary.

Preparation time: 25 minutes
Cooking time: 15 minutes

# Stracciatella
# (Italian Wedding Soup)

2 14 1/2-ounce cans clear
   chicken broth, defatted
7 cups water
1 10-ounce package frozen
   chopped spinach, thawed and
   drained
1/2 cup orzo pasta
9 egg whites
6 tablespoons freshly grated
   Parmesan cheese
1/4 cup lemon juice, fresh or
   reconstituted
Parmesan cheese

Defat chicken broth by skimming fat from top of can. Combine first four ingredients in soup kettle. Bring to a boil, stirring occasionally. Simmer 10 minutes or until pasta is fully cooked.

Meanwhile, in a small mixing bowl, combine egg whites and Parmesan cheese. Beat with a wire whisk until slightly frothy.

After pasta is cooked, gradually stir in egg-white mixture. Cook 2 additional minutes. Stir in lemon juice. Serve immediately or let cool slightly. Sprinkle individual servings with Parmesan cheese, if desired.

*This is a lower-salt version of Straciatella. The lemon juice was added for additional flavor since the sodium was reduced to about half that of the classic recipe.*

Preparation time: 15–20 minutes

# *Gazpacho Soup*

Combine all ingredients. Chill for at least 2 hours. This soup can be pureed, if desired.

*A refreshing crunchy cold soup ideal for lunch or a light supper during the summer. A crusty French bread or corn bread would be a perfect accompaniment.*

Preparation time: 20 minutes

Chill 2 hours before serving

**Yield: 14 1-cup servings**

*Per serving:*
Calories..... 63
Protein (g).. 5.7
Fat (g)...... 1.2
Sat. Fat (g). 0.6
Choles. (mg). 2
Fiber (g).... 0.6
Sodium (mg).. 289
%Cal-Fat..... 16%

*2 cups tomato sauce (no salt added)*
*2 cups tomato juice*
*1 small onion, finely chopped*
*2 cups fresh tomatoes, diced*
*1 cup minced green pepper*
*2 tablespoons fresh parsley, finely chopped*
*1 diced cucumber*
*1 teaspoon honey*
*1 clove garlic crushed*
*Juice of 1/2 lemon*
*Juice of 1 lime*
*2 tablespoons wine vinegar*
*1 teaspoon tarragon*
*1 teaspoon basil*
*Dash of ground cumin*
*1/4 teaspoon Tabasco sauce (or to taste)*
*Pepper to taste*
*1 tablespoon olive oil (optional)*

**Yield: 8 1-cup servings**

*Per serving:*
Calories...... 58
Protein (g)... 2
Fat (g)....... 0.4
Sat. Fat (g).. 0
Choles. (mg).. 0
Fiber (g)..... 2.9
Sodium (mg)... 240
%Cal-Fat...... 6%

# Cabbage Vegetable Soup

2 medium potatoes, cubed
1 16-ounce can chick peas,
  drained
4 cups cabbage, chopped
4 carrots, sliced 1/8-inch thick
2 14 1/2-ounce cans clear
  chicken broth, defatted
3 cups water
16-ounce can "no salt added"
  canned tomatoes, chopped
1/4 teaspoon celery seed
1/4 teaspoon black pepper
1/2 teaspoon basil
1 tablespoon fresh parsley,
  chopped
Salt to taste

**Yield: 10 one-cup servings,
or 6 12-ounce servings**

**Per serving:**
Calories...... 121
Protein (g)... 7
Fat (g)....... 1.9
Sat. Fat (g).. 0.3
Choles. (mg).. 0
Fiber (g)..... 5.5
Sodium (mg)... 386
%Cal-Fat...... 13%

Prepare vegetables as indicated. Drain chick peas and skim fat from top of chicken broth.

Combine all ingredients in large soup kettle. Bring to a boil and simmer 1 hour. Serve immediately.

Preparation time: 20 minutes

Cooking time: 1 hour

# Tuna Fish Sauce

Drain tuna. Combine tuna and remaining ingredients, except capers, in a food processor. Blend 2 to 3 minutes, or until sauce is smooth. Stir in capers, if desired.

Spread sauce generously over cooked and chilled chicken breasts or thin-sliced veal. Serve immediately or refrigerate for up to three days.

*This sauce is a favorite delicacy in Northern Italy. Now, with the availability of nonfat mayonnaise, it can be made nearly fat-free. The sauce, served with chilled chicken or veal, is ideal for lunch or before the main course at dinner. It is also delicious spread on crackers or bread.*

Preparation time: 15 minutes

1 3 1/2-ounce can white albacore tuna, packed in water
2 anchovy fillets
1 tablespoon brine from jar of capers
2 cloves garlic, minced
3/4 cup nonfat mayonnaise
Lemon juice to taste (about 1 teaspoon)
2 tablespoons capers (optional)

**Yield: 1 cup sauce**

**For 1 tablespoon:**
Calories...... 19
Protein (g)... 2
Fat (g)....... 0
Sat. Fat (g).. 0
Choles. (mg).. 2
Fiber (g)..... 0
Sodium (mg)... 183
%Cal-Fat...... 4%

# Bordelaise Sauce

Wash and slice mushrooms. Place in skillet with chives (no oil necessary), cover and simmer on low until mushrooms turn dark in color.

Meanwhile, remove fat from top of canned beef broth. Pour into mixing bowl. Add flour and mix with wire whisk until well blended.

Add broth mixture to mushrooms in skillet. Bring to a boil, stirring occasionally. Add remaining ingredients. Simmer 5 to 10 minutes. Serve over pork or beef.

Preparation time: 20 minutes

Cooking time: 10 minutes

3/4 cup sliced fresh mushrooms
2 tablespoons finely chopped chives or green onions
1/4 cup all-purpose flour
1 14 1/2-ounce can clear beef broth, defatted
1 teaspoon dried tarragon, crushed
1 tablespoon lemon juice
3 tablespoons dry red wine
Dash cayenne pepper (to taste)

**Yield: 2 1/4 cups**

**For 1/4 cup sauce:**
Calories...... 20
Protein (g)... 1
Fat (g)....... 0
Sat. Fat (g).. 0
Choles. (mg).. 0
Fiber (g)..... 0.2
Sodium (mg)... 165
%Cal-Fat...... 3%

# White Sauce

2 tablespoons all-purpose flour
1 cup skim milk
1/4 teaspoon salt
1/8 teaspoon white pepper

**Yield: 1 cup sauce**

**For 1/4 cup sauce:**
Calories...... 36
Protein (g)... 3
Fat (g)....... 0.2
Sat. Fat (g).. 0
Choles. (mg).. 1
Fiber (g)..... 0
Sodium (mg)... 165
%Cal-Fat...... 4%

In small bowl, combine flour and milk, mixing with a wire whisk until all lumps disappear.

Place small skillet over medium heat. Add flour/milk mixture. Add salt and pepper. Heat until sauce comes to a boil and thickens.

*For thicker sauce, increase flour to 1/4 cup; for thinner sauce, decrease flour to 1 tablespoon.*

Preparation time: 10 minutes

# Tartar Sauce

1/2 cup nonfat mayonnaise
1 tablespoon finely chopped dill
 pickle
1 teaspoon finely chopped chives
1/2 teaspoon finely chopped
 pimiento
1 teaspoon fresh parsley, finely
 chopped

**Yield: 1/2 cup sauce**

**For 1 tablespoon:**
Calories...... 13
Protein (g)... 0
Fat (g)....... 0
Sat. Fat (g).. 0
Choles. (mg).. 0
Fiber (g)..... 0
Sodium (mg)... 216
%Cal-Fat...... 0%

Combine all ingredients, mixing well. Chill at least 2 hours. Serve with fish.

Preparation time: 10 minutes

Chill 2 hours before serving

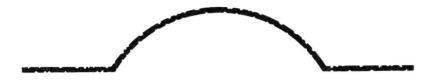

# Salads & Salad Dressings

Chicken Salad in Pineapple Boats • Curry Chicken Salad • Grilled Chicken Salad • Poached Salmon Salad • Tuna Pasta Salad • Scallop Antipasto Salad • Tuna Stuffed Tomatoes • Swiss-Style Garden Salad • Black Bean Salad • Garbanzo-Tomato Salad • Mandarin Salad • Celestial Salad • Spinach Salad with Honey Mustard Dressing • Parsley-Wheat Salad (Tabouli) • Marinated Vegetable Salad • Green Bean-Mushroom Salad • New Potato Salad • "Sour Cream" Potato Salad • Slim Waldorf Salad • Tropical Fruit Slaw • Creamy Cucumber Salad • Lemon-Tahini Salad Dressing • Fresh Cranberry Molded Salad • Cranberry Fruit Salad • Orange Mandarin Ring • Grapefruit Salad

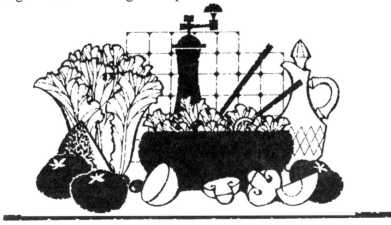

# Chicken Salad in Pineapple Boats

2 whole fresh pineapples with
 tops
2 1/2 cups cooked chicken
 breast, cubed (1 lb.)
1 cup cubed pineapple
1 cup seedless grapes, halved
1/2 cup diced celery
3/4 cup nonfat or low-fat plain
 yogurt
1/4 cup light mayonnaise
1/4 teaspoon salt
1/8 cup toasted slivered
 almonds
8 fresh strawberries for garnish
 (optional)

**Yield: 4 servings**

**Per serving:**
Calories...... 269
Protein (g)... 31
Fat (g)....... 8.6
Sat. Fat (g).. 1.8
Choles. (mg).. 83
Fiber (g)..... 1.5
Sodium (mg)... 265
%Cal-Fat...... 28%

Make pineapple boats by first slicing whole pineapples, including decorative crown, lengthwise. Cut out pineapple fruit, reserving shell and crown. Cut pineapple into bite-size pieces. Set aside.

In a large mixing bowl, combine cubed chicken, pineapple, grapes and celery. Toss.

In a small bowl, combine yogurt, mayonnaise and salt. Add to chicken mixture, tossing to coat well. Chill.

To serve chicken salad, fill pineapple boats; or, if fresh pineapple is not available, arrange lettuce on plate, top with pineapple slice, followed by chicken salad. Garnish plate with fresh strawberries.

*This dish is ideal for a refreshing spring luncheon or a light summer meal. Leftover turkey breast may be substituted for the chicken breast.*

Preparation time: 20–25 minutes (provided chicken is precooked)

# Curry Chicken Salad

Lightly toss together the chicken, rice, celery, raisins, almonds and onion.

Make dressing of yogurt, mayonnaise, curry powder, salt, lemon juice and sugar. Add dressing to chicken-rice mixture and toss until well mixed. Chill thoroughly.

Serve over pieces of Romaine lettuce. Garnish with additional almonds and/or lemon slices.

*This dish is ideal for a ladies' luncheon, served with corn bread muffins, cantaloupe slices and a light dessert.*

Preparation time: 20–25 minutes
(provided chicken and rice are precooked)

2 cups diced cooked chicken (5 chicken breast halves)
1 1/2 cups cooked white rice
3/4 cup coarsely chopped celery
1 cup raisins
2 tablespoons slivered almonds or chopped pecans
2 tablespoons finely chopped onion
1/2 cup nonfat plain yogurt
1/4 cup light mayonnaise
1 1/2 teaspoons curry powder
1/2 teaspoon salt
1 tablespoon lemon juice
2 tablespoons sugar

**Yield: 6 servings**

**Per serving:**
Calories...... 285
Protein (g)... 17
Fat (g)....... 5.9
Sat. Fat (g).. 1.1
Choles. (mg).. 38
Fiber (g)..... 2.3
Sodium (mg)... 289
%Cal-Fat...... 18%

# Grilled Chicken Salad

1 pound boneless chicken breast
1/4 to 1/2 cup no-oil Italian
  salad dressing
4 large carrots, peeled and
  sliced thin
1 large onion, sliced thin
1 bunch fresh parsley, chopped
  coarsely

Quick Low-Fat Vinaigrette
  Dressing:
5 tablespoons no-oil Italian
  dressing
1 tablespoon olive oil
3 tablespoons Balsamic vinegar

**Yield: 4 servings**

**Per serving:**
Calories...... 270
Protein (g)... 37
Fat (g)....... 7.6
Sat. Fat (g).. 1.9
Choles. (mg).. 96
Fiber (g)..... 3
Sodium (mg)... NA
%Cal-Fat...... 25%

Marinate chicken breasts in no-oil Italian salad dressing at least 2 hours. Cook on preheated grill 8 to 10 minutes per side, or until chicken is no longer pink inside. Chop into bite-size pieces.

While chicken is on grill, slice carrots and onion, and chop parsley. Set aside.

To assemble salad, place chicken pieces in bottom of 9 x 9-inch baking dish. While chicken is still warm, top with layer of sliced carrots, followed by layer of sliced onions. Sprinkle parsley over top.

Pour vinaigrette dressing evenly over top of salad. Serve within 30 minutes, or refrigerate and serve later.

*This is a quick and easy salad—perfect for an evening meal after a busy day. Serve with your favorite bread and a fruit  for dessert.*

Marinating time: 2 hours
Cooking time: 15–20 minutes
Preparation time: 15–20 minutes

# *Poached Salmon Salad*

Follow instructions for poached salmon (Recipe, page 288). Chill.

Wash Romaine and break into bite-size pieces. Place in very large salad bowl. Cut up peppers and carrot and place over top. Sprinkle sprout mix over top. Set aside until ready to serve.

To serve, divide salad equally onto four dinner plates. Top with 1-ounce chunk Farmer's cheese and 3 ounces salmon. Drizzle dressing of choice over top.

*A main-dish salad with a spectacle of color that is great for lunch or for dinner on a hot summer day. Serve with your choice of breads — French, multi-grain and/or muffins.*

Preparation time: 20 minutes
Cooking time: 15 minutes to poach salmon

1 head Romaine lettuce
1 yellow pepper, cut into thin strips
1 green pepper, cut into thin strips
1 red pepper, cut into thin strips
1 carrot, sliced julienne
1/4 cup crunchy sprout mix (bean sprouts)
4 ounces Farmer's cheese
12 ounces salmon filet, poached
Salad dressing of choice (low-fat or nonfat)

**Yield: 4 servings**

**Per serving:**
Calories...... 213
Protein (g)... 30
Fat (g)....... 6.8
Sat. Fat (g).. 1.3
Choles. (mg).. 44
Fiber (g)..... 2.5
Sodium (mg)... 65
%Cal-Fat...... 28%

# Tuna Pasta Salad

8 ounces pasta spirals
1/2 cup sliced green onions
1 green pepper, chopped
1 cup seedless cucumber, sliced
  and quartered
1 cup cherry tomatoes, halved
1 13-ounce can tuna, packed in
  water, drained
1/4 cup black olives, halved

Salad Dressing:
1 tablespoon olive oil
2 tablespoons white wine
  vinegar
2 tablespoons lemon juice
1/4 cup no-oil Italian dressing
1/4 cup Parmesan cheese
1/4 cup fresh parsley, chopped
1/4 teaspoon salt
1/4 teaspoon pepper
1/2 teaspoon garlic powder

**Yield: 6 servings**

**Per serving:**
Calories...... 286
Protein (g)... 25
Fat (g)....... 4.8
Sat. Fat (g).. 1.3
Choles. (mg).. 37
Fiber (g)..... 3
Sodium (mg)... 525
%Cal-Fat...... 15%

Prepare pasta according to package directions. Drain and immediately pour cold water over. While pasta is cooking, prepare vegetables.

In a 4- or 5-quart casserole, combine pasta, green onions, green pepper, cucumber, cherry tomatoes, tuna and olives. Mix well.

Make dressing by combining all ingredients in small mixing bowl. Beat with wire whisk. Pour over pasta mixture and mix until thoroughly blended.

Cover and refrigerate at least 8 hours before serving.

*To add extra zip, you may want to add additional no-oil Italian dressing, to taste. Also, to save time, 1/2 cup no-oil Italian dressing, plus 1/4 cup Parmesan cheese may be used as the salad dressing for this pasta salad.*

Preparation time: 25 minutes

# Scallop Antipasto Salad

Cook potatoes in boiling water until tender, about 20 minutes. Cut into quarters and place in large bowl. Cool.

Combine vinegar, olive oil, onion, parsley, mustard, dill leaves, salt and pepper. Mix well. Pour over cooled potatoes.

Rinse scallops. Place in a single layer in shallow oven-proof dish. Sprinkle with 1/4 teaspoon garlic powder. Broil on top shelf of oven until lightly browned, about 5 minutes. Toss scallops. Sprinkle with remaining 1/4 teaspoon garlic powder. Broil 5 additional minutes.

Pour scallops with juice over potato mixture. Add celery, olives and snow peas. Toss gently.

*Delicious served with baked apples and French bread.*

*For added crispness, soak snow peas in cold water in refrigerator for 1 hour. Drain. Snap in half.*

Preparation time: 30–40 minutes

1 1/2 pounds small red potatoes, unpeeled
1/4 cup red wine vinegar (preferably Balsamic vinegar)
1 tablespoon olive oil
3 tablespoons chopped red onion
3 tablespoons chopped fresh parsley
1/2 teaspoon Dijon mustard
1/4 teaspoon dill leaves
1/8 teaspoon salt
1/4 teaspoon fresh ground black pepper
1 pound bay scallops
1/2 teaspoon garlic powder
1/2 cup chopped celery
1/4 cup sliced black olives
1 cup snow peas, cut in half lengthwise

**Yield: 4 servings**

**Per serving:**
Calories...... 305
Protein (g)... 26
Fat (g)....... 5.5
Sat. Fat (g).. 0.7
Choles. (mg).. 38
Fiber (g)..... 8.5
Sodium (mg)... 377
%Cal-Fat...... 16%

1 12 1/2-ounce can tuna fish,
   in spring water
2 baby dill pickles, finely
   chopped
1/4 cup finely chopped onion
1/2 cup chopped celery
1/4 to 1/2 cup nonfat
   mayonnaise
4 large tomatoes
2 tablespoons chopped fresh
   parsley

**Yield: 4 servings**

**Per serving:**
Calories...... 172
Protein (g)... 28
Fat (g)....... 1.5
Sat. Fat (g).. 0.8
Choles. (mg).. 54
Fiber (g)..... 2.4
Sodium (mg)... 519
%Cal-Fat...... 8%

# Tuna Stuffed Tomatoes

Drain water from tuna fish. Place in large bowl. Add remaining ingredients except tomatoes and parsley. Set aside.

Cut off upper 1/3 of tomato. Scrape out pulp. Add tomato pulp to tuna mixture and stir until well blended. Fill tomatoes with tuna salad. Sprinkle with chopped parsley.

Preparation time: 15–20 minutes

2 small cucumbers, peeled, cut
   in half lengthwise, deseeded,
   and sliced 1/4-inch thick
2 medium carrots, finely
   shredded
1 11-ounce can "no salt added"
   corn, drained
1 bunch leaf lettuce, torn into
   bite-size pieces
Salad dressing of choice (low-
   fat or nonfat)

**Yield: 4 large salads**

**Per serving:**
Calories...... 129
Protein (g)... 5
Fat (g)....... 1
Sat. Fat (g).. 0.2
Choles. (mg).. 0
Fiber (g)..... 4.7
Sodium (mg)... 26
%Cal-Fat...... 9%

# Swiss-Style Garden Salad

Prepare vegetables as indicated. In 4 large individual salad bowls, place equal portions of sliced cucumbers, shredded carrots and corn, placing each in separate sections of bowl. Top with torn leaf lettuce. Pour salad dressing over top.

Preparation time: 15–20 minutes

# Black Bean Salad

Wash beans, removing any debris. Put into large pot with 8 cups cold water and soak overnight.

Drain beans in colander and rinse thoroughly. Return to pot. Add 3 cups cold water, salt and cumin. Bring to a boil, reduce heat and simmer just until tender, about 45 minutes. Remove from heat and let cool. Drain off any excess liquid.

Meanwhile, cook corn until tender. Cool.

After beans are cooled, add corn, chopped green pepper, red pepper, and onion. Toss together lightly.

To make dressing, combine vinegar, cilantro, cumin, coriander and pepper in a jar or container with a lid. Shake well to mix. Add olive oil. Shake again and pour over bean salad. Toss to combine well.

Chill for several hours or overnight. If refrigerated, salad stays fresh for at least three days.

*Four cups canned black beans may be substituted for 1 pound dried beans. Be sure to drain and rinse if using canned beans, and do not add additional salt.*

Preparation time: 25 minutes
Cooking time: 45–60 minutes (to cook beans)

1 pound dried black beans *
1 1/2 teaspoons salt
1 teaspoon cumin
2 cups corn, fresh or frozen
1 green pepper, coarsely chopped
1 red bell pepper, coarsely chopped
1 medium purple onion, finely chopped

Dressing:
1/4 cup Balsamic vinegar
1 tablespoon chopped fresh cilantro, or 1 teaspoon dried
1 teaspoon cumin
1/2 teaspoon coriander
Freshly ground pepper to taste
2 tablespoons olive oil

## Yield: 8 large salads

Per serving:
Calories...... 236
Protein (g)... 12
Fat (g)....... 4.4
Sat. Fat (g).. 0.7
Choles. (mg).. 0
Fiber (g)..... 11.6
Sodium (mg)... 415
%Cal-Fat...... 16%

# Garbanzo-Tomato Salad

1 pound cherry tomatoes, washed and dried
1 15 1/2-ounce can garbanzo beans, rinsed and drained
1 cup chopped celery
1/4 cup sliced green olives

Dressing:
3 tablespoons no-oil Italian dressing
2 tablespoons fresh lemon juice
2 teaspoons honey mustard
1/4 teaspoon salt
1/4 teaspoon freshly ground black pepper
1/4 cup chopped fresh parsley

**Yield: 6 to 8 servings**

**Per serving:**
Calories...... 129
Protein (g)... 6
Fat (g)....... 2.5
Sat. Fat (g).. 0.3
Choles. (mg).. 0
Fiber (g)..... 5.6
Sodium (mg)... 317
%Cal-Fat...... 17%

Cut tomatoes into quarters. Place in large mixing bowl. Add garbanzo beans, chopped celery and sliced olives.

To make dressing, whisk together Italian dressing, lemon juice, mustard, salt and pepper. Stir in parsley. Pour over garbanzo bean mixture. Mix well, making sure beans and vegetables are well coated. Let flavors marinate at least 2 hours before serving.

This salad may be made a day ahead of time.

Three medium-size tomatoes, chopped, may be substituted for the cherry tomatoes.

Preparation time: 20–25 minutes

# Mandarin Salad

Cook almonds and sugar in a small saucepan over medium heat, stirring constantly until sugar is dissolved and almonds are coated. Watch very carefully since the sugar can turn brown and burn. Cool to room temperature. Store in an airtight container to maintain freshness.

Make dressing by mixing all ingredients together. Chill until ready to serve.

Wash Romaine and Boston lettuce and tear into bite-size pieces. Add sliced onion and chopped celery. Just before serving, add sugared almonds and mandarin oranges. Pour dressing over and toss to coat greens evenly.

Preparation time: 30–35 minutes

1/4 cup sliced almonds
5 teaspoons sugar
1 head Romaine lettuce
1/2 head Boston lettuce
3 slices red onion, rings separated
1 cup chopped celery
1 11-ounce can mandarin oranges, drained

Salad Dressing:
2 tablespoons olive oil
1/4 cup wine vinegar
1/4 cup sugar
2 tablespoons chopped fresh parsley
1/2 teaspoon salt
Freshly ground pepper to taste
Dash of Tabasco sauce

*Yield: 8 servings*

*Per serving:*
Calories...... 108
Protein (g)... 1
Fat (g)....... 5.3
Sat. Fat (g).. 0.5
Choles. (mg).. 0
Fiber (g)..... 1.5
Sodium (mg)... 151
%Cal-Fat...... 43%

# Celestial Salad

1 head Romaine lettuce
1 11-ounce can mandarin
  oranges (drained)
1 cup seedless grapes (halved)
1/2 cup chopped green onions
1/2 cup sliced fresh mushrooms
1/4 cup sliced toasted almonds
  (optional)

Salad Dressing:
2 tablespoons olive or canola oil
1/4 cup sugar
1 teaspoon celery seeds
2 tablespoons chopped fresh
  parsley
2 tablespoons red wine vinegar
1/4 cup orange juice
1/2 teaspoon dry mustard

**Yield: 8 servings**

**Per serving:**
Calories...... 95
Protein (g)... 1
Fat (g)....... 3
Sat. Fat (g).. 0.6
Choles. (mg).. 0
Fiber (g)..... 2
Sodium (mg)... 8
%Cal-Fat...... 32%

Wash Romaine lettuce and tear into bite-size pieces. Add remaining salad ingredients, and 1/2 of the almonds, if using almonds.

To make dressing, combine all ingredients in a jar with a tight-fitting lid. Shake well. Just before serving, pour over greens. Toss lightly. Sprinkle remaining almonds over top, if desired.

*A sweet salad that is a perfect complement to a spicy or highly seasoned main dish. Spinach greens may be substituted for the Romaine, or a combination of Romaine and spinach may be used.*

Preparation time: 20–25 minutes

EAT, DRINK AND BE HEALTHY

# Spinach Salad with Honey Mustard Dressing

Wash spinach greens in cold water. Cut away the tough stems and discard. Drain leaves, wrap in paper towels, and place in plastic bag. Chill in refrigerator until ready to assemble salad.

Tear spinach leaves into bite-size pieces and place in large salad bowl. Top with sliced mushrooms and onion rings.

Make dressing by combining all ingredients in small bowl. Mix well with wire whisk. Pour over salad and toss.

*This spinach salad may also be assembled on individual salad plates with the honey mustard dressing drizzled over top.*

Preparation time: 25–30 minutes

10 to 12 ounces raw spinach
1/2 red onion, sliced thin
1 cup fresh mushrooms, sliced thin

Dressing:
1/4 cup honey
1 tablespoon Dijon mustard
1 tablespoon canola oil
2 tablespoons white wine
1/2 teaspoon Worcestershire sauce
2 teaspoons poppy seeds (optional)

**Yield: 6 servings**

**Per serving:**
Calories...... 91
Protein (g)... 3
Fat (g)....... 2.7
Sat. Fat (g).. 0.2
Choles. (mg).. 0
Fiber (g)..... 3
Sodium (mg)... 100
%Cal-Fat...... 24%

# Parsley-Wheat Salad (Tabouli)

1 cup fine or medium-grade
 bulgur
Water
1 cup finely chopped fresh
 parsley (about 1/2 bunch)
1 tablespoon minced fresh dill
 or 1 teaspoon dried
1/2 cup chopped green onions,
 including tops
2 medium tomatoes, diced
1 medium cucumber, peeled,
 deseeded, chopped
1/2 cup no-oil Italian dressing
Juice of 1/2 lemon
Freshly ground pepper to taste
Romaine lettuce leaves
Garnish: black olives, tomato
 wedges, parsley sprigs

### Yield: 4 to 6 servings

### Per serving:

Calories...... 137
Protein (g)... 5
Fat (g)....... 0.4
Sat. Fat (g).. 0
Choles. (mg).. 1
Fiber (g)..... 8.6
Sodium (mg)... 205
%Cal-Fat...... 2%

Place bulgur in large mixing bowl. Add water to cover and let stand about 1 hour or until bulgur has doubled in size and most of the liquid is absorbed. Drain well and squeeze dry.

Add parsley, dill, green onions, tomatoes and cucumber. Toss gently.

Add Italian dressing, lemon juice and pepper and toss until well mixed. Refrigerate.

To serve, line a salad bowl with Romaine leaves and mound Tabouli on top; or make individual servings by placing single piece of Romaine lettuce on plate and placing a scoop of Tabouli on top. Garnish with olives, tomato wedges and parsley sprigs.

*A delicious low-calorie version of tabouli, which is high in fiber with whole grain nutrients.*

Preparation time: 30 minutes (plus 1 hour to soak bulgur)

# Marinated Vegetable Salad

Bring about 8 cups water to a boil in large saucepan.

Meanwhile, cut up broccoli and cauliflower flowerets into bite-size pieces. Blanch vegetables by dropping into boiling water. When water returns to a second boil, drain vegetables immediately, and immerse in cold water to prevent further cooking.

Cut tomatoes in half and slice zucchini.

In a large bowl, combine all vegetables. Pour crunchy sprouts over top and mix together. Pour Italian dressing over all, and mix well, coating all vegetables.

For best results, let vegetables marinate at least 4 hours or overnight before serving.

*A colorful, nutritious, very low-fat dish which is a great accompaniment to a summer picnic meal.*

Preparation time: 20–25 minutes

Marinating time: 4–12 hours

*8 ounces broccoli flowerets (about 1 large stalk)*
*8 ounces cauliflower flowerets (about 1/2 head)*
*1 cup cherry tomatoes, halved*
*1 zucchini squash, sliced 1/8-inch thick*
*1/2 cup crunchy sprouts*
*1/2 to 3/4 cup no-oil Italian dressing*

### Yield: 6 large servings

**Per serving:**
Calories...... 37
Protein (g)... 3
Fat (g)....... 0.4
Sat. Fat (g).. 0.1
Choles. (mg).. 0
Fiber (g)..... 3.2
Sodium (mg)... 301
%Cal-Fat...... 8%

# Green Bean-Mushroom Salad

1 pound fresh green beans
1 small red onion, sliced and
   rings separated
3/4 cup sliced fresh mushrooms
12 black olives
Boston Bib or Romaine lettuce

Balsamic Vinegar Dressing:
2 tablespoons water
2 tablespoons Balsamic vinegar
1 tablespoon olive oil
1/4 teaspoon salt
Dash black pepper
1 tablespoon fresh parsley or
   basil, chopped

**Yield: 6 servings**

**Per serving:**
Calories...... 64
Protein (g)... 2
Fat (g)....... 3.4
Sat. Fat (g).. 0.5
Choles. (mg).. 0
Fiber (g)..... 3
Sodium (mg)... 174
%Cal-Fat...... 43%

Prepare Balsamic Vinegar dressing by combining all ingredients. Set aside.

To prepare beans, cut off tops. Bring water to a boil in medium saucepan. Add beans and boil for 8 minutes. Drain. Immediately immerse in ice water. Drain again. Pat dry and set aside.

Meanwhile slice red onion and separate rings. Wash mushrooms and slice.

Put beans, onion rings and mushrooms into large plastic container with an airtight lid. Pour dressing over. Marinate 1 to 2 hours. Occasionally turn over container to thoroughly cover vegetables with dressing.

Arrange lettuce leaves on salad plates. Carefully remove vegetables from marinade and place on lettuce leaves. Pour remaining dressing over individual salads. Garnish with black olives.

Preparation time: 30 minutes
Marinating time: 1 hour

# New Potato Salad

Place potatoes and enough water to cover them in medium-size saucepan. Bring to a boil. Simmer 25 minutes or until potatoes are tender. Drain and cool.

After potatoes are cooled, cut into bite-size pieces and put into large bowl. Add chopped celery, green onions and shredded carrot.

In small bowl, mix together mayonnaise, Catalina, skim milk and pickle juice. Add salt and pepper if desired. Pour over potato mixture and stir carefully until potatoes are evenly coated.

Preparation time: 20–25 minutes
Cooking time: 25 minutes (to cook potatoes)

*1 1/2 pounds new potatoes, unpeeled*
*2 ribs celery, chopped*
*1 bunch chopped green onions, including tops*
*1 carrot shredded*
*1/2 cup nonfat mayonnaise*
*2 tablespoons nonfat Catalina dressing*
*2 tablespoons skim milk*
*2 tablespoons dill pickle juice*
*Salt and pepper to taste*

### Yield: 6 servings

### Per serving:
Calories...... 124
Protein (g)... 4
Fat (g)....... 0.2
Sat. Fat (g).. 0.1
Choles. (mg).. 0
Fiber (g)..... 5.4
Sodium (mg)... 500
%Cal-Fat...... 2%

4 medium-size potatoes
1/2 cup chopped celery
3/4 cup chopped onions
1/4 cup chopped fresh parsley
1/4 cup bread and butter
  pickles, finely chopped
1 cup nonfat sour cream
1/4 cup light mayonnaise
1 teaspoon seasoned salt
1/4 teaspoon pepper
1 1/2 tablespoons fresh dillweed
  or 1 1/2 teaspoons dried
3/4 teaspoon horseradish
3 tablespoons juice from bread
  and butter pickles
2 tablespoons skim milk

**Yield: 6 servings**

**Per serving:**
Calories...... 105
Protein (g)... 1
Fat (g)....... 3.5
Sat. Fat (g).. 0.7
Choles. (mg).. 0
Fiber (g)..... 1.7
Sodium (mg)... 367
%Cal-Fat...... 30%

# "Sour Cream" Potato Salad

Boil potatoes, unpeeled, until soft, but slightly firm. Cool. Peel potatoes and cut into 1/2-inch cubes.

In large bowl, combine chopped potatoes, celery, onions, parsley and pickles.

Combine remaining ingredients in medium-size bowl. Add to potatoes and mix well. For best results, cover and refrigerate at least 4 hours before serving.

Preparation time: 25–30 minutes
Cooking time: 30 minutes (to cook potatoes)

3 apples, cored, cut into bite-
  size pieces
1/2 cup chopped celery
1/4 cup raisins
1/4 cup walnuts, coarsely
  chopped (optional)
1 cup vanilla low-fat yogurt

**Yield: 4 to 6 servings**

**Per serving:**
Calories...... 140
Protein (g)... 3
Fat (g)....... 1
Sat. Fat (g).. 0.5
Choles. (mg).. 2
Fiber (g)..... 3.4
Sodium (mg)... 41
%Cal-Fat...... 6%

# Slim Waldorf Salad

In medium-size bowl, combine apples, celery, raisins and walnuts. Stir in yogurt until well mixed.

*Omit walnuts if trying to reduce calories and fat.*

Preparation time: 15–20 minutes

# Tropical Fruit Slaw

Section oranges. Toss banana slices in orange juice and drain. In a large bowl combine fruits, cabbage and celery.

Add yogurt and toss lightly to coat. Cover and serve immediately or refrigerate for up to 3 hours before serving.

If desired, sprinkle with almonds.

Preparation time: 20–25 minutes

*2 medium oranges, peeled*
*1 medium banana, sliced*
*2 tablespoons orange juice*
*1 8-ounce can pineapple chunks, drained*
*3 cups finely shredded cabbage*
*1 cup thinly sliced celery*
*1 8-ounce carton low-fat lemon yogurt*
*2 tablespoons slivered almonds (optional)*

### Yield: 8 to 10 servings

**Per serving:**
Calories...... 67
Protein (g)... 2.2
Fat (g)....... 0.6
Sat. Fat (g).. 0.3
Choles. (mg).. 2
Fiber (g)..... 2
Sodium (mg)... 34
%Cal-Fat...... 7%

# Creamy Cucumber Salad

Wash cucumbers (peel if skin has waxy coating). Cut into slices about 1/8-inch thick. Place in large bowl and sprinkle with salt. Let soak for 1 hour. Rinse salt from cucumbers and drain well. Add chopped onion.

In small bowl, combine yogurt and sugar. Pour over cucumbers and mix well. Salad tastes best if refrigerated at least 1 hour before serving.

Preparation time: 15 minutes
Soaking time: 1 hour

*4 cups sliced cucumbers*
*1/2 teaspoon salt*
*1 tablespoon chopped onion*
*1/2 cup plain nonfat yogurt*
*2 tablespoons sugar*

### Yield: 8 servings

**Per serving:**
Calories...... 40
Protein (g)... 2
Fat (g)....... 0.2
Sat. Fat (g).. 0.1
Choles. (mg).. 0
Fiber (g)..... 1.5
Sodium (mg)... 147
%Cal-Fat...... 5%

## Lemon-Tahini Salad Dressing

1/3 cup sesame tahini
1/4 cup lemon juice
2 or 3 cloves garlic, minced
1/4 cup cold water
1/4 teaspoon salt
1/4 teaspoon pepper

**Yield: 3/4 cup salad dressing, or 6 to 8 servings**

**Per 1-tablespoon serving**
Calories...... 43
Protein (g)... 1
Fat (g)....... 3.8
Sat. Fat (g).. 0.5
Choles. (mg).. 0
Fiber (g)..... 0.7
Sodium (mg)... 47
%Cal-Fat...... 73%

Combine all ingredients in food processor. Blend until well mixed. Serve immediately, or if thicker dressing is desired, let it set overnight.

Preparation time: 15 minutes

## Fresh Cranberry Molded Salad

1 12-ounce package fresh whole cranberries
4 apples, chopped with peelings
3/4 cup sugar
1 6-ounce package lemon jello
1 1/2 cups boiling water
1 1/2 cups cold water
3/4 cup celery, chopped
1/2 cup walnuts, chopped

**Yield: 16 servings**

**Per serving:**
Calories...... 87
Protein (g)... 2
Fat (g)....... 1.4
Sat. Fat (g).. 0.1
Choles. (mg).. 0
Fiber (g)..... 2
Sodium (mg)... 42
%Cal-Fat...... 14%

Wash cranberries. Coarsely chop in food processor. Place in large mixing bowl. Core apples, cut into quarters, and chop in food processor. Add to cranberries. Add sugar. Set aside for 2 to 3 hours or overnight.

Pour package of jello into large bowl. Add 1 1/2 cups boiling water and stir until completely dissolved. Add 1 1/2 cups cold water.

Place in refrigerator until jello begins to thicken or set. Add cranberry mixture, celery and walnuts.

Spray a 6 1/2 to 8-cup jello mold with vegetable cooking spray. Pour jello into mold. Refrigerate until jello is firm, about 2 to 4 hours.

To serve, loosen edges and unmold jello onto a platter covered with lettuce leaves.

*Jello salad may be made a day before it is served. It can also be made in a 9 x 9-inch square pan and cut into squares and served on lettuce leaves.*

Preparation time: 20–25 minutes

Marinating time: 3–12 hours

# Cranberry Fruit Salad

Dissolve gelatin in boiling water. Add cold water, crushed pineapple (including juice), and cranberry sauce. Mix until well blended. Chill until partially set. Fold in celery and walnuts.

Spray a 6-cup ring mold with vegetable cooking spray. Pour jello into mold. Chill until firm. Loosen edges of jello and unmold on crisp greens.

Preparation time: 15–20 minutes

2 3-ounce packages lemon-flavored gelatin
2 cups boiling water
1 cup cold water
1 8-ounce can crushed pineapple, in its own juice
1 16-ounce can whole berry cranberry sauce
1 cup chopped celery
1/4 cup chopped walnuts (optional)

**Yield: 8 to 10 servings**

**Per serving:**
Calories...... 147
Protein (g)... 2
Fat (g)....... 0
Sat. Fat (g).. 0
Choles. (mg).. 0
Fiber (g)..... 1.5
Sodium (mg)... 76
%Cal-Fat...... 1%

**With walnuts:**
Fat (g)....... 2.3
%Cal-Fat...... 12%

# Orange Mandarin Ring

1 6-ounce package orange jello
2 cups boiling water
1 20-ounce can crushed
 pineapple, with juice
1 11-ounce can mandarin
 oranges, drained
1/2 cup orange juice
1/4 cup chopped walnuts

**Yield: 12 to 16 servings**

**Per serving:**
Calories...... 93
Protein (g)... 2
Fat (g)....... 1.2
Sat. Fat (g).. 0.l
Choles. (mg).. 0
Fiber (g)..... 1
Sodium (mg)... 34
%Cal-Fat...... 12%

Dissolve orange jello in 2 cups boiling water. Stir in crushed pineapple (with juice), mandarin oranges (drained) and orange juice. Chill until partially set. Stir in chopped walnuts.

Spray a 6 1/2-cup ring mold with vegetable cooking spray. Pour jello mixture into mold. Chill until firm. Loosen edges and unmold on crisp greens.

Preparation time: 15–20 minutes

# Grapefruit Salad

3 envelopes unflavored gelatin
3/4 cup cold water
1/4 cup orange juice
3/4 cup sugar
1 cup boiling water
3 large pink grapefruits, peeled
 and cut into sections
1 14-ounce can crushed
 pineapple, in its own juice
 (reserve juice)
1/4 cup slivered almonds

**Yield: 9 servings**

**Per serving:**
Calories...... 150
Protein (g)... 4
Fat (g)....... 2
Sat. Fat (g).. 0.2
Choles. (mg).. 0
Fiber (g)..... 2.2
Sodium (mg)... 5
%Cal-Fat...... 12%

Combine cold water and orange juice in small bowl. Soften gelatin in cold water mixture. Dissolve sugar in boiling water. In large bowl, combine gelatin and sugar water. Refrigerate until partially set.

Meanwhile, prepare grapefruits by peeling, breaking into sections, and removing filaments. Cut each section in half. Fold grapefruit sections, pineapple with juice, and almonds into gelatin-sugar mixture. Pour into an 8-inch square baking dish or a 6-cup mold. Refrigerate until set, about 3 hours.

Unmold over lettuce or cut into 2 1/2-inch squares and serve over single leaf of lettuce.

Preparation time: 35 minutes

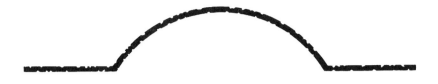

# Vegetables & Cooked Fruit

Baked Tomatoes with Spinach • Baked Tomatoes • Tomatoes with Chopped Herbs • Steamed Vegetable Medley • Mashed Potatoes with Chives • Red Potatoes with Creamy Dill Sauce • Herbed Red Potatoes • Vegetable Stir-Fry • Sweet Potato Casserole • Scrumptious Asparagus • Peas Parisienne • Beans and Mushrooms • Steamed Carrots with Onions • Green Beans Amandine • Stir-Fried Broccoli •Snow-Capped Broccoli • Sesame Broccoli • Ratatouille • Zucchini-Mushroom Casserole • Artichoke Wedges with Tomatoes • Spinach-Artichoke Casserole • Spiced Fruit Compote • Baked Apple-Date Delight

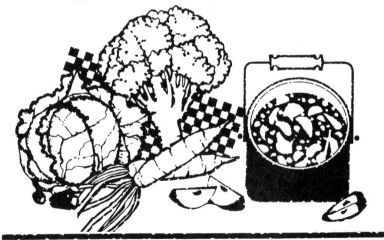

3 green onions, chopped,
  including tops
1 teaspoon olive oil
1 10-ounce package frozen
  chopped spinach
1/2 cup bread crumbs
2 egg substitutes (1/2 cup)
1/4 teaspoon salt
1/2 teaspoon thyme
1/4 teaspoon black pepper
1/4 cup grated Parmesan
  cheese, divided
4 large sun-ripened tomatoes

**Yield: 8 servings**

**Per serving:**
Calories...... 82
Protein (g)... 7
Fat (g)....... 1.8
Sat. Fat (g).. 0.7
Choles. (mg).. 4
Fiber (g)..... 2
Sodium (mg)... 190
%Cal-Fat...... 18%

# Baked Tomatoes with Spinach

Preheat oven to 350 degrees.

Sauté onions in olive oil, until tender. Thaw spinach and drain. Lightly squeeze out excess water.

Combine spinach, onions, bread crumbs, egg substitutes, salt, thyme, pepper and 2 tablespoons Parmesan cheese in a large mixing bowl. Mix until well blended.

Cut each tomato into 2 thick slices and cut out top stem. Arrange slices, cut side up, on a non-stick baking dish and top with mounds of spinach mixture. Sprinkle with remaining Parmesan cheese.

Bake at 350 degrees for 20 to 30 minutes or until tomato is slightly soft.

Preparation time: 20 minutes

Cooking time: 20–30 minutes

---

3 fresh tomatoes
2 tablespoons bread crumbs,
  plain or seasoned
1 tablespoon Parmesan cheese
Chopped fresh parsley
Parsley sprigs for garnish

**Yield: 6 servings.**

**Per serving:**
Calories...... 32
Protein (g)... 1
Fat (g)....... 0.7
Sat. Fat (g).. 0.2
Choles. (mg).. 0
Fiber (g)..... 1.5
Sodium (mg)... 40
%Cal-Fat...... 17%

# Baked Tomatoes

Cut tomatoes in half and cut out top stem. Place cut side up in a baking dish, and sprinkle with bread crumbs, Parmesan cheese and parsley.

Bake at 350 degrees for 20 minutes or until slightly soft and heated through. Garnish serving dish with fresh parsley sprigs.

Preparation time: 5–10 minutes

Cooking time: 20 minutes

# Tomatoes with Chopped Herbs

Slice tomatoes and arrange on platter. Sprinkle with herbs and pepper. Serve chilled or at room temperature.

Preparation time: 5 minutes

3 tomatoes, sliced
1 tablespoon chopped fresh parsley
1 tablespoon chopped fresh basil
Freshly ground black pepper

**Yield: 6 servings**

**Per serving:**
Calories...... 14
Protein (g)... 1
Fat (g)....... 0.1
Sat. Fat (g).. 0
Choles. (mg).. 0
Fiber (g)..... 1
Sodium (mg)... 6
%Cal-Fat...... 12%

# Steamed Vegetable Medley

Prepare vegetables: Peel carrots, cut into 3-inch lengths, cut again in half lengthwise; peel potato, cut into strips approximately the size of carrots; cut ends from green beans; cut the roots off leeks, cut each leek into 3-inch lengths and wash thoroughly (or do the same with green onions).

Arrange vegetables on steamer rack placed in a large kettle. Skim fat from top of chicken broth. Pour broth over vegetables. Cover kettle with lid, and place on stove. Bring to a boil, reduce heat and steam slowly about 20 minutes, or until vegetables are tender.

Arrange vegetables on a single platter, sprinkle immediately with *Butter Buds* and minced parsley. Garnish with sprigs of parsley.

*Other vegetables may be used in place of those given in this recipe, including rutabagas, turnips or broccoli. Cut into approximately equal-size pieces, and try to include an assortment of colors to create an eye-appealing dish.*

Preparation time: 20 minutes
Cooking time: 25 minutes

3 large carrots
1 large potato
1/2 pound fresh green beans
3 leeks or bunch green onions
1 14 1/2-ounce can clear chicken broth, defatted
Butter Buds (powdered butter flavor without fat)
Fresh parsley for garnish

**Yield: 4 or 5 servings**

**Per serving:**
Calories...... 78
Protein (g)... 2
Fat (g)....... 0.3
Sat. Fat (g).. 0
Choles. (mg).. 0
Fiber (g)..... 4.8
Sodium (mg)... 26
%Cal-Fat...... 3%

# Mashed Potatoes with Chives

4 large potatoes, peeled and cut
   into chunks
3/4 cup skim milk, heated
3 tablespoons dry nonfat milk
   powder
1 tablespoon tub margarine
1 tablespoon powdered butter
   flavoring (no fat)
1/2 teaspoon seasoned salt
1/4 teaspoon black pepper
1 tablespoon chopped chives or
   green onions
2 tablespoons finely chopped
   fresh parsley
1/4 cup Parmesan cheese

**Yield: 8 servings**

**Per serving:**
Calories...... 96
Protein (g)... 4
Fat (g)....... 2.1
Sat. Fat (g).. 0.9
Choles. (mg).. 3
Fiber (g)..... 1
Sodium (mg)... 233
%Cal-Fat...... 20%

In large pot, boil potatoes in water until soft. Drain. Transfer potatoes to large mixing bowl.

In large mixing bowl, combine potatoes, 1/2 cup warmed milk, milk powder, margarine, butter flavoring, seasoned salt and pepper. Whip with electric mixer until smooth. Add remainder of milk, if needed for proper consistency. Add green onions, parsley and Parmesan cheese. Stir until well blended.

Serve immediately, or place in covered casserole and heat up just before serving.

*It is important to heat the milk before adding to potatoes. If cold milk is added, mashed potatoes will have a rubbery texture.*

Preparation time: 15–20 minutes
Cooking time: 20–25 minutes

# Red Potatoes with Creamy Dill Sauce

Scrub potatoes. Cook in boiling water until tender, about 20 to 25 minutes.

Meanwhile, in small bowl, mix flour and skim milk with wire whisk until smooth. Pour into medium saucepan and heat on stove. Add remaining ingredients. Cook until sauce comes to a boil and thickens.

After potatoes have been cooked, drain water. Cut into quarters. Add to white sauce and mix, covering potatoes with sauce.

Preparation time: 20 minutes
Cooking time: 20–30 minutes

*2 pounds small red potatoes*
*1/4 cup flour*
*1 1/2 cups skim milk*
*2 tablespoons dry white wine*
*1 tablespoon finely chopped chives*
*1 tablespoon chopped fresh dill (or 1 teaspoon dried)*
*1/2 teaspoon salt, or to taste*
*1/4 teaspoon pepper*

**Yield: 6 servings**

**Per serving:**
Calories...... 161
Protein (g)... 7
Fat (g)....... 0.3
Sat. Fat (g).. 0.1
Choles. (mg).. 1
Fiber (g)..... 6
Sodium (mg)... 231
%Cal-Fat...... 2%

# Herbed Red Potatoes

Scrub potatoes. Cook, unpeeled, in boiling water until soft, about 30 minutes. Drain water.

Cut potatoes into quarters. Sprinkle with Butter Buds* and fresh parsley or basil. Serve immediately.

*Small red potatoes may be used instead. Before cooking, remove a 3/4-inch strip of peeling from around center of potato. Boil in water until tender, about 20 minutes. Drain, and sprinkle immediately with* Butter Buds* *and parsley.*

*Contains the natural flavor of butter without the fat.

Preparation time: 10–15 minutes
Cooking time: 20–30 minutes

*4 medium red potatoes*
*1 tablespoon Butter Buds\**
*Fresh parsley or basil, finely chopped*

**Yield: 4 servings**

**Per serving:**
Calories...... 107
Protein (g)... 4
Fat (g)....... 0.1
Sat. Fat (g).. 0
Choles. (mg).. 0
Fiber (g)..... 5.3
Sodium (mg)... 20
%Cal-Fat...... 1%

1 tablespoon reduced-sodium
  soy sauce
1 teaspoon brown sugar
2 teaspoons olive oil
1/2 pound fresh or frozen
  Chinese snow peas
1/2 cup sliced fresh mushrooms
1/2 cup fresh or canned bean
  sprouts (drained)
1/2 red pepper, cut into narrow
  2-inch strips
1 8-ounce can sliced water
  chestnuts, drained

**Yield: 4 servings**

**Per serving:**
Calories...... 87
Protein (g)... 3
Fat (g)....... 2.5
Sat. Fat (g).. 0.3
Choles. (mg).. 0
Fiber (g)..... 3.5
Sodium (mg)... 166
%Cal-Fat...... 24%

# Vegetable Stir-Fry

Prepare vegetables. Set aside.

In small bowl, combine soy sauce and sugar, stirring well.

Heat oil in sauté pan. Add snow peas, mushrooms, bean sprouts, red pepper and water chestnuts. Stir-fry for 3 minutes. Add soy sauce mixture. Stir well and sauté an additional 1 to 2 minutes, or until crisp-tender.

Preparation time: 25–30 minutes

2 medium sweet potatoes
1/4 cup reserved cooking liquid
2 tablespoons packed brown
  sugar
1 egg substitute (1/4 cup)
2 tablespoons chopped pecans

**Yield: 4 servings**

**Per serving:**
Calories...... 140
Protein (g)... 3
Fat (g)....... 3
Sat. Fat (g).. 0.3
Choles. (mg).. 0
Fiber (g)..... 2.5
Sodium (mg)... 39
%Cal-Fat...... 19%

# Sweet Potato Casserole

Peel potatoes and cut into sections. Place in medium saucepan and cover with water. Bring to a boil over high heat. Reduce heat and simmer until soft, about 15 to 20 minutes.

Drain potatoes, reserving 1/4 cup liquid. In mixing bowl, combine potatoes, cooking liquid and brown sugar. Beat at high speed with electric mixer until smooth. Add egg substitute and mix well. Stir in nuts. Add more water if too thick.

Spoon into small casserole dish. Sprinkle with brown sugar. Bake, uncovered, at 350 degrees for 30 minutes.

Preparation time: 15 minutes
Cooking time: 45–50 minutes

# Scrumptious Asparagus

Remove tough ends from fresh asparagus spears. Steam asparagus in vegetable steamer until tender, about 10 to 15 minutes.

Meanwhile, finely chop anchovy fillets, garlic and parsley.

Pour olive oil into a small saucepan. Add chopped mixture and pepper. Cook and stir occasionally over low heat for 5 minutes. Add lemon juice.

Drain asparagus thoroughly and transfer to a serving dish. Pour sauce over. Serve immediately.

*Sauce may be made ahead and heated just before serving.*

Preparation time: 20–25 minutes

2 pounds fresh asparagus
    spears or 2 10-ounce packages
    frozen
6 anchovy fillets
1 clove garlic, minced
3 sprigs fresh parsley, finely
    chopped
1 tablespoon olive oil
1/8 teaspoon white pepper
Juice of 1 lemon

**Yield: 6 to 8 servings**

**Per serving:**
Calories...... 51
Protein (g)... 5
Fat (g)....... 1.9
Sat. Fat (g).. 0.5
Choles. (mg).. 3
Fiber (g)..... 2
Sodium (mg)... 149
%Cal-Fat...... 28%

# Peas Parisienne

Combine all ingredients in medium saucepan. Simmer for 8 to 10 minutes over medium heat until peas are cooked through. Stir occasionally and add more water if peas stick to bottom.

*Spinach or other greens may be substituted for the Boston lettuce.*

Preparation time: 10 minutes

Cooking time: 10 minutes

1 16-ounce package frozen peas
2 cups Boston lettuce, shredded
1 teaspoon tub margarine
2 tablespoons water
1/4 teaspoon marjoram
1/4 teaspoon salt
1/2 teaspoon sugar

**Yield: 4 to 6 servings**

**Per serving:**
Calories...... 85
Protein (g)... 5
Fat (g)....... 1
Sat. Fat (g).. 0.2
Choles. (mg).. 0
Fiber (g)..... 4.6
Sodium (mg)... 20
%Cal-Fat...... 10%

# Beans and Mushrooms

2 10-ounce packages frozen
  French-style green beans
1/2 cup sliced fresh mushrooms
1/4 cup sliced green onions,
  including tops
2 teaspoons olive oil
1 1/2 teaspoons chopped fresh
  basil
2 tablespoons no-oil Italian
  salad dressing

Yield: 6 servings

Per serving:
Calories...... 35
Protein (g)... 2
Fat (g)....... 1
Sat. Fat (g).. 0.2
Choles. (mg).. 0
Fiber (g)..... 3.2
Sodium (mg)... 52
%Cal-Fat...... 21%

Cook beans according to package directions.

Meanwhile, in a nonstick skillet, sauté mushrooms and green onions in olive oil, stirring frequently. Sauté for about 5 minutes, or until mushrooms turn dark in color.

Add cooked beans (drained), basil and salad dressing to mushroom mixture and heat through. Serve immediately.

Preparation time: 20 minutes

# Steamed Carrots with Onions

6 large carrots, peeled and
  sliced
1 medium onion, sliced thin
2 teaspoons tub margarine

Yield: 4 to 5 servings

Per serving:
Calories...... 61
Protein (g)... 1
Fat (g)....... 1.8
Sat. Fat (g).. 0.3
Choles. (mg).. 0
Fiber (g)..... 3.4
Sodium (mg)... 56
%Cal-Fat...... 26%

Slice carrots crosswise about 1/8-inch thick. Steam in vegetable steamer, or steaming basket placed in saucepan with small amount of water, for 10 minutes or until carrots are soft.

Meanwhile, melt margarine in small sauté pan or skillet. Separate sliced onion into rings and sauté in margarine until onion is soft and translucent, but not brown.

Mix carrots with sautéed onion and serve immediately.

Preparation time: 15 minutes

# Green Beans Amandine

Wash beans and cut off ends.

Place vegetable steamer rack in large saucepan. Pour in clear chicken broth. Add water if desired, but be sure to keep water level below steamer rack. Add beans. Bring water/broth mixture to a boil. Steam beans 15 to 20 minutes or until desired tenderness.

Lift rack out of sauce pan. Pour beans into serving dish. Top with margarine and toss until all beans are coated and margarine is melted. Sprinkle with sliced almonds. Serve immediately.

Preparation time: 10–15 minutes
Cooking time: 15–20 minutes

*1 pound fresh string beans*
*14 ounces clear chicken broth, defatted*
*2 teaspoons margarine*
*2 tablespoons sliced almonds*

**Yield: 6 servings**

**Per serving:**
Calories...... 60
Protein (g)... 3
Fat (g)....... 2.9
Sat. Fat (g).. 0.5
Choles. (mg).. 0
Fiber (g)..... 2
Sodium (mg)... 238
%Cal-Fat...... 41%

# Stir-Fried Broccoli

Peel broccoli stem. Slice stem and flowerets into bite-size pieces. (Stem slices should be no more than 1/4-inch thick.)

Pour olive oil into skillet or sauté pan. Add broccoli pieces and water. Sauté, covering pan when not stirring, until crisp-tender, about 5 to 10 minutes. Sprinkle soy sauce over broccoli while sautéing. (Add additional water if necessary to keep broccoli from sticking or scorching.)

Preparation time: 10–15 minutes

*1 large stalk broccoli (3 to 4 cups chopped)*
*1 1/2 teaspoons olive oil*
*2 tablespoons water*
*1 tablespoon reduced-sodium soy sauce, or to taste*

**Yield: 4 servings**

**Per serving:**
Calories...... 33
Protein (g)... 0
Fat (g)....... 1.7
Sat. Fat (g).. 0
Choles. (mg).. 0
Fiber (g)..... 2
Sodium (mg)... 168
%Cal-Fat...... 46%

# Snow-Capped Broccoli

1 large bunch fresh broccoli, or
 2 10-ounce packages frozen
 broccoli
2 egg whites
1 tablespoon low-calorie Ranch
 dressing
2 tablespoons grated Parmesan
 cheese
1/4 cup chopped green onions,
 including tops

**Yield: Makes 6 to 8 servings**

**Per serving:**
Calories...... 37
Protein (g)... 4
Fat (g)....... 0.7
Sat. Fat (g).. 0.3
Choles. (mg).. 2
Fiber (g)..... 2.4
Sodium (mg)... 72
%Cal-Fat...... 17%

Preheat oven to 350 degrees.

Cut broccoli into spears. Steam broccoli for 10 minutes or until done.

Meanwhile, beat egg whites with an electric mixer until stiff peaks form. Gently fold in Ranch dressing, Parmesan cheese and green onions. Set aside.

Arrange cooked broccoli in a circular pattern on a 9-inch oven-proof dish or pie plate, with stem ends toward center and flowerets toward the outside.

Spoon the egg-white mixture onto the center of the platter over the broccoli stems, leaving the flowerets exposed. Sprinkle lightly with additional Parmesan cheese. Bake in 350-degree oven for 12 to 15 minutes, until topping is golden.

Preparation time: 20–25 minutes
Cooking time: 12–15 minutes

# Sesame Broccoli

1 bunch broccoli (or 2 10-ounce
 packages, frozen)
1 tablespoon tub margarine
1 tablespoon sesame seeds
Salt to taste, if desired

**Yield: 6 to 8 servings**

**Per serving:**
Calories...... 41
Protein (g)... 3
Fat (g)....... 2
Sat. Fat (g).. 0.4
Choles. (mg).. 0
Fiber (g)..... 2.5
Sodium (mg)... 40
%Cal-Fat...... 37%

Wash broccoli and separate into spears. Place in vegetable steamer and steam until broccoli is crisp-tender, about 10 to 15 minutes.

Meanwhile melt margarine in small saucepan. Add sesame seeds and sauté until lightly browned. Just before serving, sprinkle sesame seeds evenly over broccoli.

Preparation time: 10 minutes
Cooking time: 10–15 minutes

# *Ratatouille*

Preheat oven to 375 degrees.

Cut eggplant into half-inch slices. Cut again into half-inch cubes. Cut up green pepper, onion and zucchini as indicated.

Place eggplant cubes in a large baking dish or casserole. Lightly sprinkle with salt. Add separate layers of green pepper, onion and zucchini. Press down lightly with palms of hands to make more compact.

In medium-size mixing bowl, stir together chopped tomatoes, tomato sauce, and minced garlic. Pour over vegetables. Drizzle olive oil over top, if desired.

Bake, uncovered, in 375-degree oven for 1 1/4 to 1 1/2 hours. Remove from oven and wait 5 minutes before serving. Stir ratatouille well before serving.

Preparation time: 25–30 minutes
Cooking time: 1 1/4 hours

*1 eggplant, 1 to 1 1/2 pounds, unpeeled*
*1 green pepper, sliced into 1/4 x 2-inch strips*
*1 large onion, thinly sliced, rings separated*
*1 zucchini, unpeeled and sliced thin*
*16-ounces canned or fresh tomatoes, chopped coarsely*
*1 8-ounce can "no salt added" tomato sauce*
*2 cloves garlic, minced*
*2 teaspoons olive oil (optional)*
*Black pepper to taste*

### *Yield: 6 servings*

*Per serving:*
Calories...... 73
Protein (g)... 3.6
Fat (g)....... 0.4
Sat. Fat (g).. 0.1
Choles. (mg).. 0
Fiber (g)..... 6.4
Sodium (mg)... 146
%Cal-Fat...... 5%

# Zucchini-Mushroom Casserole

Vegetable cooking spray
2 medium onions, chopped
2 cloves garlic, minced
8 ounces fresh mushrooms, sliced
3 pounds zucchini (4 large zucchini), cut in half lengthwise and sliced
1 28-ounce can crushed tomatoes
2 teaspoons oregano
1 teaspoon onion powder
1 teaspoon garlic powder
1/4 cup Parmesan cheese
4 egg whites
2 tablespoons Parmesan cheese

### Yield: 8 servings

### Per serving:
Calories...... 105
Protein (g)... 7.7
Fat (g)....... 2.2
Sat. Fat (g).. 1
Choles. (mg).. 4
Fiber (g)..... 4
Sodium (mg)... 282
%Cal-Fat...... 19%

Spray large nonstick skillet with vegetable cooking spray. With lid on, sauté onions, garlic and mushrooms until tender. Add sliced zucchini to skillet and simmer, covered, over medium heat for 30 minutes.

Meanwhile, in medium-size mixing bowl, combine crushed tomatoes, oregano, onion powder and garlic powder. Add to zucchini mixture. Bring to a boil and simmer, covered, 15 minutes. Add 1/4 cup Parmesan cheese.

In small mixing bowl, combine egg whites and 2 tablespoons Parmesan cheese. Beat with wire whisk until eggs are slightly frothy. Add to skillet and cook 5 to 10 minutes or until egg whites solidify. Serve immediately.

Preparation time: 30 minutes
Cooking time: 1 hour

# Artichoke Wedges with Tomatoes

1 14-ounce can artichoke hearts, packed in water
Juice of 1 lemon
1/2 cup chopped onion
1 tablespoon olive oil
2 cloves garlic, minced
1 28-ounce can tomatoes
Pepper, to taste
2 tablespoons chopped fresh parsley

%Cal-Fat...... 28%

Drain can of artichoke hearts. Cut each artichoke into 8 equal wedges. Put into medium-size bowl along with 1 cup water and juice of lemon. Set aside.

In a 10- or 12-inch frypan, sauté chopped onion in olive oil over low heat until onion becomes translucent. Add garlic and sauté 30 seconds longer.

Break up tomato pieces with a spoon. Add to frypan, and simmer for 3 to 4 minutes.

242

Drain artichoke mixture and add to tomato mixture. Add pepper to taste.

Simmer, partially covered, 45 minutes, stirring occasionally. If mixture becomes too thick, add water. If it is too thin, boil rapidly with cover removed. Immediately before serving, add parsley and mix well.

*This is a very tasty vegetable dish. The artichokes provide an excellent source of fiber.*

Preparation time: 20–25 minutes
Cooking time: 45 minutes

**Yield: 6 to 8 servings**

**Per serving:**
Calories...... 71
Protein (g)... 3
Fat (g)....... 2.5
Sat. Fat (g).. 0.4
Choles. (mg).. 0
Fiber (g)..... 5.7
Sodium (mg)... 215

# Spinach-Artichoke Casserole

Preheat oven to 350 degrees.

Cook spinach according to package directions. Drain well, lightly squeezing out excess water.

Sauté onion in olive oil until onion becomes translucent. Drain artichoke hearts and cut into quarters.

Combine spinach, sautéed onion, artichokes, sour cream and 1/4 cup Parmesan cheese. Place in casserole dish. Sprinkle the remaining 2 tablespoons Parmesan cheese over top.

Bake at 350 degrees for 30 minutes. Serve hot.

Preparation time: 20 minutes
Cooking time: 30 minutes

*2 10-ounce packages frozen chopped spinach*
*1 tablespoon olive oil*
*1/2 cup finely chopped onion*
*1 14-ounce can artichoke hearts, packed in water*
*3/4 cup nonfat sour cream*
*6 tablespoons Parmesan cheese, divided*
*Pepper to taste*

**Yield: 8 to 10 servings**

**Per serving:**
Calories...... 79
Protein (g)... 6
Fat (g)....... 2.6
Sat. Fat (g).. 1.1
Choles. (mg).. 4
Fiber (g)..... 5.1
Sodium (mg)... 185
%Cal-Fat...... 27%

# Spiced Fruit Compote

1 16-ounce can apricot halves,
  in light syrup
1 16-ounce can peach halves, in
  light syrup
1 16-ounce can pear halves, in
  light syrup
1 8-ounce can pineapple tidbits,
  in its own juice
1/3 cup orange juice
2 tablespoons brown sugar
1 teaspoon grated orange rind
1 teaspoon grated lemon rind
4 ounces chopped dates

**Yield: 8 servings**

**Per serving:**
Calories...... 199
Protein (g)... 1.4
Fat (g)....... 0.3
Sat. Fat (g).. 0.1
Choles. (mg).. 0
Fiber (g)..... 4.9
Sodium (mg)... 9
%Cal-Fat...... 1%

Drain fruit, reserving liquid from each can. Cut apricots, peaches and pears into bite-size pieces. Combine fruits and set aside.

Combine reserved juices, orange juice, brown sugar and grated rinds in saucepan. Bring to a boil and simmer, uncovered, until liquid is reduced by half (about 10 to 15 minutes). If it's too sweet, add lemon juice to taste.

Add fruits to juice just before serving and heat through.

*If making ahead, store fruit and juices separately. Combine just before heating and serving. This makes an excellent meat accompaniment.*

Preparation time: 20 minutes
Cooking time: 20 minutes

# Baked Apple-Date Delight

8 baking apples (with skins)
1 cup chopped dates
1/2 cup firmly packed brown
  sugar
1/4 cup walnuts or pecans
1 teaspoon cinnamon
1/2 teaspoon nutmeg

**Yield: 10 servings**

**Per serving:**
Calories...... 209
Protein (g)... 1
Fat (g)....... 2.6
Sat. Fat (g).. 0.3
Choles. (mg).. 0
Fiber (g)..... 5.4
Sodium (mg)... 4
%Cal-Fat...... 10%

Preheat oven to 350 degrees.

Core apples and cut into bite-size pieces. (Do not peel.) Place in large bowl. Add remaining ingredients and mix well. Spoon into oven-proof casserole.

Bake, covered, for one hour. Check after 30 to 40 minutes and uncover if too juicy.

Preparation time: 20–25 minutes
Cooking time: 1 hour

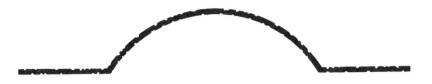

# *Poultry*

Herbed Chicken-Rice Casserole • Chicken with Wine and Mushrooms • Chicken a la King • Chicken and Dumplings • Chicken-Garbanzo Stir-Fry • Stir-Fried Chicken and Vegetables • Crunchy Chicken Casserole • Spicy Chicken and Pasta • Chicken Cordon Bleu • Breast of Chicken Beaufort • Chicken-Seafood Artichoke Casserole • Chicken Cacciatore • Beijing Chicken Stir-Fry • Chicken L'Orange • Coq au Vin • Grilled Breast of Chicken Sandwich • Barbecued Shredded Turkey Breast • Turkey Parmigiana • Stuffed Turkey Cutlets • Nonfat Turkey Gravy

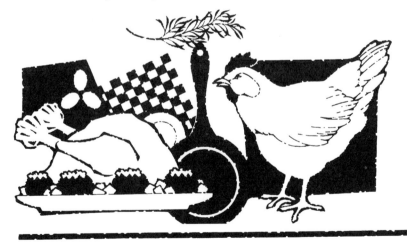

# Herbed Chicken-Rice Casserole

1 tablespoon canola oil
1/4 cup flour
2 1/2-pound fryer chicken, cut
  up, or 5 chicken breast pieces
1 cup uncooked white rice
3/8 teaspoon pepper
1/2 teaspoon garlic powder
1/2 cup finely chopped onion
1 4-ounce can sliced
  mushrooms, undrained
1 14 1/2-ounce can clear
  chicken broth, defatted
1/2 cup water
1/4 teaspoon salt
1 teaspoon margarine
  (optional)

### Yield: 5 servings

### Per serving:
Calories...... 367
Protein (g)... 32
Fat (g)....... 8.2
Sat. Fat (g).. 1.9
Choles. (mg).. 85
Fiber (g)..... 0.8
Sodium (mg)... 554
%Cal-Fat...... 20%

Preheat oven to 350 degrees.

Remove skin and visible fat from chicken pieces. Heat canola oil in nonstick sauté pan. Dip chicken pieces in flour and brown in pan.

While chicken browns, put rice, pepper and garlic in a casserole dish. Stir in chopped onion. Put in mushrooms, including juice. Arrange browned chicken pieces on top.

Skim visible fat from top of chicken broth. Pour broth into a saucepan placed over medium-high heat. Add water and salt and bring to a boil. Pour broth over chicken-rice casserole. Spread margarine over chicken pieces, if desired.

Cover and bake at 350 degrees for 1 hour.

Preparation time: 20–25 minutes
Cooking time: 1 hour

# Chicken with Wine and Mushrooms

Preheat oven to 350 degrees.

Remove all visible fat from chicken breasts and pound to flatten slightly.

In large skillet, heat olive oil.

Meanwhile, roll chicken breasts first in Parmesan cheese, then dip in egg and bread crumbs. Place in skillet and brown both sides. Remove from skillet and place in baking dish.

Pour 1 cup wine into same skillet. Bring to a boil and simmer for 3 minutes. Next add fresh mushrooms and cook 5 to 10 additional minutes. Pour wine and mushroom sauce over chicken.

Cover and bake at 350 degrees for 1 hour.

*This recipe is very tasty and goes well with the Bulgur with Steamed Vegetables. (Recipe, page 336)*

Preparation time: 25 minutes

Cooking time: 1 hour

6 to 8 boneless chicken breasts
 (about 1 1/2 pounds)
1 tablespoon olive oil
1/4 cup Parmesan cheese
3/4 cup egg substitutes,
 slightly beaten
1/2 cup bread crumbs
1 cup dry white wine
1 pint fresh mushrooms, sliced

**Yield: 6 servings**

**Per serving:**
Calories...... 316
Protein (g)... 38
Fat (g)....... 9
Sat. Fat (g).. 2.6
Choles. (mg).. 100
Fiber (g)..... 0.6
Sodium (mg)... 280
%Cal-Fat...... 26%

# Chicken a la King

1 pound chicken meat, skinless
  and visible fat removed
8 ounces fresh mushrooms,
  sliced (or 4 ounces canned
  mushrooms)
1 cup frozen peas
2 ounces chopped pimiento,
  drained
1/2 cup flour
1 14 1/2-ounce can clear
  chicken broth, defatted
3/4 cup evaporated skim milk
1/4 cup sherry
Salt and pepper to taste
8 slices whole wheat bread,
  toasted

**Yield: 4 servings**

**Per serving:**
Calories...... 494
Protein (g)... 41
Fat (g)....... 8
Sat. Fat (g).. 2.3
Choles. (mg).. 89
Fiber (g)..... 8
Sodium (mg)... 862
%Cal-Fat...... 16%

Boil chicken in water for 25 minutes. Drain and cool slightly. Cut up chicken into bite-size pieces.

Meanwhile steam mushrooms and peas until tender.

Skim fat from top of chicken broth. Pour defatted broth into medium-size bowl. Add flour and mix with wire whisk until lumps disappear.

Pour broth and flour mixture into large saucepan placed over medium heat. Add milk and sherry. Bring to a boil, stirring occasionally with wire whisk. Continue stirring until sauce thickens and has a smooth consistency. Add chicken, vegetables and drained pimiento. Heat through. Add salt and pepper to taste.

Serve over toasted bread.

*This recipe is also a great way to use up leftover turkey breast—just substitute the turkey breast for the chicken.*

Preparation time: 35 minutes

# Chicken and Dumplings

Cut all visible fat from chicken breasts. Boil chicken in water for 25 minutes. Drain and cut into bite-size pieces. Set aside.

Meanwhile, place peas, sliced carrots and onion into vegetable steamer. Steam until vegetables are tender. Set aside.

Skim fat from top of chicken broth. Pour into large saucepan placed over medium heat. Add skim milk and flour and stir with wire whisk (while still cool) until smooth. Bring to a boil, stirring occasionally. Continue stirring until sauce thickens and has a smooth consistency. Add chicken and vegetables and heat through. Season to taste. Pour into shallow casserole dish.

Preheat oven to 400 degrees.

To make dumplings:

In a medium-size bowl, combine flour, baking powder and salt. Mix well. Add milk and oil and mix just until moistened. Place heaping tablespoons of dough over top of chicken casserole.

Bake at 400 degrees, covered, for 15 minutes. Remove lid. Bake an additional 10 minutes, or until slightly brown.

Preparation time: 30–40 minutes
Cooking time: 20 minutes

1 pound boneless chicken breast
1 cup frozen peas
1 cup sliced carrots, fresh or frozen
1 large onion, cut into eighths
1/2 cup flour
1 14 1/2-ounce can clear chicken broth, defatted
1 1/4 cups skim milk
Salt and pepper to taste

Dumplings:
1 cup flour
2 teaspoons baking powder
1/2 teaspoon salt
1/2 cup milk
2 tablespoons canola oil

*Yield: 4 to 6 servings*

*Per serving:*
Calories...... 417
Protein (g)... 39
Fat (g)....... 10
Sat. Fat (g).. 1.6
Choles. (mg).. 78
Fiber (g)..... 3.7
Sodium (mg)... 745
%Cal-Fat...... 22%

# Chicken-Garbanzo Stir-Fry

1/2 to 3/4 pound boneless chicken breast, cut into bite-size pieces
1 19-ounce can garbanzo beans (chick peas), drained
2 teaspoons olive oil
1/4 cup chopped green onions, including tops
1 red or green pepper, cut into narrow bite-size pieces
3 tablespoons no-oil Italian dressing
1 tablespoon cornstarch
1/2 cup water
2 tablespoons chopped pimiento
1/4 cup slivered almonds (optional)
Reduced-sodium soy sauce or lemon juice (optional)
Rice or pasta, cooked

**Yield: 4 servings**

**Per serving:**
Calories...... 356
Protein (g)... 30
Fat (g)....... 7.4
Sat. Fat (g).. 1.4
Choles. (mg).. 48
Fiber (g)..... 6.2
Sodium (mg)... 220
%Cal-Fat...... 21%

Cut up green onions and red pepper as indicated above. Set aside. Cut up chicken.

Spray nonstick skillet or sauté pan with vegetable cooking spray. Stir-fry chicken over medium-high heat for approximately 2 minutes, or until meat turns white. Add garbanzo beans, drained, and stir-fry for an additional minute. Add olive oil, green onions and pepper. Stir-fry approximately 2 to 3 more minutes, until pepper is crisp-tender.

Meanwhile make sauce by combining Italian dressing, cornstarch and water in small mixing bowl.

Add chopped pimiento, almonds (if desired), and cornstarch mixture to skillet. Mix well and continue cooking until sauce thickens. Serve over rice or pasta and sprinkle with lite soy sauce or lemon juice.

*A tasty, quick dish that is ideal when time is limited. Protein is supplied by both the beans and chicken, thus less meat is required to get adequate protein.*

Preparation time: 25–30 minutes

# Stir-Fried Chicken and Vegetables

Cut chicken breast into bite-size pieces. Set aside. Prepare vegetables by cutting cauliflower and broccoli into bite-size pieces and cutting off ends of snow peas. Set aside.

Prepare seasoning sauce: Combine sherry, corn syrup, water, cornstarch, soy sauce and vinegar. Blend thoroughly. Set aside.

Sauté chicken pieces in non-stick sauté pan until brown (no oil necessary). Next, add three tablespoons water to sauté pan. Add snow peas, cauliflower, broccoli and minced garlic. Steam 4 to 5 minutes. Vegetables should be bright in color and slightly crispy. Add seasoning sauce and heat until sauce comes to a boil and thickens. Mix all ingredients well.

Serve over cooked rice. Sprinkle with soy sauce, if desired.

*You may substitute turkey breast for the chicken if desired.*

Preparation time: 30–35 minutes

3/4 pound boneless chicken breast
1/4 cup dry sherry
1/4 cup dark corn syrup
1/4 cup water
2 tablespoons cornstarch
3 tablespoons reduced-sodium soy sauce
2 tablespoons apple cider vinegar
3 tablespoons water
1/2 pound fresh snow peas
1/2 head cauliflower
2 large stalks of broccoli
1 clove garlic, minced
Brown or white rice
Soy sauce to taste

### Yield: 4 to 5 servings

**Per serving:**
Calories...... 365
Protein (g)... 38
Fat (g)....... 4.8
Sat. Fat (g).. 1.2
Choles. (mg).. 64
Fiber (g)..... 7
Sodium (mg)... 536
%Cal-Fat...... 12%

# Crunchy Chicken Casserole

3/4 to 1 pound boneless chicken breast
1 cup brown or white rice, uncooked
1 cup celery, diced
1/4 cup onion, diced
1 8-ounce can sliced water chestnuts, drained
1 4-ounce can sliced mushrooms, including liquid
2 tablespoons lemon juice
1/2 teaspoon salt
2 tablespoons light mayonnaise
1 1/2 cups water, divided
1 chicken bouillon cube
2 1/2 tablespoons flour
1 tablespoon tub margarine
1 3/4 cups corn flakes cereal

### Yield: 6 servings

### Per serving:
Calories...... 338
Protein (g)... 28
Fat (g)....... 7.8
Sat. Fat (g).. 1.6
Choles. (mg).. 65
Fiber (g)..... 2.9
Sodium (mg)... 583
%Cal-Fat...... 21%

Preheate oven to 350 degrees.

Cook chicken breasts by boiling in water for 30 minutes. Cut into bite-size pieces. Cook rice according to package directions. Cut up celery and onion.

In large mixing bowl, combine chicken, cooked rice, celery, onion, water chestnuts, mushrooms, including liquid, lemon juice, salt and mayonnaise. Set aside.

Dissolve chicken bouillon in medium skillet with 1 1/4 cups water. Heat on stove. Meanwhile, combine remaining 1/4 cup cold water and flour in small bowl, mixing until it becomes a smooth paste. Add flour paste to liquid in skillet, heating until it thickens and comes to a full boil.

Add gravy to other ingredients and carefully stir together until well blended. Spoon into 9 x 13-inch pan and spread evenly.

Melt margarine in medium skillet. Toss corn flakes in margarine until flakes are evenly coated. Sprinkle over top of casserole.

Bake for 35 minutes, or until heated through.

*Rice and chicken may be cooked the night before or early in the day. Remaining preparation time is then much shorter. This casserole is very moist as well as is low in fat.*

Preparation time: 30–35 minutes
Cooking time: 1 hour, divided

# Spicy Chicken and Pasta

Bring 2 quarts of water to a boil in large saucepan. Cook pasta according to package directions. Drain and set aside.

Meanwhile, heat canola oil in deep 12-inch skillet over medium heat. Add chicken breasts and brown on both sides. Cook an additional 5 minutes. Remove from skillet and cover.

Add garlic, green pepper and broccoli to skillet. Stir-fry for 2 minutes. Stir in chopped tomatoes, salt, parsley, pepper and oregano. Add chicken. Bring to a boil, reduce heat and simmer, covered, for 10 to 15 minutes, stirring occasionally. Add cooked and drained pasta, mixing well.

Transfer to a serving dish. Sprinkle with Parmesan cheese.

Preparation time: 30–40 minutes

2 teaspoons canola oil
6 chicken breasts, boneless or
  with bones, skin removed
8 ounces rotini pasta
  (corkscrew-shaped)
1 clove garlic, minced
1 green pepper, chopped
1 bunch broccoli, cut into bite-
  size pieces
2 16-ounce cans tomatoes (no
  salt added), coarsely chopped
1/2 teaspoon salt, or to taste
2 tablespoons chopped parsley
1/4 teaspoon black pepper
1 teaspoon dried oregano
2 tablespoons Parmesan cheese

**Yield: 6 servings**

**Per serving:**
Calories...... 435
Protein (g)... 46
Fat (g)....... 7.7
Sat. Fat (g).. 2.2
Choles. (mg).. 98
Fiber (g)..... 5.1
Sodium (mg)... 371
%Cal-Fat...... 18%

# Chicken Cordon Bleu

4 boneless chicken breasts
4 thin slices lean ham
4 slices Swiss cheese (1/2 oz.
   each)
1/4 cup flour
1/4 teaspoon seasoned salt
1/4 teaspoon pepper
2 teaspoons margarine, melted
1/2 pound fresh mushrooms,
   sliced
2 tablespoons lemon juice
2 tablespoons sherry
1 tablespoon Worcestershire
   sauce
1 tablespoon chopped fresh
   parsley
3 tablespoons cold water
1 1/2 tablespoons flour

### Yield: 4 servings

### Per serving:

Calories...... 312
Protein (g)... 38
Fat (g)....... 10.9
Sat. Fat (g).. 4.4
Choles. (mg).. 98
Fiber (g)..... 1.3
Sodium (mg)... 594
%Cal-Fat...... 31%

Preheat oven to 350 degrees.

Pound chicken breasts to 1/4-inch thickness. On each flattened piece of chicken, place one slice of ham and one slice of Swiss cheese. Roll and secure with a toothpick.

Combine flour, salt and pepper. Roll the breasts in the flour mixture. Brown the rolled chicken breasts in margarine in a medium-size skillet. After browned on all sides (about 10 minutes), place in an 8- or 9-inch square baking dish.

Meanwhile, sauté sliced mushrooms in lemon juice, sherry and Worcestershire sauce until tender. Add chopped parsley. Mix 1 1/2 tablespoons of flour with cold water until a smooth paste. Add to the mushroom mixture. Stir over medium heat until sauce thickens. Pour sauce over chicken breasts.

Bake at 350 degrees for 25 to 30 minutes until hot and bubbly. Serve with seasoned rice.

Preparation time: 25–30 minutes
Cooking time: 25–30 minutes

# *Breast of Chicken Beaufort*

Preheat oven to 350 degrees.

Pound chicken breasts to 1/4-inch thickness. Combine next ten ingredients to make stuffing. Place 1/6 of stuffing on each flattened chicken breast. Roll and secure with toothpicks. Place in 9-inch square baking dish. Bake, covered, in 350 degree oven for 30 minutes. Drain juices from baking dish.

To make sauce, combine flour and chicken broth in small saucepan. Mix with wire whisk until all lumps disappear. Heat until sauce comes to a boil and thickens. Add remaining ingredients and mix well until smooth. Pour over chicken breasts and bake an additional 30 minutes, uncovered.

To serve, transfer chicken breasts to serving platter. Pour sauce over.

Preparation time: 30 minutes
Cooking time: 1 hour

*6 boneless chicken breasts*
*2 ounces lean ham, finely chopped*
*1/4 cup finely chopped onion*
*1/4 cup egg substitute*
*1 cup soft bread crumbs*
*1 tablespoon chopped fresh parsley*
*1 tablespoon dry sherry*
*1/2 teaspoon salt*
*Dash cayenne pepper*
*1 clove garlic, minced*
*7 ounces backfin crabmeat*

*Sauce:*
*1 14 1/2-ounce can clear chicken broth, defatted*
*1/4 cup flour*
*1 teaspoon lemon juice*
*1/2 cup dry sherry*
*3 tablespoons tomato paste*

**Yield: 6 servings**

**Per serving:**
Calories...... 280
Protein (g)... 40
Fat (g)....... 6.3
Sat. Fat (g).. 1.4
Choles. (mg).. 111
Fiber (g)..... 0.6
Sodium (mg)... 785
%Cal-Fat...... 17%

# Chicken-Seafood Artichoke Casserole

1 14-ounce can artichokes, drained
1 pound boneless chicken breast, cooked
1 pound shrimp, cooked and cleaned
3/4 pound fresh mushrooms, sliced

Sauce:
1 1/2 cups milk
1/4 cup flour
1/4 cup sherry
1 1/2 teaspoons Worcestershire sauce
1/2 teaspoon salt
1/4 teaspoon pepper
3 tablespoons Parmesan cheese
Paprika
2 tablespoons chopped fresh parsley
6 cups cooked rice

**Yield: 8 servings**

**Per serving:**
Calories...... 463
Protein (g)... 40
Fat (g)....... 4.4
Sat. Fat (g).. 1.5
Choles. (mg).. 161
Fiber (g)..... 5.1
Sodium (mg)... 416
%Cal-Fat...... 9%

Preheat oven to 350 degrees.

Cut artichokes lengthwise into quarters and arrange in bottom of 9-inch square baking dish. Cut up cooked chicken into bite-size pieces. Arrange cooked shrimp and chicken evenly in baking dish.

In large skillet, sauté sliced mushrooms until tender. (No oil needed, but keep lid on to prevent sticking.) Drain. Spread mushrooms evenly over top of casserole.

Meanwhile, make sauce: Pour milk and flour into a medium-size skillet. Stir briskly with a wire whisk until all lumps disappear. Bring to a boil over medium heat, stirring frequently, until sauce thickens. Add sherry, Worcestershire sauce, salt and pepper.

Pour sauce over casserole. Sprinkle with Parmesan cheese, paprika and parsley.

Bake, uncovered, for 40 minutes.

Serve over rice.

*Backfin crabmeat may be substituted for the shrimp, if desired.*

Preparation time: 35–40 minutes (if shrimp are already cleaned)

Cooking time: 40 minutes

# Chicken Cacciatore

Spray large nonstick skillet with vegetable cooking spray. In skillet, over medium heat, brown chicken breast pieces. Remove chicken.

Add 2 tablespoons water to skillet. Add cut up vegetables, green peppers, onions, garlic and mushrooms. Steam until tender but not brown. Check frequently to make sure water doesn't boil away. Add more if necessary. Return chicken to skillet.

Meanwhile, roughly chop canned tomatoes in food processor. Pour into medium-size bowl. Add tomato sauce, pepper, oregano and celery seed. Mix well. Pour over chicken and vegetables in skillet. Cover and simmer 30 minutes.

Stir in 1/4 cup dry white wine. Cook chicken, uncovered, 15 minutes longer, or until desired consistency. Stir occasionally.

Meanwhile, cook pasta according to package directions. Drain. Mix small amount of tomato sauce into pasta to keep from sticking.

To serve, spoon chicken cacciatore over pasta. Sprinkle with Parmesan cheese.

Preparation time: 30 minutes
Cooking time: 45 minutes

*1 pound boneless chicken breast, cut into bite-size pieces*
*Vegetable cooking spray*
*2 tablespoons water*
*2 green peppers, cut into 1/2 x 1-inch pieces*
*2 medium onions, sliced*
*2 cloves garlic, minced*
*1/2 pound fresh mushrooms, sliced, or 4 oz. canned*
*1 16-ounce can tomatoes, chopped*
*1 8-ounce can tomato sauce*
*1/4 teaspoon pepper*
*1 teaspoon dried oregano or basil*
*1/2 teaspoon celery seed*
*1/4 cup dry white wine*
*1 pound pasta, preferable flat noodles*
*Parmesan cheese*

### Yield: 4 servings

### Per serving:
Calories...... 647
Protein (g)... 45
Fat (g)....... 6.5
Sat. Fat (g).. 1.9
Choles. (mg).. 72
Fiber (g)..... 5.6
Sodium (mg)... 309
%Cal-Fat...... 9%

# Beijing Chicken Stir-Fry

3/4 pound boneless chicken breast

2 tablespoons cornstarch, divided

3 tablespoons reduced-sodium soy sauce, divided

2 tablespoons dry sherry

1 clove garlic, minced

1 tablespoon sesame seeds, toasted

1 cup water

3 teaspoons olive oil, divided

1 16-ounce can bean sprouts or 1/2 pound fresh bean sprouts

1 bunch green onions and tops, cut into 2-inch lengths

1 8-ounce can water chestnuts, drained

12 ounces "eggless" egg noodles, cooked

**Yield: 4 servings**

**Per serving:**
Calories...... 388
Protein (g)... 34
Fat (g)....... 9
Sat. Fat (g).. 1.6
Choles. (mg).. 72
Fiber (g)..... 4.7
Sodium (mg)... 548
%Cal-Fat...... 22%

Cut chicken breast into narrow strips. Combine 1 tablespoon cornstarch, 1 tablespoon soy sauce, sherry and minced garlic in medium bowl. Stir in chicken and let stand for 10 minutes.

Meanwhile, spray small nonstick skillet with vegetable cooking spray. Place over medium heat. Add sesame seeds and heat, stirring occasionally, until seeds turn light brown. Remove from heat and set aside.

Combine water, remaining 1 tablespoon cornstarch and 2 tablespoons soy sauce in small bowl. Set aside.

Heat 2 teaspoons olive oil in wok or nonstick sauté pan until hot. Add chicken and stir-fry 3 minutes, or until chicken strips are fully cooked. Remove.

Add remaining 1 teaspoon olive oil to pan and stir-fry bean sprouts, green onions and water chestnuts for 3 minutes. Add about 2 tablespoons water if vegetables stick to pan.

Stir in chicken, soy sauce/water mixture and toasted sesame seeds. Cook and continue stirring until mixture comes to a boil and thickens. Serve immediately over hot pasta.

Preparation time: 30–35 minutes

# Chicken L'Orange

Preheat gas or charcoal grill on medium heat.

Lightly sprinkle lemon pepper on both sides of chicken breasts. Place aluminum foil on grill, spray with cooking spray, and place chicken breasts on foil. Grill 8 to 10 minutes on each side, or just until meat is no longer pink in middle. Do not overcook. (Chicken breasts may also be prepared in a non-stick skillet, sprayed with cooking spray.)

Meanwhile, make sauce. In small saucepan, combine sugars, salt and cornstarch. Slowly stir in juice until smooth. Stir in mustard with a wire whisk. Place over medium heat and bring to a boil. Simmer until transparent and thickened, about 3 minutes. Stir in drained mandarin oranges, and, if desired, orange liqueur. Heat slightly, but do not boil.

To serve, place chicken breasts on serving platter and spoon sauce over top.

*Mandarin Orange Sauce is also delicious served over fish, especially orange roughy or red snapper.*

Preparation time: 25 minutes

4 boneless chicken breasts
Lemon-pepper seasoning, to taste
Vegetable cooking spray

Mandarin Orange Sauce:
1/3 cup brown sugar
1/3 cup granulated sugar
1/4 teaspoon salt
1 tablespoon cornstarch
1 cup orange juice
1 teaspoon Dijon mustard
11-ounce can mandarin oranges in light syrup, drained
1 to 2 tablespoons orange liqueur (optional)

**Yield: 4 servings**

**Per serving:**
Calories...... 344
Protein (g)... 28
Fat (g)....... 4
Sat. Fat (g).. 1.1
Choles. (mg).. 73
Fiber (g)..... 1.6
Sodium (mg)... 223
%Cal-Fat...... 10%

# Coq au Vin

4 boneless chicken breast halves
2 teaspoons olive oil
12 whole mushrooms, scrubbed
12 small white onions, peeled
2/3 cup sliced green onion,
    including tops
1 clove garlic, crushed
2 cups Burgundy wine
1 cup canned condensed chicken
    broth, undiluted
1/4 cup flour
1/2 teaspoon seasoned salt
1/2 teaspoon dried thyme
1/8 teaspoon black pepper
8 small red potatoes, scrubbed
    (1 1/4-inch diameter)
Fresh parsley for garnish

### Yield: 4 servings

### Per serving:
Calories...... 367
Protein (g)... 30
Fat (g)....... 6.5
Sat. Fat (g).. 1.4
Choles. (mg).. 65
Fiber (g)..... 4
Sodium (mg)...539
%Cal-Fat...... 16%

Remove skin from chicken and pound to 1/4-inch thickness.

Heat olive oil in Dutch oven. Add chicken and brown on both sides. Remove and set aside.

Add mushrooms and white onions to Dutch oven. Cook until slightly browned. (You may need to add 1 to 2 tablespoons water if they begin to stick. If so, cover pan while browning.) Remove and set aside.

Add green onions and crushed garlic to Dutch oven. Sauté 2 minutes. (Add additional water, if necessary.) Immediately add Burgundy and begin to heat.

Meanwhile, with wire whisk, mix flour into condensed chicken broth until lumps disappear. Add broth mixture, salt, thyme and pepper to Dutch oven. Bring to a boil. Stir until sauce thickens.

Remove from heat. Return chicken, mushrooms and onions to Dutch oven. Cover and refrigerate for 2 hours or overnight.

Preheat oven to 375 degrees. Just before baking, add potatoes to chicken mixture. Bake, covered, about 1 hour and 50 minutes, or until chicken and potatoes are tender. Garnish with parsley.

Preparation time: 30–35 minutes
Cooking time: 1 hour, 50 minutes
Marinating time: 2–12 hours

# Grilled Breast of Chicken Sandwich

4 boneless chicken breast
    halves
1/2 cup no-oil Italian dressing
Honey mustard (to taste)
Lettuce
Tomato, sliced
4 large hamburger buns

Remove all visible fat from chicken breasts. Pound to 1/4-inch thickness. Place chicken breasts in mixing bowl and pour salad dressing over, evenly covering meat. Marinate at least 2 hours or overnight.

Preheat outdoor grill. Place aluminum foil on grill, spray with vegetable cooking spray, and cook chicken breasts over medium heat approximately 8 minutes per side. Do not overcook. Transfer to platter.

To assemble sandwich, place chicken breast on bun, top with honey mustard (or catsup), tomato and lettuce.

*This provides a tasty alternative to hamburgers or hotdogs cooked on a grill. The big bonus is that it is much lower in fat and just as easy to prepare.*

Preparation time: 10–15 minutes
Cooking time: 15–20 minutes
Marinating time: 2 hours

*Yield: 4 servings*

*Per serving:*
Calories...... 281
Protein (g)... 31
Fat (g)....... 5.6
Sat. Fat (g).. 1.5
Choles. (mg).. 73
Fiber (g)..... 1.8
Sodium (mg)... NA
%Cal-Fat...... 19%

# Barbecued Shredded Turkey Breast

Cook turkey breast in a covered pot of boiling water for 3 hours. Remove from water and allow to cool slightly. Remove meat from bone and shred. Set aside.

Combine remaining ingredients (except sandwich rolls) in 4-quart saucepan. Add shredded turkey breast and let simmer for 30 minutes or longer over low heat, stirring occasionally.

Serve on sliced hard rolls or hamburger buns.

*The liquid left over from cooking the turkey breast makes an excellent stock for chicken or turkey soup, or it can be used for cooking rice. To defat it, let it cool in the refrigerator, then remove the fat from the top. It can be refrigerated for several days or frozen until ready to use.*

Preparation time: 30 minutes
Cooking time: 3 hours, 30 minutes

*1 6- to 7-pound whole turkey breast (2 1/2 to 3 pounds turkey meat)*
*1 3/4 cups brewed strong coffee*
*1 1/4 cups Worcestershire sauce*
*1/2 cup water*
*1 1/2 cups catsup*
*5 tablespoons light margarine*
*1/4 cup packed brown sugar*
*2 teaspoons garlic powder*
*2 teaspoons onion powder*
*1 to 2 teaspoons black pepper*
*16 to 18 sandwich rolls*

*Yield: 16 to 18 servings*

*Per serving:*
Calories...... 290
Protein (g)... 28
Fat (g)....... 5.3
Sat. Fat (g).. 1.3
Choles. (mg).. 68
Fiber (g)..... 1.6
Sodium (mg)... 843
%Cal-Fat...... 17%

# Turkey Parmigiana

1 pound turkey breast slices,
  about 1/4-inch thick
2 teaspoons olive oil
1/2 cup crushed cornflake
  crumbs
1/4 cup grated Parmesan
  cheese
1 egg substitute
1 8-ounce can no-salt added
  tomato sauce
1/2 teaspoon dried oregano,
  crushed
1/2 teaspoon sugar
Dash garlic powder
2 thin slices mozzarella cheese,
  halved (2 ounces)

**Yield: 4 servings**

**Per serving:**
Calories...... 324
Protein (g)... 44
Fat (g)....... 8.6
Sat. Fat (g).. 3.6
Choles. (mg).. 110
Fiber (g)..... 1.1
Sodium (mg)... 411
%Cal-Fat...... 24%

Pound turkey breast slices with meat pounder to tenderize. Set aside.

In a medium-size bowl, combine crushed cornflake crumbs, Parmesan cheese and a dash of pepper. Pour egg substitute into a small bowl.

Heat olive oil in large skillet or sauté pan.

Dip turkey breast slices first in egg, then in crumb mixture. Place in sauté pan and brown on both sides. Cook for 20 minutes longer.

Meanwhile, in small saucepan, combine tomato sauce, oregano, sugar and garlic powder. Heat to boiling, stirring occasionally. Pour sauce over meat. Top with cheese.

Turn on oven broiler. Transfer meat to an oven-proof serving dish. Broil close to heat until cheese bubbles and turns golden, about 3 to 4 minutes. Serve immediately.

*If time is short, cheese can be melted on top of chicken in sauté pan, by putting the lid on for about 4 to 5 minutes, rather than transferring to another dish and broiling. Chicken breasts, pounded to 1/4-inch thickness, may be substituted for turkey breast.*

Preparation time: 30 minutes
Cooking time: 30 minutes

# Stuffed Turkey Cutlets

Preheat oven to 350 degrees.

Pound turkey breast cutlets slightly to tenderize. Combine stuffing mix, carrot, egg substitute and cooking oil in a small mixing bowl.

To assemble, lay turkey cutlets flat and spoon 1/4 of stuffing on one end of each cutlet. Fold other end over and secure with a toothpick. Place in a 9-inch square baking dish. Bake, covered, in 350 degree oven for 30 minutes.

Meanwhile, make sauce. Place chicken bouillon cube and 1 cup water in medium-size skillet. Heat until bouillon cube is dissolved. In a small bowl, mix flour and 1/2 cup cold water with a wire whisk until all lumps disappear. Add to skillet and stir until sauce thickens. Add lemon juice, wine and parsley and mix well.

Pour 1/2 of sauce (one cup) over turkey cutlets and bake, uncovered, for an additional 30 minutes. Transfer cutlets to a platter and spoon remaining sauce (warmed) over top.

Preparation time: 25–30 minutes
Cooking time: 1 hour

4 turkey breast cutlets (1 pound total)
1 cup herb-seasoned stuffing mix
1 medium carrot, shredded
1 egg substitute
2 tablespoons canola oil

Sauce:
1 cup water
1 chicken bouillon cube
1/4 cup flour
1/2 cup cold water
1 teaspoon lemon juice
1/2 cup Chablis wine
2 teaspoons minced parsley

**Yield: Serves 4**

**Per serving:**
Calories...... 256
Protein (g)... 27
Fat (g)....... 9.3
Sat. Fat (g).. 0.9
Choles. (mg).. 66
Fiber (g)..... 1
Sodium (mg)... 372
%Cal-Fat...... 24%

# *Nonfat Turkey Gravy*

Meat juices from roasted whole
  turkey or turkey breast
  (defatted) *
1/4 cup flour
1/2 cup cold water
1/4 teaspoon salt (or to taste)
Pepper to taste

**Yield: 2 cups gravy, or 6
servings**

**Per serving:**
Calories...... 27
Protein (g)... 2
Fat (g)....... 0.4
Sat. Fat (g).. 0.1
Choles. (mg).. 0
Fiber (g)..... 0
Sodium (mg)... NA
%Cal-Fat...... 5%

Add enough water to meat juices to make 1 1/2 cups liquid.
Pour into medium-size frypan and heat.

Meanwhile, in a small bowl, using a wire whisk, stir flour into
cold water until all lumps disappear.

Gradually add flour mixture to meat juices, stirring constantly
with a wire whisk. Bring to a boil. Reduce heat and simmer 5
to 10 minutes. Season to taste.

*\*To defat turkey juices, pour all the drippings into a tall, narrow container.
Wait 1 to 2 minutes for fat to settle to the top. Carefully skim fat away
with a spoon. Meat drippings from other types of roasts may be defatted
using same method.*

*An alternate method is especially good if you cook whole turkey or turkey
breast often. You simply save the meat juices from one turkey for the next
turkey's gravy. By not using the juices immediately, you can chill the
drippings in the refrigerator, which makes if much easier to remove the fat.*

*Prepare the drippings as follows: Pour the meat juices into an airtight
plastic container. Refrigerate overnight. The next morning, remove the
congealed fat from the top. Freeze the defatted meat juices and use in making
gravy the next time you serve turkey.*

Preparation time: 10–15 minutes

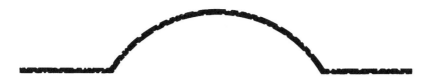

# Beef, Pork & Veal

Round Steak Chile • Beef Stew • Beef Bourguignon • Marinated Beef Stir-Fry • Swiss Steak • Pepper Steak • Marinated Beef Tenderloin • Beef-Bean Burger • Apple-Date Stuffed Tenderloin • Pork Medallions with Mushroom Sauce • Stir-Fry Gingered Pork • Pork Tenderloin with Mustard Sauce • Pork Tenderloin Florentine • Pork Marengo • Veal Saltimbocca • Veal Piccata with Mushrooms • Veal Rolls Divan

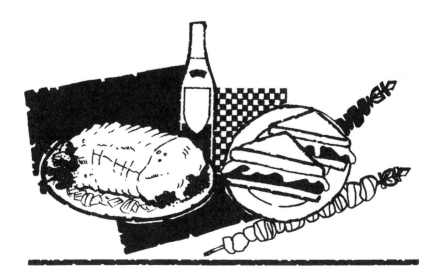

# Round Steak Chile

1/2 pound round steak, ground
(all visible fat removed)
Vegetable cooking spray
1 cup chopped onion
1 green pepper, chopped
1 16-ounce can tomatoes,
broken up
2 16-ounce cans dark red
kidney beans, drained and
rinsed
1 8-ounce can tomato sauce, no
salt added
1/4 teaspoon salt, optional
2 teaspoons chili powder, or to
taste
2 bay leaves

**Yield: 4 servings**

**Per serving:**
Calories...... 365
Protein (g)... 31
Fat (g)....... 6
Sat. Fat (g).. 1.9
Choles. (mg).. 47
Fiber (g)..... 11.2
Sodium (mg)... 881
%Cal-Fat...... 14%

Have butcher grind round steak or grind it yourself in food processor.

Spray heavy skillet with vegetable cooking spray. Add ground meat, onion and green pepper. Cook until meat is lightly browned and vegetables are tender. Stir in remaining ingredients. Simmer, covered, for 30 minutes to 1 hour.

Remove bay leaves and serve immediately.

*The amount of fat in this recipe is greatly reduced over traditional chile recipes by using round steak rather than ground beef, and by using less beef and more kidney beans.*

Preparation time: 20 minutes
Cooking time: 30 minutes–1 hour

# Beef Stew

Preheat oven to 350 degrees.

Spray large skillet with vegetable cooking spray. Brown meat cubes on stove over medium heat. Transfer meat and meat juices to large oven-proof casserole. Add next seven ingredients to casserole dish.

In medium-size bowl, combine beef broth, wine, Worcestershire sauce and pepper. Add flour, mixing with a wire whisk until all lumps are gone. Pour over meat and vegetables. Stir to mix.

Cover and bake in 350 degree oven 2 1/2 to 3 hours. Stir occasionally.

Preparation time: 35–40 minutes
Cooking time: 2 1/2–3 hours

*1 1/2 pounds round steak, all visible fat removed, cut into 1-inch cubes*
*Vegetable cooking spray*
*1 15 1/2-ounce can Northern beans, drained and rinsed*
*1 16-ounce can tomatoes, chopped*
*4 small onions, quartered*
*4 carrots, cut into 1/2-inch slices*
*4 small potatoes, cut into bite-size pieces*
*1 cup celery, chopped*
*1/2 pound fresh mushrooms, sliced*
*1 cup clear beef broth, defatted*
*1 cup dry white wine*
*2 tablespoons Worcestershire sauce*
*1/4 teaspoon ground pepper*
*1/4 cup flour*

**Yield: 6 servings**

**Per serving:**
Calories...... 423
Protein (g)... 43
Fat (g)....... 7.4
Sat. Fat (g).. 2.5
Choles. (mg).. 78
Fiber (g)..... 9
Sodium (mg)... 508
%Cal-Fat...... 17%

# Beef Bourguignon

2 pounds round steak, all
 visible fat removed, cut into
 1-inch cubes
Vegetable cooking spray
2 cups chopped onion
4 medium carrots, cut into
 bite-size chunks
2 celery stalks, chopped
1 clove garlic, minced
2 cups Burgundy wine
1 14 1/2-ounce can clear beef
 broth, defatted
1 tablespoon catsup
2 tablespoons Worcestershire
 sauce
1/2 teaspoon salt, or to taste
1/4 teaspoon pepper, or to taste
1/2 teaspoon thyme
1/4 cup flour
1/2 cup water
1 8-ounce can sliced
 mushrooms, drained
1 pint pearl onions, parboiled
 and peeled
1/4 cup chopped fresh parsley
1 pound dumpling pasta or egg
 noodles

**Yield: 6 to 8 servings**

**Per serving:**
Calories...... 533
Protein (g)... 43
Fat (g)....... 7.9
Sat. Fat (g).. 2.6
Choles. (mg).. 78
Fiber (g)..... 5.8
Sodium (mg)... 723
%Cal-Fat...... 13%

Preheat oven to 350 degrees.

Spray large skillet with vegetable cooking spray. Sauté beef cubes until thoroughly browned. With slotted spoon, transfer beef cubes to large oven-proof casserole. In same skillet, sauté chopped onion, carrots, celery and garlic until onion becomes translucent. Add to meat in casserole.

In same skillet, combine wine, beef broth, catsup, Worcestershire sauce, salt, pepper and thyme. In small bowl, mix flour and water with wire whisk until smooth. Add to wine mixture, stirring constantly, until it comes to a boil. Pour over casserole. Add mushrooms and whole onions to casserole.

Cover and bake at 350 degrees for 3 hours, or until meat and vegetables are tender.

Just before serving, sprinkle chopped parsley over casserole.

Meanwhile prepare pasta according to package directions. Serve the Beef Bourguignon over pasta.

Preparation time: 45–50 minutes
Cooking time: 3 hours

# Marinated Beef Stir-Fry

Cut beef on the bias into bite-size pieces 1/8-inch thick. (To make slicing easier, partially freeze beef in freezer about 45 minutes prior to cutting.)

Prepare marinade by combining all ingredients in small mixing bowl. Add beef and marinate at room temperature 30 minutes or in refrigerator for 2 hours. Stir occasionally.

Meanwhile, cut up green onions, bok choy and carrots as directed.

Preheat a wok or large skillet over medium-high heat. Add olive oil. Add onions and bok choy; stir-fry for 2 minutes. Add carrots and bamboo shoots; stir-fry about 3 minutes or until vegetables are crisp-tender. Remove vegetables from pan.

Add beef and marinade to skillet and stir-fry for 3 to 4 minutes or until meat is cooked. Add vegetables and heat through. Serve immediately over rice.

*To slice bok choy, first cut each celery-like stalk in half lengthwise, including dark green top. Next, cut stalk as you would chop celery, about 1/4-inch thick. Coarsely chop leafy greens at top of stalk.*

Preparation time: 30–40 minutes
Marinating time: 30 minutes–2 hours

*3/4 pound round steak, all visible fat removed*
*1/2 cup diagonally sliced green onions (1-inch slices)*
*4 cups sliced bok choy (about 5 stalks) ***
*2 carrots, shredded*
*1 8-ounce can bamboo shoots, drained*
*2 teaspoons olive oil*
*Hot cooked rice (3 to 4 cups)*

*Marinade:*
*2 tablespoons reduced-sodium soy sauce*
*2 tablespoons dry sherry*
*1 tablespoon hoisin sauce (hot bean sauce)*
*2 teaspoons grated gingerroot*
*1 clove garlic minced*

**Yield: 6 servings**

**Per serving:**
Calories...... 354
Protein (g)... 24
Fat (g)....... 7.5
Sat. Fat (g).. 2.2
Choles. (mg).. 55
Fiber (g)..... 4.3
Sodium (mg)... 352
%Cal-Fat...... 20%

# Swiss Steak

1 1/2 pounds round or flank
  steak, cut 1-inch thick
1/4 cup flour
1/2 teaspoon salt
1/8 teaspoon black pepper
2 teaspoons canola oil
1 cup chopped onion
3 fresh tomatoes, or 1 16-ounce
  can tomatoes, chopped finely
2 carrots, peeled and chopped
  finely
1 tablespoon chopped fresh
  thyme or 1 teaspoon dried

**Yield: 6 servings**

**Per serving:**
Calories...... 263
Protein (g)... 35
Fat (g)....... 8
Sat. Fat (g).. 2.5
Choles. (mg).. 78
Fiber (g)..... 1.8
Sodium (mg)... 263
%Cal-Fat...... 29%
Trim meat of all visible fat.

Combine flour, salt and pepper. Pound flour into meat using a meat mallet or the dull edge of a large knife.

In large skillet or Dutch oven, brown meat on both sides in hot oil.

In a medium-size mixing bowl, combine chopped onion, tomatoes and carrots. Pour over meat. Cover, bring to a boil and reduce heat. Simmer over low heat for 1 1/2 hours or until tender. Turn meat once or twice during cooking time.

Remove meat to a warm platter and slice, diagonally, into 1/4-inch thick slices. Pour the vegetable sauce over the slices of meat. Some sauce may be reserved for passing at the table. Serve immediately.

*If desired, you can puree the sauce in a food processor. There is enough sauce not only for the meat, but for whatever side dish of rice, potatoes or polenta you choose to serve with it.*

Preparation time: 20–25 minutes
Cooking time: 1 1/2 hours

# *Pepper Steak*

Cut steak across the grain into 1/8-inch strips (or have this done by butcher). Cut up peppers and tomatoes as indicated; cover, and set aside.

Spray large nonstick skillet with vegetable cooking spray. Brown meat strips over medium-high heat, until browned on all sides. Add minced garlic and stir-fry 1/2 minute longer. Add beef broth. Bring to a boil, reduce heat and simmer, covered, 30 to 40 minutes, or until meat is tender.

Add green or red peppers and simmer, covered, about 8 minutes. Add tomatoes and simmer an additional 5 minutes.

Meanwhile, in small mixing bowl, combine soy sauce, sherry, water and cornstarch. Add to center of skillet and bring to a boil without stirring. Cook 1 minute longer, stirring until mixture thickens and thoroughly coats meat and vegetables.

Serve immediately over hot rice. Sprinkle with additional soy sauce, if desired.

*\*If you prefer, tomatoes may be peeled.*

  Preparation time: 30–35 minutes
  Cooking time: 45–50 minutes

*1 pound round or flank steak, trimmed of all visible fat*
*2 green peppers (or 1 red and 1 green pepper), cut into 1/2 x 1-inch strips*
*2 large tomatoes, cut into small wedges\**
*Vegetable cooking spray*
*1 clove garlic, minced*
*1 cup beef broth, fat skimmed from top*
*2 tablespoons reduced-sodium soy sauce*
*1 tablespoon sherry*
*2 tablespoons water*
*1 tablespoon cornstarch*
*3 to 4 cups prepared rice*

**Yield: 4 servings**

**Per serving:**
Calories...... 520
Protein (g)... 42
Fat (g)....... 11.6
Sat. Fat (g).. 3.8
Choles. (mg).. 108
Fiber (g)..... 2.6
Sodium (mg)... 564
%Cal-Fat...... 20%

# Marinated Beef Tenderloin

1 beef tenderloin (about 4 to 6 pounds), trimmed
1/2 cup reduced-sodium soy sauce
1/4 cup dry sherry
1 tablespoon Worcestershire sauce
1 clove garlic, minced
1 tablespoon sugar
1/2 teaspoon ground ginger
1/4 teaspoon black pepper

**Yield: Approximately 16 4-ounce servings (cooked)**

**Per serving:**
Calories........ 245
Protein (g)... 32
Fat (g)....... 11.5
Sat. Fat (g).. 4.1
Choles. (mg).. 96
Fiber (g).... 0
Sodium (mg)... NA
%Cal-Fat..... 39%

**With pork tenderloin:**
Fat(g)............ 5.3
%/Cal-Fat..... 24%

Remove all visible fat and connective tissue from tenderloin.

Prepare marinade by mixing together soy sauce, sherry, Worcestershire sauce, garlic, sugar, ginger and pepper.

Pour marinade over tenderloin. Cover and refrigerate 2 to 8 hours, or overnight (the longer the better).

Preheat oven to 425 degrees.

Remove tenderloin from marinade. Place on rack in open pan. Tuck small end under so meat will cook evenly. Roast in 425-degree oven 45 minutes to 1 hour, or until internal temperature of beef is 145 degrees (medium-rare). Cook longer if you prefer tenderloin to be cooked to medium. Wait 5 minutes before slicing.

*If a whole tenderloin is too much meat, ask your butcher to cut a half tenderloin for you. Prepare as indicated above and roast at 425 degrees for 45 to 50 minutes.*

*This marinade is also excellent for pork tenderloin. Prepare as above and bake at 375 degrees for 30 to 40 minutes, or until internal temperature reaches 160 degrees. It may also be baked in a shallow pan with the marinade, if the marinating time is short, or if a stronger flavor is desired.*

Preparation time: 10–15 minutes
Cooking time: 45–60 minutes
Marinating time: 2–24 hours

# Beef-Bean Burger

In medium-size bowl, combine ground round and chopped onion.

Place drained black-eyed peas and catsup into food processor. Process until pureed. Add to ground round mixture along with remaining ingredients. Mix well. (Burgers are easier to form if the meat-bean mixture is refrigerated at least 30 minutes.)

Spray large skillet with vegetable cooking spray. Form meat mixture into 5 or 6 patties, depending on preferred size. Fry over medium heat approximately 8 minutes per side. Serve on hamburger buns or hard rolls.

*These burgers taste like a cross between a soy burger and a beef burger. You still get the taste of beef, but the texture is different from standard beef burgers. The big benefit of these burgers is the much lower fat quantity and the addition of fiber and other nutrients from the beans.*

Preparation time: 15–20 minutes
Cooking time: 15 minutes

*1/2 pound extra-lean ground round*
*1 small onion, chopped*
*1 15-ounce can black-eyed peas, drained and rinsed*
*2 tablespoons catsup*
*1/2 cup dry bread crumbs*
*1 egg substitute (1/4 cup)*
*1/2 teaspoon cumin*
*1/4 teaspoon salt (optional)*

**Yield: 5 to 6 patties**

**Per serving:**
Calories...... 250
Protein (g)... 25
Fat (g)....... 5.2
Sat. Fat (g).. 1.7
Choles. (mg).. 40
Fiber (g)..... 5.2
Sodium (mg)... 374
%Cal-Fat...... 19%

# Apple-Date Stuffed Tenderloin

1 1/4 to 1 1/2 pounds pork
  tenderloins, trimmed of all
  visible fat
1/4 cup dry white wine
2 tablespoons Worcestershire
  sauce
3/4 cup chunky applesauce
1/3 cup chopped dates
3 tablespoons brown sugar
1/4 teaspoon salt
1/2 teaspoon cinnamon
Sprigs of parsley for garnish

**Yield: 5 servings**

**Per serving:**
Calories...... 276
Protein (g)... 33
Fat (g)....... 5.5
Sat. Fat (g).. 2
Choles. (mg).. 106
Fiber (g)..... 1.6
Sodium (mg)... 280
%Cal-Fat...... 18%

Form a "pocket" in the pork tenderloin(s) by cutting a slit lengthwise down the center, about 3/4 of the way through to the other side. Be careful not to slit the other side. Open up slit tenderloin(s) and lay flat in a shallow baking dish.

Combine wine and Worcestershire sauce. Pour over pork tenderloin(s) and marinate, covered, for 1 to 3 hours in refrigerator, or 30 minutes at room temperature.

Preheat oven to 375 degrees. Spray a 7 1/2 x 11 x 2-inch baking dish with vegetable cooking spray.

In a small bowl, combine applesauce, dates, brown sugar, salt and cinnamon. Spoon mixture into pocket(s) of tenderloin(s). Close pockets loosely with wooden toothpicks. Place in prepared baking dish.

Bake at 375 degrees for approximately 30 to 40 minutes or until meat thermometer reads 157 to 160 degrees. (Do not overcook.) Let meat stand 5 minutes before slicing. Garnish with sprigs of fresh parsley.

*Quick Preparation Method: Do not marinate tenderloin, but instead lightly salt "pocket." Prepare applesauce mixture, stuff pocket, and bake as instructed above.*

Preparation time: 20–25 minutes
Cooking time: 30–40 minutes
Marinating time: 30 minutes–3 hours

# Pork Medallions with Mushroom Sauce

Cut tenderloin(s) into six equal pieces. Pound or press each tenderloin slice to 3/4-inch thickness.

Spray large skillet with vegetable cooking spray. Place over medium-high heat and brown tenderloin slices for about 2 minutes on each side. Transfer tenderloin to platter and keep warm.

Add mushrooms, water, onion, rosemary, pepper and garlic to skillet. Cover and sauté for 5 minutes or until mushrooms turn dark brown.

In a separate bowl, combine sherry, soy sauce, lime juice and sugar. Add to mushroom mixture in skillet.

Return tenderloin slices to skillet. Spoon mushroom sauce over slices. Cover and simmer for 15 to 20 minutes, turning meat over after 8 to 10 minutes. (Meat should have *no* pink inside.) Place pork tenderloin slices on serving plate. Cover with mushroom mixture. Garnish with sprigs of fresh rosemary, if desired.

Preparation time: 30–35 minutes
Cooking time: 15–20 minutes

*1 1/2 pounds pork tenderloin(s), trimmed of all visible fat*
*Vegetable cooking spray*
*8 ounces sliced fresh mushrooms*
*2 tablespoons water*
*1/4 cup finely chopped onion*
*1 teaspoon chopped fresh rosemary, or 1/2 teaspoon dried rosemary*
*1/4 teaspoon pepper*
*1/4 teaspoon garlic powder*
*6 tablespoons dry sherry*
*3 tablespoons reduced-sodium soy sauce*
*1 1/2 tablespoons lime juice*
*1 1/2 teaspoons sugar*
*Fresh rosemary sprigs (for garnish)*

### Yield: 6 4-ounce servings

*Per serving:*
Calories...... 230
Protein (g)... 34
Fat (g)....... 5.7
Sat. Fat (g).. 2
Choles. (mg).. 106
Fiber (g)..... 0.7
Sodium (mg)... 482
%Cal-Fat...... 22%

# Stir-Fry Gingered Pork

1 pound pork tenderloin,
   trimmed of visible fat, cut
   into thin, bite-size strips
1/4 cup dry sherry
2 tablespoons reduced-sodium
   soy sauce
2 tablespoons water
1 teaspoon sugar
1 cup clear beef broth, defatted
4 teaspoons cornstarch
2 teaspoons canola oil
2 teaspoons grated gingerroot
4 green onions including tops,
   finely diced
2 medium carrots, cut into
   julienne strips
1/2 pound fresh spinach,
   washed and coarsely chopped
1 8-ounce can bamboo shoots,
   drained
4 cups hot cooked rice
Soy sauce to taste

**Yield: 4 to 6 servings**

**Per serving:**
Calories...... 446
Protein (g)... 34
Fat (g)....... 7.1
Sat. Fat (g).. 1.9
Choles. (mg).. 85
Fiber (g)..... 4.3
Sodium (mg)... 510
%Cal-Fat...... 14%

Cut pork tenderloin on the bias into thin bite-size strips. In small mixing bowl, combine sherry, soy sauce, water and sugar. Add pork, stirring to coat well. Cover and marinate at room temperature 30 minutes or 2 hours in the refrigerator, stirring occasionally.

Drain pork, reserving marinade. Add beef broth and cornstarch to marinade. Stir until well blended. Set aside.

Heat oil in wok or heavy skillet over medium-high heat. Stir-fry gingerroot for 20 seconds. Add pork and stir-fry 3 to 4 minutes or until pork is no longer pink. Remove pork, keeping warm. Add green onions and carrots; stir-fry 2 minutes. Add chopped spinach and stir-fry an additional 3 minutes, or until vegetables are crisp-tender and spinach has wilted. Add bamboo shoots and heat through.

Return pork to skillet. Add marinade mixture. Cook and stir until it comes to a boil and thickens. Mix to evenly coat meat and vegetables. Serve immediately over rice.

Preparation time: 35–45 minutes
Marinating time: 30 minutes–2 hours

# Pork Tenderloin with Mustard Sauce

Preheat oven to 375 degrees.

In small bowl, combine honey mustard and water. Microwave on low for 15 seconds. Mix well until it becomes a smooth paste.

Spray roasting rack or broiler pan with non-stick cooking spray. Place trimmed tenderloin on prepared rack. Sprinkle lightly with salt and pepper, if desired. Spread half the honey mustard over top. Roast at 375 degrees for 20 minutes. Spread remaining honey mustard on tenderloin and cook an additional 10 to 20 minutes or until meat thermometer registers 157 to 160 degrees. (Avoid overcooking.) Let meat stand 5 minutes before serving.

To serve, cut into serving pieces and place on a platter. Garnish with fresh sprigs of parsley. Additional honey mustard sauce may be passed at the table, if desired.

*This is a very simple meat dish to prepare, perfect when time is limited. It can also be cooked on a preheated outdoor grill over medium heat. Place aluminum foil on the cooking rack, spray with vegetable cooking spray to avoid sticking, and cook approximately the same length of time as indicated above. Use a meat thermometer to be sure meat has been thoroughly cooked on the inside.*

*A good accompaniment for this dish is Rice-Mushroom Casserole (Recipe, page 334), a steamed vegetable of choice and a fresh green salad.*

Preparation time: 10 minutes
Cooking time: 30–40 minutes

*1 1/2 pounds pork tenderloin(s), trimmed of visible fat*
*Salt and pepper to taste (optional)*
*1/4 cup prepared honey mustard*
*1 tablespoon water*

**Yield: 6 4-ounce servings**

**Per serving:**
Calories...... 216
Protein (g)... 33
Fat (g)....... 5.7
Sat. Fat (g).. 2
Choles. (mg).. 71
Fiber (g)..... 0
Sodium (mg)... 140
%Cal-Fat...... 24%

# Pork Tenderloin Florentine

1 1/2 pounds pork tenderloins
2 10-ounce packages frozen
    chopped spinach, thawed and
    drained (squeeze lightly to
    remove excess water)
2 cups soft bread crumbs
    (about 3 slices)
1/4 cup finely chopped fresh
    parsley
1/2 cup grated Parmesan
    cheese
1 teaspoon minced garlic
2 egg substitutes (1/2 cup)
1 teaspoon lemon pepper
1/4 teaspoon salt

**Yield: 6 servings**

**Per serving:**
Calories...... 297
Protein (g)... 43
Fat (g)....... 7.6
Sat. Fat (g).. 3.5
Choles. (mg).. 109
Fiber (g)..... 2.9
Sodium (mg)... 502
%Cal-Fat...... 23%

Preheat oven to 375 degrees.

Slit the pork tenderloins lengthwise down the center, cutting about 3/4 of the way through to the other side. (If you have 2 tenderloins, do the same with both.) Open up slit tenderloin(s) and lay flat.

In large mixing bowl, combine thawed and drained spinach with remaining ingredients to make spinach pesto stuffing. Spoon mixture evenly over pork tenderloin(s), mounding slightly. Place on shallow baking pan, sprayed with vegetable cooking spray.

Bake at 375 degrees for approximately 30 to 40 minutes or until meat thermometer reads 157 to 160 degrees. Cut into six equal portions. Serve immediately.

Preparation time: 25–30 minutes
Cooking time: 30–40 minutes

# Pork Marengo

Trim all visible fat from tenderloin and cut into 3/4-inch cubes. Spray large nonstick skillet with vegetable cooking spray. Add meat cubes and sauté until light gray. Remove from skillet with slotted spoon.

Add onion, celery and garlic to meat juices in skillet. Sauté until onion becomes translucent, about 5 minutes.

Stir in 1/2 cup wine, tomato sauce, bay leaves, oregano, rosemary, salt, pepper, parsley and sautéed pork. Bring to a boil. Reduce heat and simmer, covered, 1 1/2 hours. Remove bay leaves.

Meanwhile, slice mushrooms. Toss with lemon juice. In covered medium-size skillet, sauté mushrooms until tender, about 5 to 10 minutes. Add remaining 1/2 cup wine and sautéed mushrooms to pork mixture.

Mix flour and cold water to make a paste. Add to skillet. Simmer, covered, 15 minutes longer. Meanwhile, prepare pasta according to package directions. Drain and toss with 1 tablespoon margarine to prevent pasta from sticking together.

Transfer pork mixture to a serving dish. Sprinkle with parsley. Serve over pasta.

*Recipe can be made ahead and refrigerated. Reheat in 350-degree oven for 30 to 40 minutes.*

Preparation time: 1 hour
Cooking time: 1 3/4 hours

*2 3/4 pounds pork tenderloin, trimmed of visible fat, cut into 3/4- inch cubes*
*Vegetable cooking spray*
*1 cup chopped onion*
*1 cup chopped celery*
*1 clove garlic, minced*
*1 cup dry white wine, divided*
*2 8-ounce cans tomato sauce*
*2 bay leaves*
*1 teaspoon dried oregano*
*1/2 teaspoon rosemary*
*1 teaspoon salt*
*1/2 teaspoon pepper*
*2 sprigs parsley, chopped finely*
*1 pound mushrooms, sliced*
*2 tablespoons lemon juice*
*1 tablespoon flour*
*2 tablespoons cold water*
*2 tablespoons fresh parsley, finely chopped*
*20 ounces dumpling pasta, or egg noodles*
*1 tablespoon tub margarine*

### Yield: 8 to 10 generous servings

**Per serving:**
Calories...... 525
Protein (g)... 48
Fat (g)....... 8.3
Sat. Fat (g).. 2.6
Choles. (mg).. 130
Fiber (g).... 5
Sodium (mg).. 646
%Cal-Fat..... 14%

# Veal Saltimbocca

6 veal cutlets pounded 1/8-inch
   thick
3 slices lean ham, halved
   (about 3 ounces total)
1 medium tomato, peeled and
   chopped
2 tablespoons finely chopped
   green onion
3 ounces grated mozzarella
   cheese (part-skim)
1/2 teaspoon ground sage
1/3 cup dry bread crumbs
1/4 cup grated Parmesan
   cheese
2 tablespoons fresh chopped
   parsley
1 egg substitute (1/4 cup)

**Yield: 6 servings**

**Per serving:**
Calories...... 225
Protein (g)... 31
Fat (g)....... 8.4
Sat. Fat (g).. 4.2
Choles. (mg).. 85
Fiber (g)..... 0.6
Sodium (mg)... 451
%Cal-Fat...... 33%

Preheat oven to 350 degrees.

Pound veal until it reaches desired thickness. Place the six veal cutlets on a flat surface. Top each with slice of ham (cut to size of cutlet), chopped tomato and green onion. Sprinkle mozzarella cheese and ground sage over top.

Fold in sides and roll up like a jelly roll. Secure with toothpicks.

Combine bread crumbs, Parmesan cheese and parsley. Dip veal rolls first in egg substitute, then bread crumb mixture. Place in shallow, oblong casserole dish. Bake, covered, at 350 degrees for 1 hour. Remove lid for last 10 minutes of baking.

Place on serving dish and remove toothpicks. Garnish with fresh sprigs of parsley.

Preparation time: 30 minutes
Cooking time: 1 hour

# Veal Piccata with Mushrooms

Combine mushrooms, wine and lemon juice in saucepan. Bring to a boil, reduce heat and simmer, uncovered, about 10 minutes, until mushrooms are tender. Set aside.

Meanwhile, pound veal cutlets until 1/2 original thickness. (Use a rolling pin or smooth side of meat mallet.) Sprinkle lightly with salt and pepper. Dredge with flour.

Heat olive oil in large nonstick saucepan. Place floured veal cutlets in pan and brown on both sides. Add chicken broth and simmer 3 minutes. Add mushroom mixture and cook, uncovered, 5 to 10 minutes, or until sauce begins to thicken and is reduced by approximately one-half.

Sprinkle with chopped parsley during last minute of cooking time. Transfer to a serving platter. Garnish with lemon wedges. Serve immediately.

*You may also use veal cutlets, cut 1/8-inch thick by the butcher. In this case there is no need to pound them thinner. However, they are usually more tender if pounded.*

Preparation time: 35–40 minutes

8 ounces fresh mushrooms, sliced
1/2 cup dry white wine
Juice of 1/2 lemon
3/4 pound veal cutlets, sliced 1/4-inch thick *
1/4 teaspoon salt
1/8 teaspoon pepper
1/4 cup flour
2 teaspoons olive oil
1 cup clear chicken broth, defatted
2 tablespoons chopped fresh parsley

**Yield: 4 servings**

**Per serving:**
Calories...... 231
Protein (g)... 28
Fat (g)....... 6.8
Sat. Fat (g).. 0.5
Choles. (mg).. 75
Fiber (g)..... 1.1
Sodium (mg)... 374
%Cal-Fat...... 15%

# Veal Rolls Divan

6 veal cutlets (about 3 ounces
    each), pounded 1/8-inch thick
1 tablespoon olive oil
1/2 cup chopped onion
1 1/2 cups packaged cornbread
    stuffing mix
1/4 cup plus 2 tablespoons hot
    water
1/4 cup egg substitute
Vegetable cooking spray
2 10-ounce packages frozen
    broccoli spears, thawed
1/3 cup all-purpose flour
1/2 cup skim milk
1 14-ounce can clear chicken
    broth (or from own stock)
3 tablespoons dry white wine
1/4 cup grated Parmesan
    cheese
Garnish with cherry tomatoes
    or radish roses (optional)

**Yield: 6 servings**

**Per serving:**
Calories...... 309
Protein (g)... 35
Fat (g)....... 8
Sat. Fat (g).. 3.2
Choles. (mg).. 83
Fiber (g)..... 3.7
Sodium (mg)... 566
%Cal-Fat...... 23%

Preheat oven to 350 degrees.

Pound veal cutlets to desired thickness.

Sauté onion in olive oil, until soft but not brown.

Make stuffing: In large mixing bowl, combine stuffing mix, hot water, egg substitute and sautéed onion. Mix until will blended. Place about 1/3 cup stuffing on each cutlet. Roll veal loosely, starting at narrow end. (Since cutlets generally overlap sufficiently, there is seldom a need to fasten with toothpicks. However, if veal tends to unfold, use toothpicks to fasten.)

Spray large skillet with vegetable cooking spray. Brown veal rolls on all sides. Simmer an additional 10 minutes, covered. Remove veal from skillet and set aside.

Meanwhile, thaw broccoli spears in microwave. Set aside.

Using a wire whisk, blend flour into skim milk until all lumps disappear. Pour into same skillet used for cooking veal. Immediately add chicken broth. Stir constantly and bring to a boil over medium heat. After mixture thickens, stir in wine.

Assemble dish: Place thawed broccoli spears crosswise in 11 x 7 1/2 x 2 1/2-inch baking dish. Top with veal rolls. Pour half the sauce over broccoli and veal. Cover and bake at 350 degrees for 30 minutes. Remove from oven.

Add Parmesan cheese to remaining sauce. Pour cheese sauce over veal dish. Broil 3 to 5 minutes or until sauce is lightly browned. Serve immediately. Garnish plates with cherry tomatoes or radish roses.

Preparation time: 40 minutes
Cooking time: 35 minutes

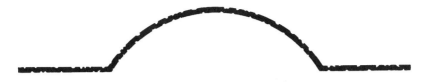

# *Fish & Seafood*

Orange Roughy with Mushroom Sauce • Kiwi Orange Roughy • Grilled Swordfish with Anchovy Sauce • Stuffed Flounder • Poached Salmon • Marinated Salmon • Salmon Stir-Fry • Salmon Teriyaki • Light Fried Fish Fillets • Dijon/ Onion-Topped Fish • Crab Cakes • Scallops Florentine • Artichoke-Scallop Linguine • Pasta with Scallops and Wine • Scallops Teriyaki • Scallops en Brochette • Shrimp Sukiyaki • Shrimp Jambalaya • Shrimp Cacciatore • Shrimp Creole

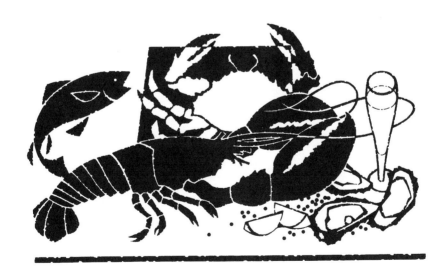

# Orange Roughy
# with Mushroom Sauce

1 to 1 1/2 pounds orange
  roughy fish fillets
8 ounces fresh mushrooms,
  sliced
1/2 cup water
1/2 cup dry sherry
1/4 cup low-sodium soy sauce
1/4 cup lime juice, divided
2 teaspoons sugar
1/4 cup flour
1 tablespoon olive oil
1/2 bunch green onions,
  chopped
2 cloves garlic, minced
1/2 teaspoon black pepper

### Yield: 4 large servings

### Per serving:

Calories...... 316
Protein (g)... 35
Fat (g)....... 8.8
Sat. Fat (g).. 1.3
Choles. (mg).. 82
Fiber (g)..... 1.4
Sodium (mg)... 704
%Cal-Fat...... 25%

Slice mushrooms in food processor. Place in medium-size covered skillet (no oil necessary) and cook on low until mushrooms darken. Drain mushrooms, reserving liquid. Set aside.

In a medium-size mixing bowl, combine juice from mushrooms, 1/2 cup water, sherry, soy sauce, 2 tablespoons lime juice and sugar. Set aside.

Rinse fish and pat dry. Rub fish with remaining 2 tablespoons lime juice. Next, rub flour evenly over both sides of fish.

Heat olive oil in large, heavy skillet, preferably nonstick. When oil is hot, place fish in skillet and sear each side for 2 to 3 minutes. Carefully transfer fish to a platter.

Add mushrooms, chopped green onions, minced garlic and pepper to hot skillet. Cook for 1 1/2 minutes. Reduce heat. Add sherry mixture and fish fillets, and bring to a boil. Cover and simmer an additional 5 to 10 minutes, until fish is opaque and flakes easily with a fork.

Transfer fish to a serving platter and pour mushroom sauce over. Serve immediately.

*This recipe is also excellent with red snapper.*

Preparation time: 35–40 minutes

Cooking time: 15–20 minutes

# Kiwi Orange Roughy

Preheat oven to 350 degrees. Wash fish fillets and pat dry.

Combine garlic powder, pepper and oregano. Sprinkle over fillets. Place fillets in a 12 x 8 x 2-inch non-stick baking dish.

Combine *Butter Buds* and lime juice. Rub canola oil over fish. Drizzle with lime juice mixture.

Cover and bake at 350 degrees for 20 minutes or until fish flakes easily with a fork.

Transfer fillets to serving platter. Carefully arrange 3 or 4 kiwi fruit slices on top of each fillet. Sprinkle with slivered almonds, if desired.

*The kiwi fruit adds interesting color and flavor to the fish.*

*Contains natural butter flavor without the oil or cholesterol. Available at most food stores.*

Preparation time: 15 minutes
Cooking time: 20 minutes

4 orange roughy fillets (1 1/2 pounds)
1/4 teaspoon garlic powder
1/4 teaspoon pepper
1/4 teaspoon dried oregano flakes
1 tablespoon Butter Buds *
1/4 cup lime juice
2 teaspoons canola oil
2 kiwi fruit, peeled and sliced
1/4 cup slivered almonds (optional)

**Yield: 4 servings**

**Per serving:**
Calories...... 240
Protein (g)... 33
Fat (g)....... 8.6
Sat. Fat (g).. 0.7
Choles. (mg).. 82
Fiber (g)..... 1.4
Sodium (mg)... 140
%Cal-Fat...... 32%

# Grilled Swordfish with Anchovy Sauce

*1 1/2 to 2 pounds swordfish steaks (sliced 3/4 to 1-inch thick)*

*Anchovy Sauce:*
*2 teaspoons olive oil*
*1 2-ounce can anchovy fillets in olive oil, drained and chopped finely*
*2 cloves garlic, minced*
*3 sprigs fresh parsley, finely chopped*
*1/4 teaspoon white pepper*
*Juice of 1 lemon*
*1/4 cup flour*
*1 1/2 cups skim milk*
*2 tablespoons whole capers*

**Yield: 4 or 5 6-ounce servings**

**Per serving:**
Calories...... 306
Protein (g)... 43
Fat (g)....... 9.7
Sat. Fat (g).. 2.9
Choles. (mg).. 82
Fiber (g)..... 0.3
Sodium (mg)... 636
%Cal-Fat...... 30%

Preheat gas grill or set oven control to broil.

Make anchovy sauce: Pour olive oil into small saucepan. Add chopped anchovy fillets, garlic, parsley and pepper. Cook and stir occasionally over low heat for 5 minutes. Add lemon juice. Set aside.

In a medium-size saucepan, whisk together flour and milk until all lumps disappear. Place over medium heat. Bring to a boil, stirring frequently, and continue cooking until sauce thickens. Add anchovy mixture and heat almost to a boil. Stir in capers. Keep warm until ready to serve.

Meanwhile, wash swordfish steaks and pat dry. Grill or broil approximately 5 minutes per side, or until fish flakes easily with a fork. (Grill over hot coals, or broil on lightly greased broiler rack, placed 4 inches from heat.)

To serve, place swordfish steaks on serving platter, and spoon anchovy sauce over each steak.

*To remove excess oil from anchovy fillets, pat dry with a paper towel. This sauce is also excellent over other firm-flesh fish, including salmon, shark and red snapper.*

Preparation time: 30–35 minutes

# Stuffed Flounder

Preheat oven to 400 degrees.

In saucepan, sauté onion and green pepper in olive oil until tender. Add crabmeat, breadcrumbs, egg substitute, parsley, salt and pepper. Mix well.

Wash flounder and pat dry. Place 1/4 of stuffing mixture on each fillet. Roll fillets and place seam side down in 12 x 7 1/2 x 2-inch baking dish.

Make sauce: Using a wire whisk, mix together flour and skim milk in mixing bowl until all lumps disappear. Pour into skillet placed over medium heat. Add salt, wine and 2 tablespoons Parmesan cheese. Bring to a boil, continually stirring until mixture thickens.

Pour sauce over fish. Sprinkle with paprika and 1 tablespoon Parmesan cheese. Bake in 400-degree oven for 35 minutes, or until fish flakes easily with fork. Transfer fish to serving dish. Spoon excess sauce from pan over fish. Serve immediately.

Preparation time: 30 minutes
Cooking time: 35 minutes

2 teaspoons olive oil
1/4 cup finely chopped onion
2 tablespoons finely chopped
  green pepper
1 cup fresh or canned
  crabmeat, drained and shell
  fragments removed
1/2 cup dry bread crumbs
3 tablespoons egg substitute
1 tablespoon finely chopped
  fresh parsley
1/2 teaspoon seasoned salt
1/4 teaspoon pepper
4 fresh flounder fillets (about 1
  1/2 pounds total weight)

Sauce:
1/4 cup flour
1 1/2 cups skim milk
1/2 teaspoon seasoned salt
1/3 cup dry white wine
2 tablespoons Parmesan cheese
1/2 teaspoon paprika
1 tablespoon Parmesan cheese

Yield: 4 servings

Per serving:
Calories...... 360
Protein (g)... 48
Fat (g)....... 6.5
Sat. Fat (g).. 2.1
Choles. (mg).. 117
Fiber (g)..... 1.1
Sodium (mg)... 741
%Cal-Fat...... 18%

# Poached Salmon

1 pound salmon, steaks or fillet
4 cups water
2 tablespoons lemon juice
1 teaspoon salt
1 bay leaf

**Yield: 4 servings**

**Per serving:**
Calories...... 163
Protein (g)... 22
Fat (g)....... 7.2
Sat. Fat (g).. 1.1
Choles. (mg).. 62
Fiber (g)..... 0
Sodium (mg)... 292
%Cal-Fat...... 38%

In a large skillet or saucepan, combine water, lemon juice, salt and bay leaf. Bring to a boil. Carefully place salmon in pan and bring to a second boil. Simmer for 10 minutes. Remove from pan with a spatula. Chill.

*If pan is not large enough to cook salmon in one layer, cook half at a time. Same water mixture can be used again.*

Preparation time: 10 minutes
Cooking time: 10 minutes

# Marinated Salmon

1 1/2 to 2 pounds salmon fillets
1/2 cup no-oil Italian dressing

**Yield: 4 or 5 6-ounce servings**

**Per serving:**
Calories...... 216
Protein (g)... 36
Fat (g)....... 9.1
Sat. Fat (g).. 1.0
Choles. (mg).. 94
Fiber (g)..... 0
Sodium (mg)... NA
%Cal-Fat...... 38%

Wash salmon fillets and pat dry. Place in shallow baking dish. Pour Italian dressing over top and marinate for 4 to 6 hours.

Remove fillets from marinade. Broil 4 inches from heat on lightly greased broiler rack or grill over hot coals until fish flakes easily with a fork. (Generally, allow about 5 minutes per side for fish 1-inch thick. Adjust the time, based on intensity of heat and thickness of fish.)

Preparation time: 5–10 minutes
Cooking time: 10 minutes
Marinating time: 4–6 hours

# Salmon Stir-Fry

Prepare vegetables: Cut off tops of snow peas; slice mushrooms and red pepper; and drain water chestnuts. Set aside.

Drain salmon, reserving liquid. Break salmon into chunks. Set aside.

Heat olive oil in large skillet or sauté pan. Stir-fry vegetables and minced garlic for 5 minutes.

Add water to reserved salmon liquid to make 1/2 cup liquid. Mix in cornstarch and cayenne. Pour liquid over vegetables and cook until it begins to boil. Add chunks of salmon and toss until well coated.

Serve over brown rice. Sprinkle with soy sauce or lemon juice.

Preparation time: 25–30 minutes
Cooking time: 50 minutes (for brown rice)

1 can (16 ozs.) salmon
1/2 pound fresh or frozen Chinese snow peas
1 cup sliced fresh mushrooms
1 red or green pepper, cut into narrow strips
1 8-ounce can sliced water chestnuts, drained
1 clove garlic, minced
2 teaspoons olive oil
2 teaspoons cornstarch
1/4 teaspoon cayenne pepper
Brown rice (4 cups cooked)
Reduced-sodium soy sauce or lemon juice

*Yield: 4 servings*

*Per serving:*
Calories...... 444
Protein (g)... 30
Fat (g)....... 11.8
Sat. Fat (g).. 2.7
Choles. (mg).. 50
Fiber (g)..... 5
Sodium (mg)... 621
%Cal-Fat...... 25%

# *Salmon Teriyaki*

*1 to 1 1/2 pounds salmon fillets*
*2 tablespoons reduced-sodium*
  *soy sauce*
*1/4 cup Chablis wine*
*1/4 teaspoon paprika*
*1 1/2 teaspoons sugar*

***Yield: 4 servings***

***Per serving:***
Calories...... 255
Protein (g)... 30
Fat (g)....... 9
Sat. Fat (g).. 1.2
Choles. (mg).. 88
Fiber (g)..... 0
Sodium (mg)... NA
%Cal-Fat...... 36%

Wash salmon fillets and pat dry.

Prepare marinade by combining soy sauce, wine, paprika and sugar. Place fillets in shallow container and pour marinade over. Marinate for 30 minutes at room temperature, or 1 to 2 hours in refrigerator.

Meanwhile, set oven control to broil.

Spray broiler rack with vegetable cooking spray. Remove salmon from marinade and place on rack. Spoon 2 tablespoons of marinade over top of fish. Broil approximately 4 to 6 inches from heat, skin side down, for 8 to 10 minutes, or until fish flakes easily with a fork.

Place on platter and serve immediately. Garnish with lemon wedges.

Preparation time: 10–15 minutes
Cooking time: 10 minutes
Marinating time: 30 minutes–2 hours

# Light Fried Fish Fillets

Rinse fish and pat dry.

In a small bowl, combine egg substitutes and sherry.

On a platter or paper plate, place bread crumbs.

Heat olive oil in a large nonstick fry pan. Dip fish first in egg mixture, then in bread crumbs. Place in preheated frypan. Fry 4 to 6 minutes per side, or until fish flakes easily with a fork. Avoid overcooking, which dries out the fish.

Transfer fish to serving platter. Garnish with fresh sprigs of parsley and lemon slices. Squeeze fresh lemon over fish, or serve with nonfat tartar sauce (Recipe, page 208), or seafood cocktail sauce.

Preparation time: 15 minutes
Cooking time: 10 minutes

*1 to 1 1/2 pounds fish fillets: flounder, sole, orange roughy, red snapper, or catfish*
*2 egg substitutes (1/2 cup)*
*1 tablespoon sherry*
*1/2 cup Italian style bread crumbs*
*2 teaspoons olive oil*
*Lemon slices and fresh sprigs of parsley for garnish*

### Yield: 4 servings

### Per serving:
Calories...... 270
Protein (g)... 40
Fat (g)....... 7.6
Sat. Fat (g).. 2.3
Choles. (mg).. 87
Fiber (g)..... 0.4
Sodium (mg)... 379
%Cal-Fat...... 27%

# Dijon/Onion-Topped Fish

6 small fish steaks, 1-inch
  thick (1 1/2 to 2 pounds)
Dash pepper
2 egg whites
2 tablespoons grated Parmesan
  cheese
2 tablespoons Dijon-style
  mustard
2 tablespoons chopped green
  onions (including tops)

Yield: 6 servings

Per serving (using flounder or
sole):
Calories...... 135
Protein (g)... 24
Fat (g)....... 3.3
Sat. Fat (g).. 0.7
Choles. (mg).. 56
Fiber (g)..... 0
Sodium (mg)... 214
%Cal-Fat...... 22%

Rinse fish and pat dry.

Set oven control to broil and/or 550 degrees. Sprinkle fish steaks with pepper. Place fish on lightly greased broiler rack placed about 4 inches from heat. Broil until light brown, about 5 minutes. Turn, and broil for an additional 5 minutes, or until fish flakes easily with a fork.

Meanwhile, beat egg whites until stiff but not dry. Fold in Parmesan cheese, mustard and onions. Spread mixture over fish. Broil until topping is golden brown, about 1 1/2 minutes. Serve immediately.

*This sauce is excellent with salmon or halibut steaks, but is also good on a variety of other fish. Garnish with fanned green onion tops.*

Preparation time: 15–20 minutes

Cooking time: 10–15 minutes

# Crab Cakes

1 pound lump crabmeat
1 egg substitute (1/4 cup)
3/4 cup evaporated skim milk
1 1/4 cups dry bread crumbs
1/4 teaspoon cayenne pepper
3/4 teaspoon dry mustard
1 teaspoon seasoned salt
2 teaspoons Worcestershire
  sauce
1 tablespoon tub margarine,
  melted

Preheat oven on broil setting.

Carefully look over crabmeat and remove shells. Combine all ingredients, except margarine, mixing thoroughly.

Spray cookie sheet with vegetable cooking spray. Press crab mixture into 8 patties, about 3/4-inch thick. Place on cookie sheet. Brush tops of cakes with melted margarine. Broil, with oven door open, 5 inches from heat source, about 4 minutes on each side, or until lightly browned.

Preparation time: 20–25 minutes
Cooking time: 8 minutes

*Yield: 8 crab cakes*

*Per serving:*
Calories...... 152
Protein (g)... 16
Fat (g)....... 2.5
Sat. Fat (g).. 0.5
Choles. (mg).. 52
Fiber (g)..... 0.6
Sodium (mg)... 498
%Cal-Fat...... 17%

# Scallops Florentine

Wash scallops in cold water. Drain and pat dry. Set aside.

Microwave spinach to thaw completely. Lightly squeeze excess moisture from spinach. (Do not squeeze completely dry.)

Combine flour, salt and pepper in medium-size mixing bowl. Toss scallops in flour mixture to coat completely.

Heat olive oil in large nonstick skillet. Add minced garlic. When garlic oil becomes hot, add scallops and sauté about 5 minutes, or until scallops become firm and opaque. (Do not overcook scallops or they will become rubbery.) Add spinach and toss until heated through, about 4 to 5 additional minutes. Serve immediately.

*This dish is delicious with a rice casserole, crusty French bread and a crisp green salad.*

Preparation time: 25 minutes
Cooking time: 10 minutes

1 1/2 pounds fresh bay or sea
  scallops
1 10-ounce package frozen
  chopped spinach
1/4 cup all-purpose flour
1/2 teaspoon salt
1/4 teaspoon pepper
1 1/2 tablespoons olive oil
4–6 cloves garlic, minced

*Yield: 4 to 6 servings*

*Per serving:*
Calories...... 200
Protein (g)... 25
Fat (g)....... 5.3
Sat. Fat (g).. 0.7
Choles. (mg).. 45
Fiber (g)..... 1.7
Sodium (mg)... 481
%Cal-Fat...... 24%

# Artichoke-Scallop Linguine

2 teaspoons olive oil
4 green onions, chopped
(including tops)
2 cloves garlic, minced
2 tablespoons fresh basil,
minced, or 2 teaspoons dried
1/2 teaspoon salt
Dash red pepper
1 16-ounce can tomatoes
1/2 cup dry white wine
2 tablespoons tomato paste
1 pound bay scallops, rinsed
and drained
1 14-ounce can artichoke
hearts, cut lengthwise into
quarters
8 ounces linguine
2 tablespoons slivered almonds,
toasted
Parmesan cheese (optional)

**Yield: 4 servings**

**Per serving:**
Calories...... 453
Protein (g)... 31
Fat (g)....... 6.8
Sat. Fat (g).. 0.8
Choles. (mg).. 37
Fiber (g)..... 6.4
Sodium (mg)... 770
%Cal-Fat...... 14%

In a heavy skillet, heat olive oil over medium heat. Add green onions and minced garlic. Saute 2 minutes. Add basil, salt, pepper, tomatoes, wine and tomato paste. Bring to a boil, breaking tomatoes up into small chunks with a spoon. Cover. Simmer for 20 minutes.

Add scallops and quartered artichoke hearts to tomato mixture. Cook until scallops are cooked, about 5 minutes.

Meanwhile, cook linguine according to package directions and drain. Toss with scallop mixture, mixing well. Transfer to shallow bowl or platter. Sprinkle with slivered almonds and Parmesan cheese, if desired.

Preparation time: 25 minutes
Cooking time: 25 minutes

# Pasta with Scallops and Wine

Cut large scallops in half and set aside. (Do not cut small scallops.)

In large saucepan cook onion in olive oil until tender but not brown. Stir in wine, bouillon cube, basil and pepper. Bring to a boil over medium heat. Simmer, uncovered, for 12 to 15 minutes, or until liquid is reduced to about 1/2 the original amount. Add scallops and chopped tomatoes. Cover and simmer about 5 minutes or just until scallops are cooked. (They will be white and more firm when cooked.)

Meanwhile, cook pasta according to package directions. Toss pasta with scallop mixture, Parmesan cheese and parsley until ingredients are well blended. Serve immediately. Sprinkle with Parmesan cheese if desired.

*Twelve ounces of medium-size fresh or frozen shrimp may be substituted for the scallops. This is a delicious meal to serve on a special occasion. Scallop mixture may be made a day ahead of time, and heated up at last minute, before tossing with pasta, cheese and parsley.*

Preparation time: 30–35 minutes

*12 ounces fresh sea scallops, drained and rinsed*
*2 teaspoons olive oil*
*1 cup chopped onion*
*1 cup dry white wine*
*1 chicken bouillon cube*
*1 tablespoon fresh basil, finely chopped, or 1 teaspoon dried*
*1/8 teaspoon freshly ground pepper*
*1 1/2 cups chopped tomato (fresh or canned)*
*12 ounces dumpling pasta or "eggless" egg noodles, cooked*
*1/4 cup grated Parmesan cheese*
*1/2 cup fresh minced parsley*

### Yield: 4 servings

### Per serving:
Calories...... 332
Protein (g)... 22
Fat (g)....... 6.9
Sat. Fat (g).. 1.9
Choles. (mg).. 33
Fiber (g)..... 3
Sodium (mg)... 455
%Cal-Fat...... 19%

1 pound sea scallops
1 medium onion, sliced and
    quartered
1 green or red pepper, chopped
    in 1/4 x 1-inch pieces
1 8-ounce can sliced water
    chestnuts, drained
2 tablespoons sherry

*Seafood Teriyaki Marinade:*
1/2 cup reduced-sodium soy
    sauce
2 teaspoons lemon juice
2 tablespoons brown sugar
2 cloves garlic, minced
1 teaspoon ground ginger
1 tablespoon olive oil
1 tablespoon sherry

**Yield: 4 servings**

**Per serving:**
Calories...... 241
Protein (g)... 22
Fat (g)....... 4.5
Sat. Fat (g).. 0.4
Choles. (mg).. 38
Fiber (g)..... 2.2
Sodium (mg)...0
%Cal-Fat...... 18%

# Scallops Teriyaki

Rinse scallops. Prepare marinade by mixing together soy sauce, lemon juice, brown sugar, garlic, ginger, olive oil and 1 tablespoon sherry. Pour marinade over scallops and refrigerate 1 to 3 hours.

Meanwhile, chop onion and pepper as specified. Drain water chestnuts and set aside.

Spray nonstick frypan or sauté pan with vegetable cooking spray. Add onions and peppers and sauté over medium heat 3 minutes. (Add 2 tablespoons water if vegetables stick.)

Remove scallops from marinade. Add to frypan. Cook over medium heat, stirring frequently until scallops are firm and opaque (about 5 minutes). Add water chestnuts, 2 tablespoons sherry and heat through. Serve with side dish of rice.

Preparation time: 30–35 minutes
Cooking time: 5–10 minutes
Marinating time: 1–3 hours

# Scallops en Brochette

Preheat gas or charcoal grill.

Wash scallops in cold water. Drain and pat dry. Prepare vegetables (cherry tomatoes, green peppers and onion). Set aside.

Combine honey mustard and egg substitute in small bowl.

Dip scallops first in egg mixture, next in bread crumbs.

Thread scallops and vegetables on 8 skewers, starting with green pepper square, followed by cherry tomato, onion and

1 pound fresh sea scallops
2 tablespoons honey mustard
1 egg substitute (1/4 cup)
1/2 cup Italian bread crumbs
1 pint cherry tomatoes
2 green peppers, cut into 1-inch
    squares
1 large onion, cut into bite-size
    pieces
Salt and pepper to taste

scallop. Repeat until skewers are full. End with green pepper square.

Grill over medium heat for 10 to 15 minutes, until scallops are lightly browned.

Serve with plain or seasoned rice.

Preparation time: 40–45 minutes
Cooking time: 10–15 minutes

Yield: 4 servings

Per serving:
Calories...... 202
Protein (g)... 24
Fat (g)....... 2.6
Sat. Fat (g).. 0.4
Choles. (mg).. 38
Fiber (g)..... 2.4
Sodium (mg)... 407
%Cal-Fat...... 12%

# Shrimp Sukiyaki

Cook rice according to package directions.

Meanwhile, clean shrimp (thaw, if frozen). Prepare onion, spinach, green onions and mushrooms as indicated. Set aside.

In small mixing bowl, combine 1/4 cup soy sauce, 1 tablespoon cornstarch, 1/2 cup water and brown sugar. Set aside.

Blend remaining 1 tablespoon soy sauce and 1 tablespoon cornstarch in a small bowl. Stir in shrimp until well coated.

Heat olive oil in large skillet. Add shrimp and stir-fry for 3 minutes. Remove.

Add 2 tablespoons water and onion to skillet; cook 1 minute. Add spinach, green onions, mushrooms and soy sauce mixture. Cover and cook until spinach wilts, stirring occasionally. Return shrimp to skillet. Cook 5 to 7 minutes or until vegetables are tender and shrimp is pink.

Serve immediately over rice. Sprinkle with lemon juice or additional soy sauce if desired.

Preparation time: 50–60 minutes

Cooking time: 10–15 minutes

*12 ounces medium-size raw shrimp, peeled and deveined*
*1 medium onion, thinly sliced*
*3/4 pound fresh spinach, trimmed, washed and drained*
*1 bunch green onions and tops, cut into 2-inch lengths*
*1/4 pound fresh mushrooms, sliced*
*5 tablespoons reduced-sodium soy sauce, divided*
*2 tablespoons cornstarch, divided*
*1/2 cup water*
*2 tablespoons brown sugar, firmly packed*
*1 tablespoon olive oil*
*2 tablespoons water*
*1 cup uncooked brown or white rice*

Yield: 4 servings

Per serving:
Calories...... 384
Protein (g)... 27
Fat (g)....... 6.3
Sat. Fat (g).. 1.1
Choles. (mg).. 165
Fiber (g)..... 6.5
Sodium (mg)... 850
%Cal-Fat...... 14%

# Shrimp Jambalaya

1 tablespoon olive oil

2–3 cloves garlic, minced

1 green pepper, chopped

1 medium onion, chopped fine

1 16-ounce can whole tomatoes, chopped

1 tablespoon Worcestershire sauce

1 pound fresh or frozen shrimp, cleaned

2 cups water

1/2 teaspoon salt or to taste

1/4 teaspoon thyme

1/8 teaspoon pepper

1/4–1/2 teaspoon cayenne pepper, or to taste

1 cup uncooked long-grain rice

**Yield: 6 1-cup servings**

**Per serving:**
Calories...... 237
Protein (g)... 19
Fat (g)....... 4
Sat. Fat (g).. 0.6
Choles. (mg).. 172
Fiber (g)..... 2.1
Sodium (mg)... 449
%Cal-Fat...... 15%

Cut up green pepper and onion as indicated above.

Heat olive oil in heavy 10-inch skillet. Add minced garlic, green pepper and onion. Sauté 5 minutes. Add chopped tomatoes and Worcestershire sauce to skillet.

Thaw shrimp, if frozen, and drain. Add shrimp to skillet along with water and seasonings. Bring to a boil. Stir in rice. As soon as mixture returns to a boil, reduce heat. Simmer, covered, about 30 minutes, or until all liquid is absorbed.

*For a variation, substitute 2 to 3 cups cooked chicken or turkey meat. Another delicious variation is to use 1/2 pound shrimp and 1/2 pound scallops. Corn bread provides a nice complement to this meal.*

Preparation time: 25 minutes
Cooking time: 30 minutes

# Shrimp Cacciatore

Place sliced mushrooms and chopped onion and pepper in large frypan. Cover and sauté until vegetables are tender. (No cooking oil necessary.)

Chop tomatoes coarsely in food processor. Add to vegetables in frypan. Also add prepared spaghetti sauce, oregano, basil, garlic powder, pepper and white wine. Bring to a boil and simmer, uncovered, 20 minutes or until sauce thickens slightly. Stir in cleaned shrimp and bring to a boil. Simmer 5 minutes.

Meanwhile, cook spaghetti according to package directions. Drain.

To serve, place desired portion of spaghetti on individual plates. Top with tomato-shrimp sauce. Sprinkle with Parmesan cheese.

*To prevent spaghetti from sticking together, add 1/4 cup tomato sauce to spaghetti immediately after it is drained.*

Preparation time: 25–30 minutes (if shrimp are already cleaned)

Cooking time: 25 minutes

1/4 pound fresh mushrooms, sliced
1 medium onion, chopped
1 green pepper, coarsely chopped
1 15-ounce can "no-salt-added" tomatoes, chopped
2 cups prepared spaghetti sauce
1/2 teaspoon dried oregano
1 tablespoon fresh basil or 1 teaspoon dried
1/2 teaspoon garlic powder
1/4 teaspoon black pepper
1/4 cup dry white wine
1 1/2 pounds fresh shrimp, shelled and deveined
1 pound spaghetti, uncooked
Parmesan cheese

### Yield: 6 servings

**Per serving:**
Calories...... 514
Protein (g)... 36
Fat (g)....... 5.5
Sat. Fat (g).. 1
Choles. (mg).. 172
Fiber (g)..... 6.8
Sodium (mg)... 618
%Cal-Fat...... 10%

# Shrimp Creole

1 large onion, chopped
1/2 cup finely chopped celery
1 green pepper, chopped finely
3 to 4 cloves garlic, chopped
2 teaspoons olive oil
1 28-ounce can tomatoes,
  chopped
1 teaspoon sugar
1/2 teaspoon chili powder
1/4 teaspoon black pepper
1 tablespoon Worcestershire
  sauce
1/4 teaspoon basil
1/4 teaspoon thyme
Tabasco sauce to taste
1 pound fresh medium-size
  shrimp, peeled and deveined
2 tablespoons fresh parsley,
  chopped
1 teaspoon cornstarch
2 teaspoons water
Rice (3 to 4 cups cooked)

### Yield: 4 servings

### Per serving:
Calories...... 444
Protein (g)... 31
Fat (g)....... 5.4
Sat. Fat (g).. 0.9
Choles. (mg).. 172
Fiber (g)..... 4.2
Sodium (mg)... 572
%Cal-Fat...... 11%

In large saucepan, cook onion, celery, green pepper and garlic in olive oil until tender, but not brown. Add chopped tomatoes, sugar, chili powder, pepper, Worcestershire sauce, basil, thyme and Tabasco sauce. Simmer, covered, 30 to 45 minutes.

Add shrimp and parsley to saucepan. Bring to a boil, and simmer an additional 20 minutes.

Mix cornstarch with water in small bowl. Stir into sauce and continue stirring until mixture thickens. Serve over rice.

Preparation time: 35 minutes (if shrimp already cleaned)
Cooking time: 50–60 minutes

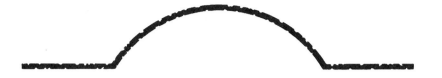

# *Meatless Main Dishes*

Vegetarian Chili • Bean Stroganoff • Lentil Burritos • Puerto Rican Black Beans and Rice • Hearty Bean Stew over Pasta • Black-Eyed Peas, Artichoke Hearts and Linguine • Vegetarian Chow Mein • Egyptian Pocket Sandwich • Beanburgers • Carolyn's Barbecued Beans • Stuffed Baked Potatoes • Spinach Frittata • Egg Foo Yong • Vegetable-Pasta Stir-Fry • Spinach-Noodle Casserole • Vegetarian Lasagna • Eggplant Parmesan • Deep-Dish Sicilian Pizza

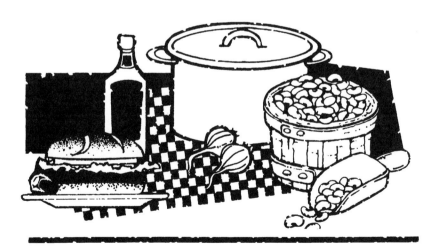

# Vegetarian Chili

3 cans (15 ounces) kidney
  beans, drained and rinsed
1 cup water
1 vegetable bouillon cube
1 cup raw bulgur
1/2 teaspoon minced garlic
1 1/2 cups chopped onion
1 cup chopped carrots
1 cup chopped green peppers
1 tablespoon olive oil
3 large fresh tomatoes, or 1 15-
  ounce can tomatoes, chopped
2 8-ounce cans tomato sauce
2 tablespoons dry red wine
Juice of 1/2 lemon
2 teaspoons chili powder (or
  more, to taste)
Water as needed, at least one
  cup
Salt to taste

**Yield: 6 to 8 servings**

**Per serving:**
Calories...... 309
Protein (g)... 14
Fat (g)....... 3.4
Sat. Fat (g).. 0.7
Choles. (mg).. 0
Fiber (g)..... 12.6
Sodium (mg)... 764
%Cal-Fat...... 9%

Drain and rinse kidney beans in a colander. Set aside.

Bring water to a boil. Add bouillon cube and stir until dissolved. Pour over raw bulgur. Cover and let stand at least 15 minutes.

In large skillet, sauté garlic, onions, carrots and green peppers in olive oil until tender (about 10 minutes).

Add kidney beans, bulgur and remaining ingredients to skillet and simmer 45 minutes or longer. Add water as needed for desired consistency.

*A hearty chili which tastes great with Millet Bread (Recipe, page 343). It is also very good served over pasta, with or without the bulgur.*

Preparation time: 25–30 minutes
Cooking time: 45 minutes

# Bean Stroganoff

In large skillet, sauté mushrooms and onions in olive oil.

In medium-size mixing bowl, mix flour and beef broth with a wire whisk until smooth. Add to skillet. Add remaining ingredients except yogurt and pasta. Bring to a boil and simmer 30 minutes to blend flavors.

Remove from heat and stir in yogurt. Serve over dumpling pasta or egg noodles.

*Vegetable bouillon dissolved in 2 cups boiling water may be substituted for the beef broth.

Preparation time: 35–40 minutes
Cooking time: 30 minutes

1 large onion, minced
16 ounces fresh mushrooms, sliced
2 teaspoons olive oil
5 tablespoons flour
1 14 1/2-ounce can clear beef broth, defatted*
2 tablespoons tomato paste
2 teaspoons prepared mustard
1 teaspoon Worcestershire sauce
1/4 teaspoon pepper
1/2 teaspoon sugar
1/4 teaspoon garlic powder
1/2 cup sherry
3 16-ounce cans pinto beans, drained and rinsed
3/4 cup plain nonfat yogurt
16 ounces dumpling pasta, or "eggless" egg noodles

### Yield: 8 servings

### Per serving:
Calories...... 460
Protein (g)... 20
Fat (g)....... 3.2
Sat. Fat (g).. 0.5
Choles. (mg).. 0
Fiber (g)..... 13.7
Sodium (mg)... 634
%Cal-Fat...... 7%

# Lentil Burritos

1 1/2 cups dried lentils
3 1/2 to 4 cups water
1 bay leaf
1 clove garlic, minced
1/2 teaspoon salt
1/4 teaspoon dried thyme
1 small onion chopped (1/4 to
  1/2 cup)
1/2 cup chili salsa
6 10-inch flour tortillas
1 medium tomato, chopped
2 ounces reduced-calorie
  cheddar cheese, shredded

**Yield: 6 10-inch burritos**

**Per serving:**
Calories...... 290
Protein (g)... 19
Fat (g)....... 4.7
Sat. Fat (g).. 1.7
Choles. (mg).. 10
Fiber (g)..... 6.5
Sodium (mg)... 417
%Cal-Fat...... 15%

Wash lentils. Combine lentils, 3 1/2 cups water, and next four ingredients in saucepan. Bring to a boil, reduce heat, and simmer 1 1/2 hours. Stir occasionally and add additional water if necessary. Remove bay leaf.

Add chopped onion and chili salsa to saucepan. Cook bean mixture, uncovered, over medium heat 5 minutes, stirring frequently.

Meanwhile, wrap tortillas tightly in aluminum foil; heat in a 350-degree oven 10 minutes, or until warmed. (If not wrapped tightly, they will dry out and become hard.)

To assemble burrito, spoon 1/6 of the bean mixture (about 1/3 cup) on each tortilla near one edge. Top with chopped tomato and shredded cheese. Fold the edge nearest the filling over the top of the filling, just covering it. Fold in the two sides, like an envelope, then roll up. Serve immediately.

Preparation time: 20–25 minutes
Cooking time: 1 1/2 hours

# Puerto Rican
# Black Beans and Rice

Wash beans and soak 8 hours or overnight. Drain.

Sauté onion, green pepper and garlic in olive oil until vegetables are tender.

In a large kettle, combine drained beans, sautéed vegetables, water, tomatoes, vinegar, sugar, salt and Tabasco sauce. Bring to a boil. Cover and simmer about 2 hours or until beans are tender.

Meanwhile, prepare rice according to package directions (without added salt or margarine).

To serve, spoon black beans over rice. Sprinkle with green onions. Top with salsa, if desired.

Preparation time: 25–30 minutes
Cooking time: 2 hours

1 pound dried black beans
1 cup chopped onion
1 green pepper, chopped
2 cloves garlic, minced
1 tablespoon olive oil
3 cups water
1 16-ounce can tomatoes, chopped
1 tablespoon wine vinegar
1/2 teaspoon sugar
1 teaspoon salt
1/8 teaspoon Tabasco sauce
5 to 6 cups cooked rice (1 1/2 cups uncooked)
1/4 cup chopped green onions
Salsa (optional)

*Yield: 6 to 8 servings*

*Per serving:*
Calories...... 486
Protein (g)... 20
Fat (g)....... 3.5
Sat. Fat (g).. 0.7
Choles. (mg).. 0
Fiber (g)..... 14.1
Sodium (mg)... 368
%Cal-Fat...... 7%

# Hearty Bean Stew over Pasta

1 16-ounce can red kidney
  beans, rinsed and drained
1 19-ounce can garbanzo
  beans, rinsed and drained
3 large carrots, peeled and cut
  into 1/4-inch slices
1/2 cup chopped onion
1 16-ounce can diced tomatoes,
  or whole tomatoes, chopped
1 16-ounce can (no salt added)
  tomatoes, chopped
1 8-ounce can tomato sauce
1/2 cup water
1/2 cup dry white wine
1 tablespoon olive oil
2 teaspoons chili powder
2 tablespoons fresh parsley,
  finely chopped
1/2 teaspoon garlic powder
1/4 teaspoon pepper
1 10-ounce package frozen
  chopped spinach, thawed
  (optional)
12 ounces dumpling pasta, or
  "eggless" egg noodles
Parmesan cheese (optional)

### Yield: 6 servings

### Per serving:
Calories...... 491
Protein (g)... 22
Fat (g)....... 5
Sat. Fat (g).. 0.8
Choles. (mg).. 0
Fiber (g)..... 11.5
Sodium (mg)... 636
%Cal-Fat...... 9%

In a Dutch oven or large saucepan, combine all ingredients except spinach, pasta and Parmesan cheese. Bring to a boil, reduce heat, and simmer, covered, 1 hour or until vegetables are tender.

Thaw spinach in microwave. Lightly squeeze out excess water. Add to stew. Cook 10 additional minutes. Add water to stew if you prefer more liquid.

Meanwhile, cook pasta according to package directions. Drain. Serve bean stew over pasta in pasta bowls. Sprinkle with Parmesan cheese, if desired.

Preparation time: 25–30 minutes
Cooking time: 1 hour

# Black-Eyed Peas, Artichoke Hearts and Linguine

Heat olive oil in large saucepan. Add chopped carrot, onions and garlic. Sauté 5 minutes.

Meanwhile, blanch dried tomatoes by placing in boiling water for 2 minutes. Drain and chop coarsely. Add to carrot-onion mixture.

Add remaining ingredients to saucepan, except linguine and Parmesan cheese. Bring to a boil, reduce heat and simmer 30 minutes.

Meanwhile, cook linguine according to package directions. Drain and put into serving dish. Spoon 1/2 of the bean mixture over the linguine. Mix well. Spoon remaining sauce over top of linguine and sprinkle with Parmesan cheese.

Preparation time: 20–25 minutes
Cooking time: 30 minutes

2 teaspoons olive oil
1 carrot, peeled and chopped
1/2 cup chopped onions
2 cloves garlic, minced
1 1/2 ounces sun-dried tomatoes (optional)
1 16-ounce can black-eyed peas, rinsed and drained
1 14-ounce can artichoke hearts, drained and quartered
1/4 cup black olives, sliced
1 16-ounce can diced tomatoes, or whole tomatoes, chopped
1/2 cup water
1/4 cup chopped parsley
12 ounces linguine, broken in half
1/4 cup grated Parmesan cheese

**Yield: 4 servings**

**Per serving:**
Calories...... 612
Protein (g)... 28
Fat (g)....... 8
Sat. Fat (g).. 2.2
Choles. (mg).. 5
Fiber (g)..... 14.2
Sodium (mg)... 616
%Cal-Fat...... 12%

# Vegetarian Chow Mein

1/4 cup dry white wine
3 tablespoons reduced-sodium
    soy sauce
2 tablespoons cornstarch
1 teaspoon instant chicken
    bouillon granules
1 cup cold water
2 teaspoons olive oil
1 teaspoon grated ginger root
2 medium carrots, cut julienne
    style
1/2 cup sliced onions, rings
    separated
2 medium zucchini, halved
    lengthwise and sliced 1/4-inch
    thick
1 4-ounce can mushrooms,
    drained
8 ounces fresh bean sprouts (or
    16-ounce can, drained)
1 16-ounce can pinto beans,
    rinsed and drained
1 8-ounce can sliced water
    chestnuts, drained
Hot cooked rice (about 4 cups)
Soy sauce to taste

**Yield: 4 to 6 servings**

**Per serving:**
Calories...... 398
Protein (g)... 13
Fat (g)....... 3
Sat. Fat (g).. 0.5
Choles. (mg).. 0
Fiber (g)..... 7
Sodium (mg)... 866
%Cal-Fat...... 7%

Combine wine, soy sauce, cornstarch, bouillon granules and water. Set sauce aside.

Cut up vegetables (carrots, onion, and zucchini) as indicated. Set aside.

In a wok or large skillet, preheat olive oil over medium-high heat. Stir-fry ginger root for 15 seconds. Add carrots, onions, zucchini and mushrooms; stir-fry about 4 to 6 minutes or until vegetables are crisp-tender. Stir in bean sprouts; stir-fry 1 minute.

Stir sauce. Add to center of wok or skillet. Cook and stir until thickened. Add pinto beans and water chestnuts. Stir until vegetables and beans are evenly coated with sauce. Cover and cook 1 minute longer. Serve immediately over hot cooked rice. Sprinkle with soy sauce, if desired.

*For a variation, 8 ounces fresh tofu (bean curd), cut into 1/2-inch cubes, may be substituted for the pinto beans. Add tofu at the same time as the pinto beans.*

Preparation time: 35–40 minutes

Cooking time: 10–15 minutes

# Egyptian Pocket Sandwich

Cut large pita bread slices in half and open up to make a pocket. Cover and set aside.

In medium saucepan, combine drained fava beans, garlic powder, cumin and water. Bring bean mixture to a boil over medium heat. Reduce heat and simmer, partially covered, for 30 minutes. Mixture should not be watery, but about the consistency of a light paste. Add more water if too thick.

Make salad mixture by combining chopped cucumbers, chopped tomato, parsley, olive oil, and lemon juice. Set aside.

Make Tahini-Lemon Sauce:

Combine all ingredients in food processor. Blend until smooth. Sauce may be served immediately.( If stored in refrigerator, it will stay fresh for several weeks. It will thicken slightly after chilling overnight in refrigerator.)

Assemble pocket sandwich: First put approximately 1/4 cup fava bean mixture into pocket, followed by 1/4 cup salad mixture. Top with 1 tablespoon Tahini-Lemon Sauce. Serve immediately. (Pita bread may be warmed in microwave before filling, if desired.)

Preparation time: 35–45 minutes

Cooking time: 30 minutes

3 large slices pita bread
1 16-ounce can fava beans, drained
1/2 teaspoon garlic powder
1/2 teaspoon cumin
1/4 cup water
2 small cucumbers, peeled and chopped
1 tomato, chopped
1 tablespoon fresh parsley, minced
1 tablespoon olive oil
1 tablespoon lemon juice

Tahini-Lemon Sauce:
1/3 cup sesame tahini
1/4 cup lemon juice
2 to 3 cloves garlic, minced
1/4 cup cold water
1/4 teaspoon salt
1/4 teaspoon pepper

**Yield: 6 large 1/2-pocket sandwiches**

**Per serving:**
Calories..... 272
Protein (g).. 13
Fat (g)...... 7
Sat.Fat (g).. 0.9
Choles. (mg).. 0
Fiber (g)..... 6.1
Sodium (mg)... 414
%Cal-Fat...... 23%

# *Beanburgers*

3/4 cup dry lentils
3 cups water
1 medium onion, chopped finely
1/2 cup dry bread crumbs
1 egg substitute (1/4 cup)
2 tablespoons chopped walnuts
1/4 cup chili sauce
1/2 teaspoon prepared mustard
1/2 teaspoon salt
Dash cayenne
1 tablespoon olive oil
5 large buns

### *Yield: 5 burgers*

### *Per serving:*
Calories...... 337
Protein (g)... 16
Fat (g)....... 7.2
Sat. Fat (g).. 1.3
Choles. (mg).. 0
Fiber (g)..... 5.9
Sodium (mg)... 634
%Cal-Fat...... 19%

Rinse lentils. Place lentils and water in saucepan. Bring to a boil and simmer, covered, 45 to 50 minutes, or until tender. Drain. Transfer to mixing bowl and mash with a fork.

Add onion, bread crumbs, egg substitute, walnuts, chili sauce, mustard, salt and cayenne to mixing bowl. Mix well. Shape into 5 patties, about 1/2 to 3/4-inch thick.

Pour olive oil into skillet. Cook beanburgers in olive oil over medium heat about 4 minutes per side, or until lightly browned.

Serve on a bun with condiments and garnishes of choice: mayonnaise (fat-free or light), catsup, mustard, pickles, green onions and/or sliced tomatoes.

*The beanburger mix can be made ahead and stored in the refrigerator for up to 4 days. If a longer storage time is desired, make into patties and freeze.*

Preparation time: 20 minutes
Cooking time: 55 minutes

# Carolyn's Barbecued Beans

Wash beans. Soak overnight or at least 6 hours.* Drain.

In large kettle, place presoaked beans. Pour in enough water to make water level 2 inches above beans. Add salt and onion. Cook 1 to 1 1/2 hours or until tender. Drain, reserving 1 1/2 cups of bean broth. Add remaining ingredients, including reserved broth. Bring to a boil and simmer for 30 minutes.

*Instead of soaking beans overnight, an alternate method may be used: Place beans in large kettle and cover with water, 2 inches above level of beans. Heat until boiling. Boil 2 minutes and remove from heat. Let beans sit, covered, for at least 1 hour before draining. (Beans may soak this way all day long.)

Add fresh water (2 inches above level of beans), onion and salt. Cook beans 45 to 60 minutes, or until they are tender. Drain, reserving 1 1/2 cups of bean broth. Add remaining ingredients, including reserved broth, and simmer 30 minutes.

Preparation time: 20–30 minutes
Cooking time: 1 1/2–2 hours

1/2 cup black beans, dry
1/2 cup lima beans, dry
1/2 cup red kidney beans, dry
1/2 cup black-eyed peas, dry
1 cup navy beans, dry
2 teaspoons salt
1/2 cup chopped onion
1 carrot, chopped
1 apple with peel, cored and diced
2 tablespoons molasses
1/2 cup catsup
1/2 cup spicy barbecue sauce
2 tablespoons firmly packed brown sugar
1 teaspoon prepared mustard

**Yield: 8 servings**

**Per serving:**
Calories...... 242
Protein (g)... 12
Fat (g)....... 1.2
Sat. Fat (g).. 0.2
Choles. (mg).. 0
Fiber (g)..... 10.6
Sodium (mg)... 757
%Cal-Fat...... 4%

# Stuffed Baked Potatoes

4 large baking potatoes
1 16-ounce can vegetarian
   baked beans
1/2 cup chopped scallions or
   chives
2 ounces reduced-calorie
   cheddar cheese, shredded
Nonfat sour cream (optional)

**Yield: 4 servings**

**Per serving:**
Calories...... 339
Protein (g)... 11
Fat (g)....... 3.1
Sat. Fat (g).. 1.2
Choles. (mg).. 6
Fiber (g)..... 8.1
Sodium (mg)... 398
%Cal-Fat...... 3%

Bake potatoes in oven or microwave until soft. (Bake for about 1 hour at 350 degrees in oven, or 15 to 18 minutes in microwave on high setting.)

Heat baked beans on stove.

To serve, slash potatoes across top, spread open, and fill with baked beans. Sprinkle scallions and cheddar cheese on top, and if desired, nonfat sour cream.

*This is a quick, nutritious, low-fat meal. It is popular with children because they can assemble it themselves. Serve with your favorite bread and a crisp fruit salad, such as Slim Waldorf Salad. (Recipe, page 226)*

Preparation time: 10 minutes
Cooking time: 1 hour (18 minutes microwave)

# Spinach Frittata

2 teaspoons canola oil
1 10-ounce package frozen
   chopped spinach, thawed and
   drained
1 small zucchini, coarsely
   chopped
1 small onion, finely chopped
1 teaspoon minced garlic
6 egg substitutes (1 1/2 cups)
1/4 cup skim milk
1/4 teaspoon pepper
1/4 teaspoon dried oregano
1/4 teaspoon dried basil
1/4 teaspoon salt
1/2 cup grated Parmesan
   cheese
7 cherry tomatoes, halved

Thaw spinach and squeeze lightly to remove excess water.

Heat oil in large skillet. Add spinach, zucchini, onion and garlic to skillet and sauté until vegetables are tender, about 5 to 10 minutes. Remove from heat and let cool slightly.

In large mixing bowl, beat egg substitutes and milk with a wire whisk. Add pepper, oregano, basil and salt. Stir in Parmesan cheese and vegetables.

Spray 9-inch pie pan with vegetable cooking spray. Pour egg mixture into pie pan. Arrange cherry tomatoes, cut side up, on top of frittata. Bake in 350-degree oven for 25 to 30 minutes or until puffed and slightly browned. Serve hot.

*This frittata may be baked a day in advance and stored in the refrigerator. Heat just before serving, either in the oven, covered, or in the microwave. This is an excellent choice for a brunch.*

Preparation time: 25–30 minutes
Cooking time: 25–30 minutes

*Yield: 8 servings*

*Per serving:*
Calories...... 89
Protein (g)... 11
Fat (g)....... 3.2
Sat. Fat (g).. 1.2
Choles. (mg).. 6
Fiber (g)..... 1.8
Sodium (mg)... 302
%Cal-Fat...... 32%

# Egg Foo Yong

In a medium-size mixing bowl, combine egg substitutes and flour. Mix with a wire whisk until all lumps disappear. Add Oriental vegetables, green onions, seasoned salt and pepper. Mix until well blended.

Spray a 10-inch nonstick skillet or sauté pan with a vegetable cooking spray. Place over medium-high heat. Add 1/4 cup egg mixture; press down with spatula until about 4 inches in diameter. (Cook 2 or 3 at a time in skillet.)

Cook the egg foo yong 1 to 2 minutes, or until it starts to lightly brown on bottom; turn with spatula and cook other side, about 1 to 2 minutes. Transfer to warmed serving platter. Repeat with remaining mixture.

Serve immediately with Duck Sauce or Hot Sweet Mustard Sauce.

*For a variation, 6 ounces of crabmeat or 3/4 cup diced shrimp, chicken or turkey may be added.*

Preparation time: 20–25 minutes

*4 egg substitutes (1 cup)*
*1/4 cup all-purpose flour*
*1 16-ounce can mixed Oriental vegetables, drained*
*1/4 cup minced green onions*
*1/2 teaspoon seasoned salt*
*1/8 teaspoon black pepper*
*Vegetable cooking spray*

*Yield: 6 small servings*

*Per serving:*
Calories...... 60
Protein (g)... 6
Fat (g)....... 1.4
Sat. Fat (g).. 0.3
Choles. (mg).. 0
Fiber (g)..... 1
Sodium (mg)... 163
%Cal-Fat...... 21%

# Vegetable-Pasta Stir-Fry

1 pound linguine
1 tablespoon canola oil
2 cloves garlic, minced
1 medium eggplant, cut into
    1/2-inch cubes
1 red pepper, cut into 1-inch
    strips
1 medium onion, chopped
1/4 cup Burgundy wine
1/2 teaspoon salt
1 16-ounce can garbanzo
    beans, drained and rinsed
4 medium tomatoes, chopped
1/4 cup pitted ripe olives, sliced
1/2 cup fresh parsley, chopped
2 teaspoons tub margarine
1/4 cup grated Parmesan
    cheese
Parmesan cheese (optional)

**Yield: 6 servings**

**Per serving:**
Calories...... 338
Protein (g)... 14
Fat (g)....... 7.6
Sat. Fat (g).. 1.5
Choles. (mg).. 3
Fiber (g)..... 8.4
Sodium (mg)... 425
%Cal-Fat...... 20%

Prepare vegetables (eggplant, red pepper, onion, tomatoes, olives and parsley) by cutting/chopping as indicated. Set aside.

Cook linguine in boiling water according to package directions.

Meanwhile, preheat oil in wok or large skillet over medium-high heat; add garlic and stir-fry for 15 seconds. Add eggplant, red pepper and onion; stir-fry 3 minutes. Add wine and salt, and mix well. Steam for 5 minutes.

Add beans, tomatoes, olives and parsley. Cover and cook 5 additional minutes.

After pasta is cooked, drain, and place in large bowl. Add vegetables, margarine and Parmesan cheese. Toss gently until well mixed. Serve immediately. Sprinkle additional Parmesan cheese over top, if desired.

Preparation time: 35–45 minutes

# Spinach-Noodle Casserole

Preheat oven to 375 degrees.

Cook noodles according to package directions. Drain. Set aside.*

Meanwhile, spray skillet or sauté pan with vegetable cooking spray. Sauté mushrooms and onions until vegetables are tender. Stir in spinach. Pour in wine. Steam until wine evaporates (about 2 minutes).

In large mixing bowl, stir together egg substitutes, cottage cheese, 1/2 cup Parmesan cheese and seasoned salt. Add mushroom-spinach mixture. Add cooked noodles and wheat germ. Spread in 9 x 13-inch pan. Sprinkle remaining Parmesan cheese over top.

Bake at 375 degrees for 30 minutes, covered; and an additional 15 minutes, uncovered.

*If cooked noodles need to be held awhile before mixing them with other ingredients, they should be placed over steaming hot water in a colander. Steam will keep them hot without further cooking, and stickiness will be minimized.

Preparation time: 30–35 minutes
Cooking time: 45 minutes

8 ounces "eggless" egg noodles, uncooked
Vegetable cooking spray
1/2 pound fresh mushrooms, sliced
1 medium onion, chopped
1 10-ounce package frozen chopped spinach, thawed and pressed dry
1/4 cup dry white wine
3 egg substitutes (3/4 cup)
3 cups low-fat cottage cheese
1/2 cup Parmesan cheese
1 teaspoon seasoned salt
2 tablespoons wheat germ
2 tablespoons Parmesan cheese

**Yield: 8 servings**

**Per serving:**
Calories...... 257
Protein (g)... 23
Fat (g)....... 4.8
Sat. Fat (g).. 2.3
Choles. (mg).. 10
Fiber (g)..... 3
Sodium (mg)... 690
%Cal-Fat...... 17%

# Vegetarian Lasagna

1 cup chopped onion
2 teaspoons olive oil
1 10-ounce package frozen
  chopped spinach, thawed and
  squeezed dry
1 cup all-purpose flour
3 cups skim milk
1/2 cup Parmesan cheese
3/4 teaspoon seasoned salt
1/4 teaspoon pepper
1 teaspoon dried oregano,
  crushed
8 ounces lasagna noodles,
  cooked and drained
1/4 cup Parmesan cheese
2 ounces part-skim mozzarella
  cheese, shredded

**Yield: 4 to 6 servings**

**Per serving:**
Calories...... 455
Protein (g)... 25
Fat (g)....... 9.6
Sat. Fat (g).. 4.6
Choles. (mg).. 21
Fiber (g)..... 4.2
Sodium (mg)... 643
%Cal-Fat...... 19%

Preheat oven to 350 degrees.

In a large, covered skillet, cook chopped onion in olive oil until onion is tender but not brown. Add chopped spinach and mix together.

In large mixing bowl, combine flour with milk using a wire whisk until all lumps disappear. Pour into skillet. Add 1/2 cup Parmesan cheese, seasoned salt, pepper and oregano. Cook over medium heat, stirring occasionally, until mixture comes to a boil and thickens. Simmer, covered, over low heat until ready to assemble lasagna.

Meanwhile cook lasagna noodles according to package directions.

Drain and pat dry with paper towels.

Arrange a single layer of lasagna noodles in the bottom of a lightly greased 12 x 7 1/2 x 2-inch baking dish. Top with 1/3 of the spinach mixture. Repeat the layers two more times. Sprinkle 1/4 cup Parmesan cheese over top, followed by mozzarella cheese.

Bake, uncovered, for 30 to 35 minutes, or until cheese is lightly browned on top. Let stand 10 minutes before serving.

Preparation time: 30–35 minutes
Cooking time: 35 minutes

# Eggplant Parmesan

Preheat oven to 425 degrees.

Spray large cookie sheet with vegetable cooking spray. Cut eggplant (unpeeled) into 1/4-inch-thick slices. Dip each slice first in egg substitutes and then bread crumbs. Place in single layer on cookie sheet. Bake at 425 degrees 10 minutes. Turn over and bake an additional 10 minutes.

Meanwhile, make tomato sauce by combining prepared spaghetti sauce and tomato sauce (no salt added) in small bowl. Season to taste.

Reduce oven heat to 350 degrees.

Assemble Eggplant Parmesan in a 2 to 3-quart casserole dish. Place 2 or 3 tablespoons tomato sauce on bottom of baking dish. Next arrange layer of eggplant slices on top of sauce. Top with 1/3 of sauce and 1/3 of Parmesan cheese. Repeat layers three times or until all ingredients are used up, ending with sauce and Parmesan cheese on top. Cover with thin layer of mozzarella cheese.

Bake, covered, at 350 degrees 20 minutes. Broil, uncovered, an additional 3 to 5 minutes or until cheese is lightly browned.

Preparation time: 30 minutes
Cooking time: 30 minutes

1 large eggplant
2 egg substitutes (1/2 cup)
3/4 cup Italian bread crumbs
1 cup prepared light spaghetti sauce
1 cup tomato sauce (no salt added)
1/4 cup Parmesan cheese
2 1/2 ounces part-skim mozzarella cheese

**Yield: 6 large servings**

*Per serving:*
Calories...... 159
Protein (g)... 11
Fat (g)....... 3.6
Sat. Fat (g).. 2.3
Choles. (mg).. 10
Fiber (g)..... 3
Sodium (mg)... 485
%Cal-Fat...... 20%

# Deep-Dish Sicilian Pizza

1 pound frozen bread dough, white or whole wheat
1 1/4 cups spaghetti sauce, or seasoned tomato sauce
1 14-ounce can artichoke hearts in water, drained and chopped
1 medium onion, sliced thin, rings separated
1/2 green pepper, sliced in 2-inch narrow strips
1/4 cup Parmesan cheese
2 ounces (1/2 cup) shredded mozzarella cheese (optional)

**Yield: 1 14-inch pizza, or 8 slices**

**Per slice:**
Calories...... 231
Protein (g)... 8
Fat (g)....... 4.2
Sat. Fat (g).. 1.1
Choles. (mg).. 2.5
Fiber (g)..... 4
Sodium (mg)... 597
%Cal-Fat...... 16%

**With mozzarella:**
Fat (g)........5.4
%Cal-Fat.....20%

Thaw dough overnight in refrigerator or at room temperature for 2 hours.

Place dough in greased bowl, cover, and let rise in warm place until it has doubled in size (about 45 to 60 minutes).

Spray 14-inch deep-dish pizza pan with vegetable cooking spray. Punch dough down. On floured surface, roll out into large circle. Place in pizza pan. Spread with fingers to make dough fit to edges of pan. Cover dough and let rise in warm place 45 to 60 minutes.

Preheat oven to 400 degrees.

Pour spaghetti sauce over dough. Arrange vegetables on top. (Other toppings may be substituted, depending on individual preferences.) Sprinkle Parmesan cheese and, if desired, mozzarella cheese over top.

Bake at 400 degrees 20 to 25 minutes, or until cheese melts and crust turns light brown.

Preparation time: 15–20 minutes
Cooking time: 20–25 minutes (plus 1 1/2–2 hours for dough to rise)

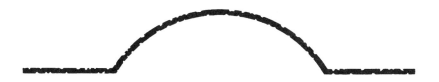

# *Pasta, Rice & Grains*

Fettucine with Artichokes in White Sauce • Pasta with Red Clam Sauce • Pasta with White Clam Sauce • Baked Ziti • Tuna Fettuccine • Spaghetti and Meatballs • Quick Marinara Sauce with Pasta • Ziti with Creamy Mushroom Sauce • Linguine with Chicken and Vegetables • Fettucine with Shrimp and Mussels •Spaghetti Putanesca • Parmesan Rice • Wild Rice Baked Casserole • Saffron Rice • Spanish Rice • Rice-Mushroom Casserole • Green Rice Casserole • Baked Bulgur with Fruit • Bulgur with Steamed Vegetables • Polenta • Potato Gnocchi

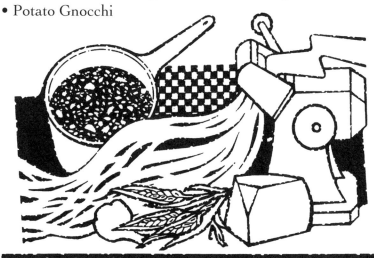

# Fettucine with Artichokes
# in White Sauce

3 tablespoons flour
1 1/2 cups chicken stock, or 1
   14 1/2-ounce can clear
   chicken broth, defatted
3 cloves of garlic, crushed, or 1
   teaspoon minced garlic
1 1/2 tablespoons fresh lemon
   juice
Freshly ground pepper, to taste
1 14-ounce can artichoke
   hearts in water, drained and
   cut into bite-size pieces
12 ounces fettucine or linguine,
   uncooked
1/4 cup fresh parsley, minced
1/4 cup Parmesan cheese
1 tablespoon tub margarine

**Yield: 6 servings**

**Per serving:**
Calories...... 246
Protein (g)... 11
Fat (g)....... 3.8
Sat. Fat (g).. 0.9
Choles. (mg).. 3
Fiber (g)..... 5.3
Sodium (mg)... 289
%Cal-Fat...... 14%

In a large heavy skillet, combine flour and chicken broth, mixing with a wire whisk until all lumps disappear. Cook over medium heat, stirring occasionally, until mixture comes to a boil and thickens.

Add garlic, lemon juice and pepper to skillet. Cook, uncovered, for 5 minutes over low heat, stirring occasionally. Add artichoke hearts and cook, uncovered, for an additional 8 minutes. Meanwhile, cook fettucine according to package directions, and drain.

Pour fettucine into large serving dish. Immediately add artichoke sauce, parsley, Parmesan cheese and margarine. Toss until well mixed. Serve immediately.

Pass additional Parmesan cheese to sprinkle over top.

*A delicious lower-fat alternative to Fettucine Alfredo, which contains large amounts of butter and cream.*

Preparation time: 20–30 minutes

Cooking time: 15–20 minutes

# *Pasta with Red Clam Sauce*

Drain clams. Set aside.

Sauté chopped onion in olive oil in medium-size skillet until onions are soft. Add wine and clams. Cook until liquid is reduced by one-half.

Chop tomatoes in food processor. Add to skillet along with prepared spaghetti sauce. Simmer, uncovered, for 15 to 30 minutes.

Meanwhile, prepare pasta as directed on package. Drain. Place in large serving bowl. Spoon clam sauce over top. Sprinkle with Parmesan cheese.

Preparation time: 15–20 minutes
Cooking time: 20–30 minutes

3 6 1/2-ounce cans minced
  clams, drained
1 medium onion, chopped fine
2 teaspoons olive oil
1/2 cup dry white wine
1 15-ounce can tomatoes (no
  salt added)
2 cups prepared spaghetti sauce
16 ounces pasta
Parmesan cheese

*Yield: 4 to 6 servings*

*Per serving:*
Calories...... 555
Protein (g)... 38
Fat (g)....... 8
Sat. Fat (g).. 1.3
Choles. (mg).. 70
Fiber (g)..... 4.8
Sodium (mg)... 625
%Cal-Fat...... 13%

# Pasta with White Clam Sauce

3 6 1/2-ounce cans chopped
   clams, including juice
2 teaspoons olive oil
1/2 cup chopped onion
2 to 4 cloves garlic, minced
1/2 cup dry white wine
1 teaspoon dried basil
4 teaspoons cornstarch
1/4 cup Parmesan cheese
1/4 cup fresh chopped parsley
1 pound linguine or angel-hair
   pasta

**Yield: 4 to 6 servings**

**Per serving:**
Calories...... 495
Protein (g)... 29
Fat (g)....... 6
Sat. Fat (g).. 1.9
Choles. (mg).. 43
Fiber (g)..... 4
Sodium (mg)... 279
%Cal-Fat...... 11%

Heat olive oil in medium-size skillet over low heat. Add onions and sauté until they become translucent. Add garlic and sauté an additional 1/2 minute.

Meanwhile, drain juice from 2 cans of clams, reserving liquid.

Add drained clams and 1 can of clams with liquid to skillet. Add wine and basil. Bring to a boil and simmer, covered, about 10 to 15 minutes.

Add cornstarch to reserved liquid from clams. Mix well with wire whisk. Add to skillet and continue to cook, uncovered, over low heat until mixture returns to a boil and thickens.

Meanwhile, cook pasta according to package directions. Drain well.

In large bowl, combine drained pasta, clam sauce, Parmesan cheese and parsley. Toss until well mixed. Serve immediately. Sprinkle with additional Parmesan cheese, if desired.

*Garnish with open clam shells on top for a nice effect.*

Preparation time: 20–25 minutes

Cooking time: 15–20 minutes

# Baked Ziti

Spray large skillet with vegetable cooking spray. Add chopped onion and garlic and sauté until onion becomes translucent. Add 2 tablespoons water, if necessary, to keep onion from sticking.

Add crushed tomatoes, chopped tomatoes, tomato sauce, parsley, basil, fennel, wine, 1 tablespoon Parmesan cheese, pepper and sugar to skillet. Bring to a boil. Cover and simmer on low 1 to 1 1/2 hours. Add water if sauce is too thick. Salt to taste, if desired.

Meanwhile, cook pasta according to package directions. Drain. Rinse with cold water immediately to prevent pasta from sticking together.

Assemble in 9 x 13-inch pan: Spread about 1 1/4 cups sauce on bottom of pan. Top with 1/3 of the cooked ziti. Crumble 1/4 pound ricotta cheese and sprinkle 2 ounces mozzarella cheese over ziti. Repeat layers of sauce, ziti, ricotta and mozzarella. Pour about 1 1/2 cups sauce over top. Add remaining 1/3 of the ziti and the remaining sauce (about 1 1/2 cups). Sprinkle Parmesan cheese over top.

Bake, uncovered, in 350-degree oven 30 minutes, or until heated through. Remove from oven and let sit for 5 minutes before serving.

*Quick Preparation Method: Instead of layering pasta, tomato sauce and cheeses, mix all together (except Parmesan cheese) in large bowl. Spread in a 9 x 13-inch pan. Sprinkle Parmesan cheese over top. Bake as directed.*

*Baked ziti can be assembled a day in advance, covered and refrigerated until ready to bake. To bake, cover with aluminum foil and bake at 350 degrees 45 minutes, removing foil for last 20 minutes of baking.*

Preparation time: 30–35 minutes
Cooking time: 1 1/2–2 hours

## Ingredients

Vegetable cooking spray
1 medium onion, chopped
2 cloves garlic, minced
1 28-ounce can crushed tomatoes
1 16-ounce can tomatoes, finely chopped
1 8-ounce can tomato sauce
1/4 cup minced parsley
2 teaspoons dried basil
2 teaspoons fennel
1/4 cup dry white wine
1 tablespoon Parmesan cheese
1/4 teaspoon pepper
1 1/2 teaspoons sugar
Salt to taste
1 pound pasta, penne rigate or cut ziti
1/2 pound ricotta low-fat cheese
4 ounces part-skim mozzarella cheese, shredded
1/4 cup Parmesan cheese, grated

**Yield: 6 to 8 servings**

*Per serving:*
Calories...... 407
Protein (g)... 21
Fat (g)....... 7.1
Sat. Fat (g).. 3.9
Choles. (mg).. 22
Fiber (g)..... 4.6
Sodium (mg)... 557
%Cal-Fat...... 16%

# Tuna Fettuccine

12 ounces spinach fettuccine
1/2 cup sliced green onion,
  including tops
2 teaspoons olive oil
1/4 cup all-purpose flour
2 cups skim milk
1/2 teaspoon seasoned salt
1/4 cup Parmesan cheese
1 6 1/2 ounce can tuna in
  spring water, drained
1/4 cup sliced, pitted ripe olives

**Yield: 4 servings**

**Per serving:**
Calories...... 497
Protein (g)... 32
Fat (g)....... 6
Sat. Fat (g).. 2
Choles. (mg).. 15
Fiber (g)..... 4.8
Sodium (mg)... 589
%Cal-Fat...... 11%

Cook fettuccine according to package directions. Drain. To keep warm, place in colander over pot of hot water and cover.

Meanwhile, in medium skillet, sauté green onion in olive oil.

With a wire whisk, combine flour and milk in mixing bowl. Add to onions in skillet. Slowly heat until mixture comes to a boil and thickens. Add seasoned salt, Parmesan cheese, tuna (broken into chunks) and olives. Heat through.

To serve, spoon tuna mixture over fettuccine.

Preparation time: 20–25 minutes

Cooking time: 10 minutes

# Spaghetti and Meatballs

In large bowl, mix together first five ingredients until well blended.

Heat olive oil in 10-inch skillet. Form ground turkey mixture into 1 1/4-inch balls and brown in skillet.

Meanwhile, mix together in medium-size bowl the marinara sauce ingredients.

After meatballs have browned, pour sauce over. Simmer for 20 to 60 minutes.

While sauce and meatballs are simmering, cook pasta according to package directions.

To serve, drain pasta and place on large tray or in large spaghetti bowl. Stir in 1/2 cup sauce to prevent pasta from sticking together. Arrange several meatballs on top. Sprinkle with Parmesan cheese. Have additional sauce and meatballs to pass at table.

*The ground turkey commercially available at grocery stores contains both light and dark turkey meat, plus some fat and skin, which amounts to about 12 grams of fat per 3-ounce serving. Skinless turkey breast, with the fat removed, that you can grind yourself or have your butcher grind, contains only 2.5 grams of fat per 3-ounce serving. However, even the commercially available ground turkey, in most cases, contains 25% less fat than "lean" ground beef.

Preparation time: 30 minutes
Cooking time: 30–60 minutes

1 pound ground turkey breast*
2 egg substitutes (1/2 cup)
1 cup seasoned breadcrumbs
1/2 cup finely chopped onion
1 tablespoon Parmesan cheese
1 tablespoon olive oil
Marinara sauce (Recipe, page 326)
1 pound spaghetti pasta
Parmesan cheese

**Yield: 6 servings**

**Per serving:**
Calories...... 591
Protein (g)... 40
Fat (g)....... 7.5
Sat. Fat (g).. 1.6
Choles. (mg).. 67
Fiber (g)..... 4.2
Sodium (mg)... 649
%Cal-Fat...... 11%

# Quick Marinara Sauce
## with Pasta

1 16-ounce can tomatoes (no salt added), chopped finely in food processor
2 cups prepared spaghetti sauce
2 tablespoons dry white wine
1/4 cup bean paste* (optional)
Dash freshly ground black pepper
1/4 teaspoon garlic powder
1 tablespoon fresh chopped basil, or 1 teaspoon dried Parmesan cheese, to taste
16 ounces pasta

**Yield: 4 cups sauce, enough for 4 to 6 servings**

**Per serving:**
Calories...... 457
Protein (g)... 15
Fat (g)....... 4.3
Sat. Fat (g).. 0.9
Choles. (mg).. 0
Fiber (g)..... 4.8
Sodium (mg)... 521
%Cal-Fat...... 8%

To make marinara sauce, combine all ingredients except cheese and pasta in a medium-size skillet. Bring to a boil and simmer, uncovered, for at least 20 minutes.

Meanwhile, cook pasta according to package directions. Drain. Place in a large bowl. Stir in 1/4 cup marinara sauce to keep pasta from sticking together.

To serve, spoon marinara sauce over pasta and sprinkle with Parmesan cheese.

*To make bean paste, use a 16-ounce can of beans, either black-eyed peas, northern beans, garbanzo beans or kidney beans. Drain beans, reserving 2 tablespoons liquid. Puree beans and reserved liquid in food processor until smooth. Refrigerate until ready to use. Keeps in refrigerator for up to 2 weeks.

Sodium in most prepared spaghetti sauces is high. By adding "no salt added" tomatoes to a prepared sauce as this recipe specifies, the sodium content is approximately cut in half. Bean paste adds additional protein and makes the sauce slightly thicker.

Tip: Add hot taco sauce (to taste) to leftover bean paste for a delicious and nutritious dip—perfect for cold vegetables or melba rounds.

Preparation time: 15–20 minutes
Cooking time: 20–40 minutes

# Ziti with Creamy Mushroom Sauce

Cook pasta according to package directions. Drain.

Meanwhile, heat olive oil in a medium-size skillet. Add sliced mushrooms and cook until mushrooms become soft and turn dark in color.

Place a large skillet over medium heat. Pour in chicken broth.

In a small mixing bowl or measuring cup, add flour to skim milk. Stir briskly with a wire whisk until all lumps disappear. Add to chicken broth along with seasoned salt and pepper. Heat until mixture comes to a boil and thickens. Add cooked mushrooms, including juice, and heat through.

To serve, place cooked ziti in a large bowl. Pour mushroom sauce over and toss to coat. Add Parmesan cheese and mix well. Serve immediately. Add salt or additional Parmesan cheese to taste, if desired.

Preparation time: 20–25 minutes

Cooking time: 15–20 minutes

*1 pound ziti pasta*
*2 teaspoons olive oil*
*8 ounces fresh mushrooms, sliced*
*1 cup clear chicken broth, defatted*
*1 cup skim milk*
*1/3 cup flour*
*1/2 teaspoon seasoned salt*
*1/8 teaspoon white pepper*
*1/4 cup Parmesan cheese*
*Salt to taste*
*Parmesan cheese to taste*

### Yield: 6 side-dish servings

**Per serving:**
Calories...... 368
Protein (g)... 15
Fat (g)....... 4.5
Sat. Fat (g).. 1.3
Choles. (mg).. 4
Fiber (g)..... 4.4
Sodium (mg)... 412
%Cal-Fat...... 11%

# Linguine with Chicken and Vegetables

1 pound boneless chicken breasts, skinned

3 cups clear chicken broth, defatted (canned or from stock)

2 small onions, sliced and separated into rings

4 carrots, sliced into julienne strips

1/2 cup celery, chopped

12 ounces fresh mushrooms, sliced

1/4 cup fresh parsley, chopped finely

3/4 teaspoon dried tarragon

16 ounces linguine

1/2 cup minced green onions or chives

Grated Parmesan cheese

Freshly ground pepper, to taste

Salt, to taste (optional)

**Yield: 6 main-dish servings**

**Per serving:**
Calories...... 296
Protein (g)... 30
Fat (g)....... 5
Sat. Fat (g).. 1.4
Choles. (mg).. 59
Fiber (g)..... 4.6
Sodium (mg)... 369
%Cal-Fat...... 15%

Cut up chicken into strips 1/2-inch by 1 1/2-inches. Remove visible fat from top of chicken broth.

In large soup kettle, heat chicken broth over medium heat. Add chicken strips and onions. Bring to a boil and simmer, covered, 8 to 10 minutes.

Add carrots, celery, mushrooms, parsley and tarragon to soup kettle. Return to a boil and simmer, covered, an additional 8 to 10 minutes, or until vegetables are tender.

Meanwhile, cook linguine according to package directions. Drain. Add to broth mixture, after vegetables are fully cooked. Add minced green onions.

Serve in large soup bowls. Sprinkle with Parmesan cheese and freshly ground pepper. Salt to taste, if desired.

*This dish with its generous amount of "noodles" resembles an oriental soup and can serve as the entree of a hearty evening meal.*

Preparation time: 20 minutes
Cooking time: 10–15 minutes

# Fettucine with Shrimp and Mussels

Preheat oven to 325 degrees.

Clean shrimp. Set aside.

Rinse mussels and remove any debris. Place on large cookie sheet in preheated oven. Bake 5 to 10 minutes or until shells open. Remove from oven. Set aside.

Meanwhile, heat olive oil in large skillet placed over medium heat. Add minced garlic and sauté for 1 minute. Stir in flour, mixing well. Add chicken broth, stirring constantly with wire whisk until mixture comes to a boil and thickens. Stir in wine, lemon juice and pepper.

Add shrimp and mussels to skillet. Cook 3 to 4 minutes, uncovered, until shrimp turn pink in color. Stir occasionally.

Meanwhile, cook fettucine according to package directions.

Remove mussels from skillet. Set aside, keeping warm.

To assemble, place drained fettucine in large serving dish. Immediately pour shrimp mixture, parsley and Parmesan cheese over top. Add margarine, if desired. Toss until well blended. Add mussels and toss lightly. Serve immediately. Pass additional Parmesan cheese to sprinkle over top.

Preparation time: 30–40 minutes

Cooking time: 20–25 minutes

3/4 pound large fresh shrimp
18 to 24 fresh mussels (in shells)
2 tablespoons olive oil
1 teaspoon minced garlic
3 tablespoons flour
1 3/4 cups chicken stock, or one 14 1/2-ounce can clear chicken broth, defatted
1/4 cup dry white wine
1 tablespoon lemon juice
Freshly ground pepper, to taste
14 cup fresh parsley, chopped
1/4 cup grated Parmesan cheese
12 ounces fettucine or linguine
2 tablespoons tub margarine, optional

## Yield: 4 servings

### Per serving:
Calories.......... 435
Protein (g)....... 25
Fat (g).............. 10.1
Sat. Fat (g)....... 2.4
Choles. (mg)... 140
Fiber (g)........... 3
Sodium (mg).. 490
%Cal-Fat.............. 20%

# Spaghetti Putanesca

1 medium onion, chopped
8 to 10 cloves garlic, chopped
  coarsely
2 teaspoons olive oil
1 15-ounce can tomatoes (no
  salt added), chopped coarsely
2 cups prepared spaghetti sauce
  (reduced salt)
1/3 cup dry white wine
1 3/4 ounces capers, drained
  (optional)
2 ounces anchovies, packed in
  oil, drained and chopped
2 ounces pitted ripe olives, cut
  into thirds
1 teaspoon dried oregano
2 tablespoons chopped fresh
  basil, or 1 teaspoon dried
16 ounces spaghetti pasta
Parmesan cheese

**Yield: 4 to 6 servings**

**Per serving:**
Calories..... 541
Protein (g).. 18
Fat (g)...... 8.4
Sat. Fat (g). 1.1
Choles. (mg). 8
Fiber (g).... 2
Sodium (mg).. 804
%Cal-Fat..... 14%

Heat olive oil in large skillet over low heat. Add chopped onions and sauté until they become translucent. Add garlic and sauté an additional 1 minute. Add remaining ingredients in the order in which they appear, except pasta and Parmesan cheese. Cover and simmer 30 to 60 minutes.

Meanwhile, cook pasta according to package directions. Drain. Place in a large serving bowl. Spoon sauce over top. Sprinkle with freshly grated Parmesan cheese.

Preparation time: 20–25 minutes

Cooking time: 30–60 minutes

# Parmesan Rice

Cook rice according to package directions.

Meanwhile, in large casserole dish (5 quart), combine chopped green onions, red pepper, salsa, chick peas, parsley and basil.

In a medium-size mixing bowl, combine remaining ingredients, except Parmesan cheese. Beat with a wire whisk. Set aside.

Add rice to casserole dish. Mix well. Add egg mixture and Parmesan cheese. Stir until all ingredients are well mixed. Sprinkle additional Parmesan cheese lightly over top.

Bake at 350 degrees 30 minutes.

Preparation time: 30–35 minutes
Cooking time: 30 minutes

2 cups rice, uncooked
1 bunch green onions, chopped
1 red pepper, chopped
1/4 cup salsa (medium)
1 cup canned chick peas,
    drained
1/2 cup chopped fresh parsley
1 tablespoon fresh basil,
    chopped
2 egg substitutes (1/2 cup)
1/2 cup skim milk
1 teaspoon salt
1/4 teaspoon pepper
1 teaspoon garlic powder
1 tablespoon white wine vinegar
1 tablespoon sugar
1/2 cup Parmesan cheese

### Yield: 10 1-cup servings

*Per serving:*
Calories...... 208
Protein (g)... 8
Fat (g)....... 2.5
Sat. Fat (g).. 1
Choles. (mg).. 3
Fiber (g)..... 2
Sodium (mg)... 330
%Cal-Fat...... 11%

# Wild Rice Baked Casserole

1 cup wild rice, uncooked
1 tablespoon tub margarine
1 large onion, chopped
1 large stalk celery, chopped
1 cup long-grain white rice,
   uncooked
2 14-ounce cans clear chicken
   broth, defatted
2 tablespoons reduced-sodium
   soy sauce
1/4 cup dry white wine

**Yield: 8 servings**

**Per serving:**
Calories...... 191
Protein (g)... 7
Fat (g)....... 2.8
Sat. Fat (g).. 0.5
Choles. (mg).. 0
Fiber (g)..... 2
Sodium (mg)... 520
%Cal-Fat...... 13%

Preheat oven to 350 degrees.

Place wild rice in a medium saucepan and cover with about 2 inches of water. Bring to a boil and simmer 20 minutes. Drain water and set rice aside.

Meanwhile, in large skillet, melt margarine. Add chopped onion and celery. Sauté until onion becomes translucent, but not brown. Add white rice and sauté 2 to 3 minutes, or until rice is lightly browned. Stir in wild rice.

Transfer to a covered 2 1/2-quart casserole dish. (At this stage, casserole may be refrigerated for several hours or overnight.)

Before you are ready to bake casserole, combine chicken broth, soy sauce and wine in medium saucepan. Bring to a boil. Pour over rice in casserole dish. Bake in 350 degree oven 1 hour or until all liquid is absorbed.

Preparation time: 20–25 minutes
Cooking time: 1 hour

# Saffron Rice

Skim fat from top of chicken broth. Pour into medium saucepan and bring to a boil. Keep broth barely simmering over low heat.

Meanwhile, melt margarine in heavy saucepan. Add chopped onion, and sauté until onion is soft but not brown. Add the rice and sauté 2 minutes. Add wine and simmer until liquid is reduced by 1/2 (about 2 minutes).

Add half the broth and the saffron to the rice mixture, and cook, uncovered, over medium heat, stirring frequently. As the broth is absorbed, add more, about 1/2 cup at a time. Continue cooking, adding broth as needed, until rice is tender, but not soft. The total cooking time, after the broth is added, should be about 30 minutes. Stir constantly toward the end of the cooking time to avoid sticking.

Remove from heat. Stir in the Parmesan cheese. Cover until ready to serve.

*The saffron lends a delicate flavor and a beautiful soft yellow color to the rice.*

*\* To reduce sodium, use homemade chicken broth, or dilute the canned broth with water.*

Preparation time: 15–20 minutes
Cooking time: 30 minutes

*4 cups chicken broth, homemade or canned, defatted\**
*2 teaspoons tub margarine*
*1/4 cup finely chopped onion*
*1 cup uncooked white rice*
*1/4 cup dry white wine*
*Pinch of saffron*
*1/4 cup freshly grated Parmesan cheese*

### Yield: 4 servings

### Per serving:
Calories...... 263
Protein (g)... 11
Fat (g)....... 4
Sat. Fat (g).. 1.8
Choles. (mg).. 5
Fiber (g)..... 1.2
Sodium (mg)... 520
%Cal-Fat...... 14%

# Spanish Rice

1 cup uncooked white rice
2 teaspoons olive oil
1 medium onion, chopped finely
1 clove garlic, minced
1 8-ounce can tomato sauce
3 tablespoons salsa (medium or hot)
1 1/2 cups water

**Yield: 4 servings**

**Per serving:**
Calories...... 236
Protein (g)... 5
Fat (g)....... 3
Sat. Fat (g).. 0.5
Choles. (mg).. 0
Fiber (g)..... 2.3
Sodium (mg)... 198
%Cal-Fat...... 12%

Heat olive oil in large skillet. Add rice, onion and garlic, and sauté until rice turns golden brown. Add remaining ingredients and bring to a boil. Reduce heat and simmer 25 minutes or until liquid is absorbed and rice is tender.

Preparation time: 15 minutes
Cooking time: 25 minutes

# Rice-Mushroom Casserole

1 pound fresh mushrooms, sliced
2 14-ounce cans clear chicken broth, defatted
3/4 cup water
1/2 cup wild rice, uncooked
1 1/2 cups long-grain rice, uncooked
1 tablespoon tub margarine

**Yield: 8 servings**

**Per serving:**
Calories...... 187
Protein (g)... 7
Fat (g)....... 2.2
Sat. Fat (g).. 0.5
Choles. (mg).. 0
Fiber (g)..... 2.2
Sodium (mg)... 337
%Cal-Fat...... 10%

Wash mushrooms and slice. Place in skillet (no oil necessary), cover, and simmer on low until mushrooms turn dark in color. Stir occasionally. Drain, saving juice from mushrooms. Set aside.

Meanwhile, in a large saucepan, combine chicken broth, water and wild rice. Bring to a boil, and simmer for 10 minutes.

Add long-grain rice, juice from mushrooms, and margarine to saucepan. Bring to a second boil. Reduce heat and simmer for approximately 30 minutes longer, or until liquid is fully absorbed.

Stir in mushrooms. Serve immediately.

Preparation time: 30 minutes
Cooking time: 30 minutes

# Green Rice Casserole

Cook rice according to package directions. Thaw spinach in microwave. Squeeze lightly to remove excess moisture.

Combine first eight ingredients in large mixing bowl.

In small mixing bowl, mix together eggs, milk, Parmesan cheese and soy sauce with a wire whisk. Add to rice mixture, stirring until uniformly mixed.

Pour into 3-quart casserole dish. Cover. Bake at 350 degrees 30 to 40 minutes.

Preparation time: 20–25 minutes
Cooking time: 1–1 1/4 hours

*3 to 4 cups cooked long grain rice*
*1 10-ounce package frozen chopped spinach, thawed*
*1/2 cup chopped green onions with tops*
*1/4 cup minced parsley*
*1/4 cup slivered almonds*
*2 teaspoons lemon juice*
*1/4 teaspoon salt*
*1/4 teaspoon garlic powder*
*2 egg substitutes (1/2 cup)*
*3/4 cup skim milk*
*1/4 cup Parmesan cheese*
*2 tablespoons reduced-sodium soy sauce*

*Yield: 8 servings*

*Per serving:*
Calories...... 208
Protein (g)... 9
Fat (g)....... 4
Sat. Fat (g).. 1
Choles. (mg).. 3
Fiber (g)..... 2.2
Sodium (mg)... 400
%Cal-Fat...... 18%

## Baked Bulgur with Fruit

2 vegetable bouillon cubes
  (or 1 large cube)
2 cups boiling water
1 cup bulgur
1/2 teaspoon basil
1/2 cup dark raisins
1/2 cup chopped golden apple,
  with peel
1/4 cup coarsely chopped
  pecans

**Yield: 4 to 6 servings**

**Per serving:**
Calories...... 202
Protein (g)... 5
Fat (g)....... 4.4
Sat. Fat (g).. 0.5
Choles. (mg).. 0
Fiber (g)..... 7.8
Sodium (mg)... 452
%Cal-Fat...... 19%

Preheat oven to 350 degrees.

Dissolve bouillon in boiling water. Pour into 2-quart casserole. Add remaining ingredients and stir to mix. Cover and bake at 350 degrees 40 minutes.

Preparation time: 15 minutes
Cooking time: 40 minutes

## Bulgur with Steamed Vegetables

1/4 cup chopped carrots
1/4 cup chopped celery
1/4 cup chopped onion
3 tablespoons water, divided
1 cup bulgur
1 1/2 cups water
1 chicken bouillon cube
2 tablespoons chopped fresh
  parsley

**Yield: 4 to 6 servings**

**Per serving:**
Calories...... 106
Protein (g)... 4
Fat (g)....... 0.6
Sat. Fat (g).. 0.1
Choles. (mg).. 0
Fiber (g)..... 6.7
Sodium (mg)... 236
%Cal-Fat...... 5%

In a nonstick sauté pan or medium frypan, add chopped vegetables and 2 tablespoons water. Steam 2 minutes.

Add bulgur and one additional tablespoon water. Toss for 3 to 5 minutes until vegetables have softened and bulgur is golden brown.

Add 1 1/2 cups water and bouillon cube and bring to a boil. Reduce heat to medium-low. Simmer, uncovered, about 15 minutes, or until all liquid has been absorbed. Stir in chopped parsley immediately before serving.

*Excellent served with boneless chicken breasts and bright, crisp green salad or fresh tomato slices.*

Preparation time: 15–20 minutes
Cooking time: 15 minutes

# *Polenta*

Bring 3 cups water to a boil in medium-size saucepan.

Meanwhile, combine cornmeal with 1 cup cold water and salt. Add slowly to boiling water. Reduce heat and cook, stirring constantly, until cornmeal mixture returns to a boil.

Cook, uncovered, stirring frequently, about 5 to 15 minutes, depending on the coarseness of the cornmeal. The cooking is complete when the mixture thickens and the cornmeal is soft.

Serve immediately, either plain or with a small amount of margarine.

*Polenta is sometimes used as a substitute for spaghetti in Northern Italy. It is commonly served with the sauce or gravy accompanying a meat or fish dish.*

Preparation time: 15–30 minutes

Cooking time: 15–20 minutes

3 cups water
1 cup coarse yellow cornmeal
1 cup cold water
1 teaspoon salt
2 teaspoons tub margarine
    (optional)

*Yield: 4 cups or 6 servings*

*Per serving:*
Calories...... 110
Protein (g)... 3
Fat (g)....... 1
Sat. Fat (g).. 0.1
Choles. (mg).. 0
Fiber (g)..... 3.3
Sodium (mg)... 542
%Cal-Fat...... 9%

# Potato Gnocchi

3 cups water
1 cup skim milk
3 cups instant mashed potato
  flakes
2 egg substitutes (1/2 cup)
3 1/2 cups all-purpose flour,
  divided
1 teaspoon salt

**Yield: 3 pounds of dough, 8
large servings**

**Per serving:**
Calories...... 282
Protein (g)... 10
Fat (g)....... 1.2
Sat. Fat (g).. 0.2
Choles. (mg).. 0
Fiber (g)..... 2.5
Sodium (mg)... 329
%Cal-Fat...... 4%

Combine 3 cups water and 1 cup skim milk in medium saucepan. Bring to a boil. Remove from heat and stir in 3 cups instant mashed potatoes. (This makes stiff mashed potatoes.) Transfer to a large mixing bowl.

Add egg substitutes (or 3 lightly beaten egg whites), 1/2 cup flour and salt to mashed potatoes. Mix should be very sticky.

Knead in 3 cups of flour, one cup at a time. (This can be done with an electric mixer using a dough attachment.)

On a well-floured surface, roll dough into 1/2-inch-diameter tubes, about 10 inches long. Cut into 1-inch lengths. Place on a tray lined with wax paper. Separate layers of gnocchi with additional wax paper.

Add 1 tablespoon canola oil and 1/2 teaspoon salt to large pot of water. Bring to a boil. Add gnocchi, stirring frequently. Bring to a second boil and cook 10 to 12 minutes, stirring occasionally. Drain well in a colander.

Serve topped with your favorite tomato sauce or white sauce.

*Making this dough can be a fun family project on a Sunday afternoon. Allow at least one hour to make pasta. Gnocchi is a soft chewy pasta that is a favorite with many Italian families.*

Preparation time: 1–1 1/2 hours
Cooking time: 15 minutes

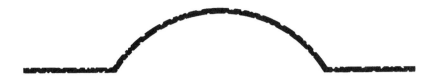

# Breads, Muffins & Brunch Foods

Honey Grain Bread • Oatmeal Bread • Hearty Bulgar Bread • Millet Bread • Quick French Bread • Italian Olive-Onion Bread • Pesto-Onion Bread • Date-Nut Bread • Lemon Tea Bread • Pumpkin Bread • Banana-Nut Bread • Orange Corn Bread • Garlic Crustinos • Oat Bran-Apple Muffins • Southern-Style Spoon Bread • Blueberry Muffins • Carrot Bran Muffins • Bran Muffins • Crustless Spinach Quiche • Make-Ahead French Toast • Cinnamon French Toast

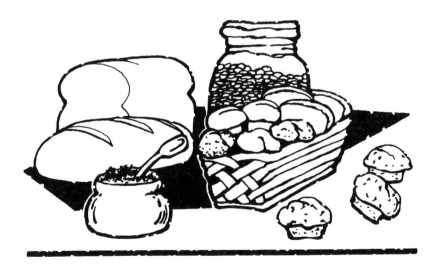

# *Honey Grain Bread*

3 cups whole wheat flour
2 cups all-purpose flour
1 cup quick-cooking oats
1/2 teaspoon salt
2 packages active dry yeast
1 1/2 cups water
1/4 – 1/2 cup honey
1/3 cup canola oil
3 egg whites or 1/2 cup egg
  substitutes
1/2 to 1 1/2 cups all-purpose
  flour

**Yield: 2 loaves or 34 1/2-inch slices**

**Per slice:**
Calories...... 118
Protein (g)... 3
Fat (g)....... 2.5
Sat. Fat (g).. 0.3
Choles. (mg).. 0
Fiber (g)..... 2
Sodium (mg)... 37
%Cal-Fat...... 19%

Place 3 cups whole wheat flour, 2 cups all-purpose flour, oats, salt and yeast in bowl. Mix well.

Combine water, honey and canola oil in saucepan; heat to 120 to 130 F. Slowly add warm liquids to flour mixture by hand or with an electric mixer or food processor (using dough attachment) until well mixed, about 1 minute.

Add egg whites. Mix well, for about 1 minute.

Add remaining flour, 1/2 cup at a time, until dough becomes elastic, or if using an electric appliance, until dough clings to attachment and cleans sides of bowl, about 3 minutes. Continue to knead for 7 to 10 minutes, by hand or machine, until dough is smooth and elastic.

Place in lightly greased bowl, turning to grease top. Cover, let rise in warm place until doubled in size, about 40 to 60 minutes.

Punch dough down. Divide dough in half. Shape each half into a loaf. Place each loaf in a nonstick 8 1/2 x 4 1/2 x 2 1/2-inch bread pan.

Bake at 350 degrees for 30 to 40 minutes. Remove from pans and cool on wire racks for 10 minutes. Cool to room temperature. Wrap to keep moist.

Preparation time: 30 minutes
Baking time: 30–40 minutes
Rising time: 40–60 minutes

# Oatmeal Bread

Pour oats into large mixing bowl. Pour boiling water over and soak oats for 1/2 hour. Add salt, molasses and canola oil.

Soften yeast in 1/3 cup lukewarm water (100 to 110 degrees). Add to mixing bowl. Add flour and raisins and knead well (about 10 minutes), either by hand or using electric mixer with dough hook. Dough should be elastic, but not sticky.

Place in large greased bowl and let rise in warm place until double in bulk, about 1 hour. Punch down. Divide dough in half, form into two loaves and place in greased 9 x 5 x 3-inch loaf pans. Let rise until double in bulk, about 30 to 40 minutes.

Bake in 325-degree preheated oven for 50 minutes, or until loaves are golden brown. Remove from pans after 15 minutes. Wrap to keep moist.

Preparation time: 40–45 minutes
Baking time: 50 minutes
Rising time: 1 1/2 hours

*1 cup rolled oats*
*2 cups boiling water*
*1 teaspoon salt*
*1/2 cup molasses*
*3 tablespoons canola oil*
*2 packages active dry yeast*
*1/3 cup lukewarm water*
*2 cups whole wheat flour*
*4 to 5 cups all-purpose or bread flour*
*1 cup raisins*

### Yield: 2 loaves or 36 1/2-inch slices

*Per slice:*
Calories...... 126
Protein (g)... 3
Fat (g)....... 1.1
Sat. Fat (g).. 0.2
Choles. (mg).. 0
Fiber (g)..... 1.3
Sodium (mg)... 73
%Cal-Fat...... 8%

# Hearty Bulgur Bread

1 cup water
1/3 cup raw bulgur
1/2 teaspoon salt
2 cups warm water (120 to 130 degrees)
2 packages active dry yeast
2 teaspoons sugar
1 cup whole wheat flour
3 to 4 cups bread flour, divided
2 teaspoons salt
1 tablespoon canola oil

**Yield: 2 loaves or 36 1/2-inch slices**

**Per serving:**
Calories..... 71
Protein (g).. 2.2
Fat (g)...... 0.4
Sat. Fat (g). 0
Choles. (mg). 0
Fiber (g).... 1.2
Sodium (mg).. 149
%Cal-Fat..... 5%

Bring 1 cup water to a boil. Add bulgur and salt, and bring to a second boil. Reduce heat, cover and simmer on low 20 to 25 minutes. Set aside and cool until warm. (If too hot, it will kill yeast.)

In a large bowl, dissolve yeast in warm water. Add sugar and let rest for 10 minutes. Add cooked bulgur, breaking up lumps with a wooden spoon. Stir in whole wheat flour.

In a medium-size bowl, mix together 3 cups bread flour and salt. Add this flour, one cup at a time, to yeast mixture. Stir with a wooden spoon until mixture is too stiff to stir. Begin kneading and continue adding additional flour until dough comes away from sides and bottom of bowl and is no longer sticky. Scrape sides of bowl and incorporate into dough. Knead an additional 5 minutes.

Spread oil on sides of bowl. Continue kneading until dough is covered with oil. Cover with a towel and let rise in warm place until double in size, about 40 to 60 minutes.

Preheat oven to 375 degrees.

Punch dough down, adding more flour if too sticky to handle. Divide in half. Shape each half into a loaf and place in a non-stick 8 1/2 x 4 1/2 x 2 1/2-inch bread pan, lightly sprayed with vegetable cooking spray. In loaf pan, flatten dough with hand. Cover and let rise 10 to 20 minutes. Make slash lengthwise in center of dough, about 1/4-inch deep.

Bake at 375 degrees, 30 to 40 minutes, until crust is light brown. Remove from pans after 15 minutes. Let cool 1 hour before cutting and bagging.

Preparation time: 30 minutes
Baking time: 30–40 minutes
Rising time: 1 1/4 hours

# Millet Bread

Bring 1 1/3 cups water to a boil. Add millet and bring to a second boil. Reduce heat, cover and simmer on low 25 to 30 minutes or until all liquid is absorbed. Set aside and cool until warm. (If too hot, it will kill yeast.)

In a large bowl, dissolve yeast in warm water. Add sugar. Add cooked millet, breaking up lumps with wooden spoon.

In a separate bowl, mix together 5 cups flour and salt. Add flour, 1 cup at a time, to millet mixture. Stir with a wooden spoon until dough pulls away from sides of bowl. Continue to add flour, kneading with hands, until dough is no longer sticky. Knead an additional 5 minutes.

Spread oil on sides of bowl, and knead until dough is covered with oil. Cover with towel and let rise in warm place until double in size, about 1 hour.

Preheat oven to 375 degrees.

Punch dough down, adding more flour if too sticky to handle. Divide in half. Shape each half into a loaf and place in a non-stick 8 1/2 x 4 1/2 x 2 1/2-inch bread pan, lightly sprayed with vegetable cooking spray. Cover and let rise 10 to 20 minutes. Make slash lengthwise in center of dough, about 1/4-inch deep.

Bake at 375 degrees 30 to 40 minutes, until light brown in color. Remove from pans after 15 minutes. Cool to room temperature. Wrap to keep moist.

*The millet makes this a wonderfully moist bread with a delicate flavor.*

Preparation time: 30 minutes
Baking time: 30–40 minutes
Rising time: 1 1/4 hours

*1 1/3 cups water*
*2/3 cup millet*
*2 cups warm water (120 to 130 degrees)*
*2 packages active dry yeast*
*2 teaspoons sugar*
*5 to 6 cups bread flour*
*2 teaspoons salt*
*2 teaspoons canola oil*

*Yield: 2 loaves or 36 1/2-inch slices*

Per slice:
Calories..... 90
Protein (g).. 2.6
Fat (g)...... 0.4
Sat. Fat (g). 0
Choles. (mg). 0
Fiber (g).... 0.8
Sodium (mg).. 119
%Cal-Fat..... 4%

# Quick French Bread

1 package active dry yeast
1 cup warm water (105 to 115 degrees)
1 tablespoon tub margarine
3 1/2 to 3 3/4 cups all-purpose flour, divided*
1 teaspoon salt

Glaze (optional):
1 egg substitute (1/4 cup)
1 tablespoon water

**Yield: 2 medium loaves (24 slices)**

**Per slice:**
Calories...... 77
Protein (g)... 2
Fat (g)....... 0.6
Sat. Fat (g).. 0.1
Choles. (mg).. 0
Fiber (g)..... 0.6
Sodium (mg)... 100
%Cal-Fat...... 8%

Dissolve yeast in warm water. Add margarine.

With steel blade in food processor bowl, add 2 cups flour and salt. Turn machine on and off to combine. Add yeast mixture and process until combined. Gradually add remaining flour and process until dough is no longer sticky and collects into a ball. The dough should be slightly stiff.

Place dough in lightly greased bowl, cover with a towel and let rise in warm place for 1 hour or until double in size.

Turn the dough out onto a lightly floured board, punch it down and knead again. Divide the dough in half and form into two loaves. Place shaped loaves on lightly greased baking sheet. Let rise until double in size, about 1 hour.

Mix egg and water to make a glaze. Brush gently over top. Bake in 375-degree oven for 20 to 25 minutes, until loaves are golden brown and sound hollow when tapped.

*If making bread by hand, without a food processor, less flour is needed.*

*This simple dough may also be used to make 2 10-inch pizza crusts.*

Preparation time: 20–25 minutes
Baking time: 20–25 minutes
Rising time: 2 hours

# Italian Olive-Onion Bread

Place wheat flour, 2 1/2 cups all-purpose flour, sugar, salt and yeast in mixing bowl. (An electric mixer, fitted with dough hook, works best.) Mix well.

Combine water and oil in small saucepan. Heat over low heat until very warm (120 to 130 degrees F.)

Gradually add warm liquid to flour mixture, mixing well. Add egg substitutes and mix until well blended.

Combine 1/2 cup flour with chopped onion and olives. Add to mixing bowl and mix until olives and onions are blended throughout.

Add remaining flour, 1/2 cup at a time, and knead until dough becomes smooth and elastic. (If using an electric mixer, dough should no longer stick to sides of bowl. Knead with dough hook for 7 to 10 minutes.)

Place in a lightly greased bowl, turning to grease top. Cover and let rise in a warm place until doubled in size, about 1 hour.

Punch dough down and divide in half. Shape each half into a loaf. Place each loaf in a nonstick 8 1/2 x 4 1/2 x 2 1/2-inch loaf pan. Bake at 375 degrees for 25 to 30 minutes or until bread is a light golden brown. Cool slightly. Remove from pans and cool on wire racks.

Preparation time: 30–35 minutes
Baking time: 25–30 minutes
Rising time: 1 hour

*2 cups whole wheat flour*
*2 1/2 cups all-purpose flour*
*2 tablespoons sugar*
*1 teaspoon salt*
*2 packages active dry yeast*
*1 1/4 cups water*
*2 tablespoons cooking oil*
*2 egg substitutes (1/2 cup)*
*1/2 to 1 1/2 cups all-purpose flour*
*1/2 cup chopped onion*
*1/3 cup green pimiento olives, coarsely chopped*
*1/3 cup black olives, coarsely chopped*

*Yield: 2 loaves, or 34 slices*

*Per 1/2-inch slice:*
Calories...... 82
Protein (g)... 3
Fat (g)....... 1.4
Sat. Fat (g).. 0.1
Choles. (mg).. 0
Fiber (g)..... 1.8
Sodium (mg)... 100
%Cal-Fat...... 16%

# Pesto-Onion Bread

Dough for "Quick French Bread"

Pesto-Onion Filling:
1 cup fresh basil (loosely packed), chopped finely, or 2 tablespoons dried
2 tablespoons egg substitutes
1 tablespoon olive oil
2 cloves garlic, crushed
1/4 teaspoon salt
1/2 cup onion, minced
3 tablespoons grated Parmesan cheese

**Yield: 2 crescent-shaped loaves (24 slices)**

*Per 1-inch slice:*
Calories...... 73
Protein (g)... 2
Fat (g)....... 1.4
Sat. Fat (g).. 0.3
Choles. (mg).. 0
Fiber (g)..... 0.6
Sodium (mg)... 130
%Cal-Fat...... 17%

Prepare dough for "Quick French Bread" (Recipe, page 344).

While dough is rising, prepare Pesto-Onion filling: Chop basil finely and combine with remaining ingredients.

After dough has risen for the first time, punch it down and knead slightly. With a rolling pin press dough into a rectangle, about 11 x 14 inches.

Spread the basil-onion mixture over the dough, up to 1 inch from the edges. Starting with a long side, roll the dough into a cylinder. Place the cylinder in a crescent shape, seam side down, on a lightly greased cookie sheet. With a sharp knife, cut half way down through the dough at 1-inch intervals. Allow the dough to rise for about 15 minutes.

Bake in preheated 400-degree oven 20 to 25 minutes or until bread is golden brown.

Place bread on a rack to cool slightly. Serve warm for the best flavor.

Preparation time: 40–45 minutes.
Baking time: 20–25 minutes
Rising time: 1 hour 15 minutes

# Date-Nut Bread

Preheat oven to 350 degrees.

Mix baking soda and dates in large mixing bowl. Add boiling water. Cool slightly.

After it cools, add sugar, salt and eggs. Mix well.

Combine all-purpose flour, wheat flour and baking powder. Add to date mixture. Stir until well blended. Add vanilla. Fold in applesauce and chopped walnuts.

Lightly spray two 8 1/2 x 4 1/2 x 2 1/2-inch nonstick loaf pans with a vegetable cooking spray. Pour batter into loaf pans. Bake at 350 degrees 55 to 60 minutes. Test for doneness by inserting toothpick into center of loaf. If toothpick comes out clean, it is done.

Preparation time: 20–25 minutes
Baking time: 55–60 minutes

*1 8-ounce package chopped dates*
*2 teaspoons baking soda*
*2 cups boiling water*
*1 1/4 cups sugar*
*1/2 teaspoon salt*
*1/2 cup egg substitutes, slightly beaten*
*2 cups all-purpose flour*
*2 cups whole wheat flour*
*2 teaspoons baking powder*
*2 teaspoons vanilla*
*1/2 cup natural applesauce*
*1/2 cup walnuts, chopped*

### Yield: 2 loaves or 34 slices

### Per 1/2-inch slice:
Calories...... 120
Protein (g)... 2
Fat (g)....... 1.5
Sat. Fat (g).. 0.2
Choles. (mg).. 0
Fiber (g)..... 1.3
Sodium (mg)... 146
%Cal-Fat...... 10%

## Lemon Tea Bread

1/2 cup whole wheat flour
1 1/2 cups all-purpose flour
3/4 cup sugar
2 1/2 teaspoons baking powder
1/4 teaspoon salt
3/4 cup skim milk
1/4 cup canola oil
2 egg substitutes (1/2 cup)
1 teaspoon grated lemon peel
1/2 cup chopped walnuts
   (optional)

Glaze:
2 teaspoons freshly squeezed
   lemon juice
1 tablespoon skim milk
Confectioners sugar

Yield: l loaf, 17 1/2-inch
slices

Per slice:
Calories...... 129
Protein (g)... 3
Fat (g)....... 3.9
Sat. Fat (g).. 0.4
Choles. (mg).. 0
Fiber (g)..... 1.1
Sodium (mg)... 99
%Cal-Fat...... 27%

Preheat oven to 350 degrees.

Combine the first five dry ingredients in large bowl. Stir until blended. Set aside.

Combine milk, canola oil and eggs in medium-size bowl. Add milk mixture to dry ingredients, mixing until well moistened. Stir in grated lemon peel, and walnuts, if desired.

Pour into nonstick loaf pan 8 1/2 x 4 1/2 x 2 1/2-inches. Bake in 350-degree oven 45 to 55 minutes or until done. Let cool for 10 minutes before removing from pan.

Meanwhile, make lemon glaze: Combine lemon juice and milk in a small bowl. Add enough powdered sugar to make a thick frosting. Spread the glaze over warm bread.

Bread may be served warm or cool. After it has reached room temperature, wrap and store in refrigerator.

Preparation time: 25 minutes
Baking time: 45–55 minutes

## Pumpkin Bread

2 1/2 cups sugar
4 egg substitutes (1 cup)
3 1/2 cups all-purpose flour
1/2 teaspoon baking powder
2 teaspoons baking soda
1/2 teaspoon salt
1 1/2 teaspoons pumpkin pie
   spice
1/4 teaspoon cinnamon
1/3 cup canola oil
2/3 cup water
1 16-ounce can pumpkin

Preheat oven to 325 degrees.

In large mixing bowl, cream together sugar and eggs.

In another bowl, combine flour, baking powder, baking soda, salt and spices, mixing well.

Add dry ingredients, oil, water and pumpkin to mixing bowl. Mix thoroughly with electric mixer.

Spray bottoms of two 9 x 5 x 3-inch loaf pans with a vegetable cooking spray. Pour batter evenly into both pans. Bake at 325 degrees for 65 to 75 minutes, or until toothpick inserted into center of loaf comes out clean. Cool. Remove from pans.

*This is a delicious sweet bread that is low in fat, very moist and high in vitamin A. It tastes great toasted.*

Preparation time: 20 minutes
Baking time: 65–75 minutes

*Yield: 2 loaves, or 54 slices*

*Per 1/3-inch slice:*
Calories...... 82
Protein (g)... 1
Fat (g)....... 1.6
Sat. Fat (g).. 0.1
Choles. (mg).. 0
Fiber (g)..... 0.4
Sodium (mg)... 63
%Cal-Fat...... 17%

# Banana-Nut Bread

Preheat oven to 350 degrees.

Spray a 9 x 5 x 3-inch loaf pan with a vegetable cooking spray.

Combine sugar, baking soda, flour and salt in large mixing bowl. Mix well.

In a small mixing bowl, combine eggs (slightly beaten), canola oil, applesauce, vanilla and milk. Add egg mixture to dry ingredients. Add pureed bananas. Stir until combined, but do not over mix. Fold in walnuts.

Pour into loaf pan and bake at 350 degrees 40 to 50 minutes, or until toothpick inserted in center of loaf comes out clean.

Preparation time: 20 minutes
Baking time: 40–50 minutes

*3/4 cup sugar*
*1 1/2 teaspoons baking soda*
*2 cups all-purpose flour*
*1/4 teaspoon salt*
*2 egg substitutes (1/2 cup)*
*1/4 cup canola oil*
*1/4 cup natural applesauce*
*1 teaspoon vanilla*
*3 tablespoons skim milk*
*3 ripe bananas, pureed*
*1/4 cup chopped walnuts*

*Yield: 1 large loaf or 27 slices (1/3-inch thick)*

*Per slice:*
Calories...... 94
Protein (g)... 2
Fat (g)....... 3
Sat. Fat (g).. 0.3
Choles. (mg).. 0
Fiber (g)..... 0.5
Sodium (mg)... 75
%Cal-Fat...... 28%

# Orange Corn Bread

1 cup all-purpose flour
1 cup yellow cornmeal
1/2 teaspoon baking soda
1 tablespoon baking powder
1/3 cup sugar
1/4 cup orange juice
2 egg substitutes (1/2 cup)
1 cup skim milk
2 tablespoons canola oil

**Yield: 16 2-inch square
pieces**

**Per serving:**
Calories...... 103
Protein (g)... 3
Fat (g)....... 2.2
Sat. Fat (g).. 0.2
Choles. (mg).. 0
Fiber (g)..... 0.8
Sodium (mg)... 106
%Cal-Fat...... 19%

Preheat oven to 425 degrees.

Combine dry ingredients in large mixing bowl. Set aside.

Combine remaining ingredients in medium-size mixing bowl. Add orange juice mixture to dry ingredients and stir until well moistened.

Pour into nonstick 9 x 9 x 2-inch pan. Bake at 425 degrees for 20 to 25 minutes. May be served warm or cold.

Preparation time: 10–15 minutes
Baking time: 20–25 minutes

# Garlic Crustinos

1 French baguette (long,
    narrow French bread)
Vegetable cooking spray
Garlic salt

**Yield: As desired**

**Per 2 slices:**
Calories...... 30
Protein (g)... 1
Fat (g)....... 0.4
Sat. Fat (g).. 0
Choles. (mg).. 0
Fiber (g)..... 0.3
Sodium (mg)... 125
%Cal-Fat...... 12%

Preheat oven to 275 degrees.

Slice bread into 1/4-inch thick slices (as many slices as desired). Place slices on cookie sheet; spray them with vegetable cooking spray and sprinkle with garlic salt.

Bake at 275 degrees for 15 minutes, or until bread becomes very crisp. Serve warm or at room temperature. After bread has cooled completely, store in air-tight container to keep crisp.

*These crustinos are delicious served with soup, especially Bouillabaisse.*

Preparation time: 5 minutes
Baking time: 15 minutes

# Oat Bran-Apple Muffins

Preheat oven to 375 degrees.

In large bowl combine oat bran, oatmeal, flour, brown sugar, cinnamon and baking powder.

In medium-size bowl, lightly beat egg substitutes. Stir in skim milk, canola oil and applesauce until well blended.

Stir milk mixture into flour mixture until just moistened. Spoon batter into muffin tins lined with paper bake cups. Bake at 375 degrees for 15 to 20 minutes, or until lightly browned.

Preparation time: 15–20 minutes
Baking time: 15–20 minutes

1 1/4 cups oat bran cereal
1 cup oatmeal
1 1/4 cups all-purpose flour
1/2 cup brown sugar
1 teaspoon cinnamon
3 teaspoons baking powder
2 egg substitutes (1/2 cup)
1 cup skim milk
2 tablespoons canola oil
1 cup chunky applesauce

## Yield: 16 to 18 muffins

### Per serving:
Calories...... 122
Protein (g)... 4
Fat (g)....... 2.9
Sat. Fat (g).. 0.4
Choles. (mg).. 0
Fiber (g)..... 1.7
Sodium (mg)... 96
%Cal-Fat...... 21%

# Southern-Style Spoon Bread

Preheat oven to 325 degrees.

Scald milk in top of double boiler. Gradually stir in corn meal with a wire whisk. Cook over medium heat until thickened, stirring frequently. Add margarine, salt, sugar and baking powder. Mix well.

Beat egg whites until stiff peaks form. Fold into cornmeal mixture. Spoon into nonstick 8 x 8-inch baking dish. Bake at 325 degrees for 30 minutes, or until mixture is set.

To serve, spoon onto plates.

*Consistency is similar to a thick pudding.*

Preparation time: 20–25 minutes
Baking time: 30 minutes

2 cups skim milk
1/2 cup yellow cornmeal
1 tablespoon tub margarine
3/4 teaspoon salt
1 tablespoon sugar
1/2 teaspoon baking powder
2 egg whites

## Yield: 6 servings

### Per serving:
Calories...... 101
Protein (g)... 5
Fat (g)....... 2.2
Sat. Fat (g).. 0.5
Choles. (mg).. 1
Fiber (g)..... 0.9
Sodium (mg)... 378
%Cal-Fat...... 20%

# Blueberry Muffins

2 cups all-purpose flour
1/2 cup sugar
3 teaspoons baking powder
1/4 teaspoon salt
1 cup skim milk
1 egg substitute (1/4 cup)
2 tablespoons canola oil
1/4 cup natural applesauce
1 cup fresh or frozen
   blueberries, unthawed

### Yield: 12 muffins

### Per serving:
Calories...... 143
Protein (g)... 3
Fat (g)....... 2.7
Sat. Fat (g).. 0.2
Choles. (mg).. 0
Fiber (g)..... 1
Sodium (mg)... 149
%Cal-Fat...... 17%

Preheat oven to 400 degrees.

Combine flour, sugar, baking powder and salt in large mixing bowl. Mix well.

Combine milk, egg substitute, canola oil and applesauce. Add all at once to flour mixture. Mix just until moistened. Carefully fold in blueberries.

Spray nonstick muffin pans with cooking spray, or line with paper bake cups. Spoon batter into 12 muffin forms, filling 2/3 full. Bake at 400 degrees for 20 minutes or until golden brown. Remove from tin after 20 minutes.

*You may also use a 15-ounce can of blueberries in syrup, drained and rinsed. However, because they are softer, when you fold them into the batter, the blue color from the blueberry juice will marble throughout the batter.*

Preparation time: 15 minutes
Baking time: 20 minutes

# Carrot Bran Muffins

Preheat oven to 400 degrees.

Grate carrots and set aside.

In large bowl combine flours, sugar, baking powder, baking soda and salt.

In medium-size bowl, lightly beat egg whites with a wire whisk or fork. Stir in milk, applesauce and canola oil until well blended.

Stir milk mixture into flour mixture just until moistened.

Fold in drained pineapple, grated carrots and raisins.

Spoon batter into nonstick muffin tins. Bake at 400 degrees for 15 to 20 minutes, or until golden brown and top springs back when touched.

*Ideal for a snack with either fruit juice or milk.*

Preparation time: 20–25 minutes
Baking time: 15–20 minutes

1 cup all-purpose flour
1 cup whole wheat flour
1/2 cup sugar
1 tablespoon baking powder
1/2 teaspoon baking soda
1/4 teaspoon salt
2 egg whites
1 cup skim milk
1/4 cup natural applesauce
1 tablespoon canola oil
1 8-ounce can crushed
  pineapple, drained (no sugar
  added)
1 cup finely grated carrot
1/2 cup raisins

**Yield: 12 to 18 muffins, depending on size**

**Per serving:**
Calories...... 128
Protein (g)... 3
Fat (g)....... 1.2
Sat. Fat (g).. 0.1
Choles. (mg).. 0
Fiber (g)..... 2
Sodium (mg)... 140
%Cal-Fat...... 8%

# Bran Muffins

1 1/2 cups 100% wheat bran
    cereal
1 1/4 cups skim milk
1 1/4 cups all-purpose flour
1/2 cup sugar
1/4 teaspoon salt
1 tablespoon baking powder
1 teaspoon cinnamon
1/2 teaspoon ground cloves
1/2 teaspoon nutmeg
1 egg substitute (1/4 cup)
2 tablespoons canola oil
1/2 cup natural applesauce
1/2 to 3/4 cup raisins

*Yield: 16 muffins*

*Per serving:*
Calories...... 120
Protein (g)... 3
Fat (g)....... 2
Sat. Fat (g).. 0.2
Choles. (mg).. 0
Fiber (g)..... 3.1
Sodium (mg)... 196
%Cal-Fat...... 15%

Preheat oven to 375 degrees.

Combine cereal and milk in large mixing bowl. Let soak 5 to 10 minutes, or until cereal softens.

Meanwhile, stir together flour, sugar, salt, baking powder, cinnamon, cloves and nutmeg.

Add egg substitute, canola oil and applesauce to cereal mixture. Mix well. Add dry ingredients and mix just until moistened. Stir in raisins.

Prepare muffin tins by spraying with cooking spray or line with paper bake cups. Fill each muffin tin 2/3 full. Bake in preheated 375-degree oven for 15 to 20 minutes, or until golden brown.

*For variety, raisins may be omitted, or other fruits may be substituted for the raisins, such as drained crushed pineapple or chopped dates.*

Preparation time: 20 minutes
Baking time: 15–20 minutes

# Crustless Spinach Quiche

Preheat oven to 350 degrees.

Combine egg substitutes, milk, salt, pepper and nutmeg in large mixing bowl. Beat slightly. Set aside.

Heat olive oil in medium-size saucepan. Add onion and sauté until onion becomes translucent. Mix thawed and drained spinach with sautéed onion. Add to egg mixture.

Toss grated cheese with flour.

Sprinkle cheese evenly into two greased and floured 9-inch pie pans. Pour egg mixture over top.

Bake at 350 degrees for 40 to 45 minutes.

*Other ingredients may be added or substituted, such as lean ham, mushrooms, etc.*

Preparation time: 20 minutes
Baking time: 40–45 minutes

8 egg substitutes (2 cups)
1 12-ounce can evaporated skim milk
1/2 teaspoon salt
1/8 teaspoon cayenne pepper
1/2 teaspoon ground nutmeg
2 teaspoons olive oil
1/4 cup chopped onion
2 10-ounce packages frozen chopped spinach, thawed and drained (squeezed dry)
1 cup (4 ounces) shredded Swiss or Cheddar cheese (reduced-calorie)
2 tablespoons flour

**Yield: 16 servings (8 servings per pie)**

**Per serving:**
Calories...... 80
Protein (g)... 7
Fat (g)....... 3
Sat. Fat (g).. 1
Choles. (mg).. 1
Fiber (g)..... 1
Sodium (mg)... 215
%Cal-Fat...... 33%

## Make-Ahead French Toast

4 egg substitutes (1 cup)
1/2 cup orange juice
1/4 cup skim milk
1/4 cup sugar
1/2 teaspoon vanilla
1/4 teaspoon ground nutmeg
8 slices French or Italian bread
  (3/4-inch thick)
Butter-flavored vegetable spray

**Yield: 8 slices French toast**

**Per serving:**
Calories...... 143
Protein (g)... 7
Fat (g)....... 2
Sat. Fat (g).. 0.4
Choles. (mg).. 1
Fiber (g)..... 0.6
Sodium (mg)... 199
%Cal-Fat...... 13%

Combine first six ingredients in medium-size bowl.

Arrange slices of bread in a single layer in a 9 x 13-inch pan or a jelly-roll pan. Pour egg mixture over the bread. Cover and refrigerate overnight.

The next morning, preheat oven to 400 degrees.

Spray a 9 x 13-inch pan or jelly-roll pan with a butter-flavored cooking spray. Transfer soaked bread slices to pan, arranging in a single layer.

Bake at 400 degrees for 20 minutes. Turn bread slices. Bake an additional 5 minutes.

Serve with lite syrup or warmed, cooked fruit over top.

*An ideal make-ahead breakfast for Sunday mornings or when entertaining out-of-town guests for the weekend.*

Preparation time: 10–15 minutes
Baking time: 25 minutes

## Cinnamon French Toast

4 egg substitutes (1 cup)
1/2 cup skim milk
1 teaspoon sugar
1/2 teaspoon cinnamon
8 slices whole wheat bread
Vegetable cooking spray

**Yield: 8 slices**

**Per serving:**
Calories...... 104
Protein (g)... 7
Fat (g)....... 2.3
Sat. Fat (g).. 0.6
Choles. (mg).. 0
Fiber (g)..... 2.1
Sodium (mg)... 250
%Cal-Fat...... 19%

Spray skillet or griddle with cooking spray and place on stove at medium setting.

Combine egg substitutes, milk, sugar and cinnamon in shallow mixing bowl. Mix well.

Dip slices of bread in egg mixture and fry in preheated skillet or griddle until brown on both sides. Serve hot with syrup and if desired, a small scraping of margarine.

Preparation time: 10–15 minutes
Cooking time: 5 minutes

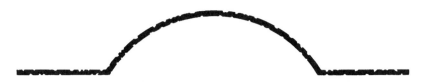

# *Desserts*

Chocolate Brownie Pudding Cake • Chocolate Chip Bundt Cake with Chocolate-Coffee Frosting • Chocolate Angel Food Cake • Amaretto Fudge Cake • New Orleans Bread Pudding • Carrot Cake with Cream Cheese Frosting • Steamed Date-Nut Pudding • Mock Cherry Cheesecake • Lemon Custard Delight • Hamilton Pie • Strawberry Shortcake • Frozen Yogurt Charlotte • Ice Cream Cake Roll with Blueberry Sauce • Blueberry Sauce • Bananas Foster • Blueberry Meringue Tortes • Strawberry Russe • Brownie Baked Alaska • Fresh Pineapple with Orange Liqueur • Peach-Raspberry Supreme • Peaches in Wine • Custard Pie • Granola Apple Cobbler • Frosted Apple Cookies • Baked Rice Pudding • Rice Pudding (Stovetop) • Oatmeal Crispies • Lemon-Glazed Spice Bars • Low-Fat Lemon Bars • Guilt-Free Tiramisu • Brandy Sauce • Hard Sauce • Amaretto Custard Sauce • Yogurt Dessert Topping

# Chocolate Brownie Pudding Cake

2 1/2 cups all-purpose flour
1 1/2 cups sugar
1 teaspoon baking soda
1 teaspoon baking powder
1/2 teaspoon salt
3 tablespoons cocoa powder
2 egg whites, slightly beaten
1 1/4 cups skim milk
1 1/2 teaspoons lemon juice
3/4 teaspoon vanilla
1/2 cup chopped pecans
Amaretto Custard Sauce
  (Recipe, page 385)

**Yield: 8 to 10 servings**

**Per serving:**
Calories...... 262
Protein (g)... 5
Fat (g)....... 4.3
Sat. Fat (g).. 0.5
Choles. (mg).. 0
Fiber (g)..... 1.6
Sodium (mg)... 227
%Cal-Fat...... 14%

Combine first six ingredients (dry ingredients) in a large mixing bowl. Stir to blend evenly. Add slightly beaten egg whites and skim milk, stirring until dry ingredients are moistened and batter is smooth. You may use an electric mixer. Stir in lemon juice, vanilla and pecans.

Spray a 1 1/2-quart pudding mold* with a vegetable cooking spray. Pour batter into mold and cover tightly with lid; or pour batter into a well-greased heat-proof bowl and cover with a double layer of aluminum foil. Secure with string.

Position mold on a 1-inch rack in a large kettle placed over medium heat. Add boiling water, filling kettle one-third full. Cover and steam 2 1/4 hours. Water should boil gently during this time. Add more boiling water if necessary.

Lift mold from kettle. Remove lid to allow steam to escape. After 15 minutes, loosen sides with a knife and invert onto serving dish. Serve warm or cold with Amaretto Custard Sauce.

*A pudding mold is a metal dome-shaped mold with a lid that fastens down with clamps. It can be purchased at most kitchen accessory stores.

Preparation time: 20–25 minutes
Cooking time: 2 1/4 hours

# Chocolate Chip Bundt Cake

Preheat oven to 350 degrees. Spray a 10-inch nonstick bundt pan with vegetable cooking spray.

Combine first six ingredients (dry ingredients) in a large mixing bowl. Mix well. Add remaining ingredients except chocolate chips. Beat at high speed for 2 minutes. Batter will be thin.

Pour into bundt pan. Sprinkle chocolate chips over top. Stir in slightly, letting some chips sink into batter. Bake at 350 degrees 40 to 50 minutes, or until toothpick inserted into center of cake comes out clean. Cool for 15 minutes before removing from pan. Cool completely before frosting with Chocolate-Coffee Frosting.

*Chocolate-Coffee Frosting:* In small bowl, melt margarine in microwave. Dissolve coffee grounds in melted margarine.

In mixing bowl, combine powdered sugar, margarine mixture, cocoa powder and 3 tablespoons skim milk. Beat until smooth. Add more milk as needed until desired consistency.

*Note: To make cupcakes, preheat oven to 375 degrees. Prepare batter as above, except omit chocolate chips. Pour batter into cupcake tins lined with foil bake cups, filling 2/3 full. Bake at 375 degrees for 18 to 20 minutes, or until cupcakes spring back when touched lightly on top. Cool and frost. Makes 24 to 30 cupcakes.*

Preparation time: 30 minutes
Cooking time: 45 minutes

*2 1/2 cups all-purpose flour*
*2 cups sugar*
*1 cup cocoa powder*
*2 teaspoons baking soda*
*2 teaspoons baking powder*
*1/2 teaspoon salt*
*5 egg whites*
*1 1/3 cups skim milk*
*1 cup boiling water*
*2/3 cup applesauce*
*2 1/2 teaspoons vanilla*
*1/4 cup mini-chocolate chips (2 ounces)*

*Chocolate-Coffee Frosting:*
*2 tablespoons light margarine, melted*
*1/2 teaspoon instant coffee grounds*
*2 cups powdered sugar*
*1/4 cup cocoa powder*
*Skim milk as needed (3 to 4 tablespoons)*

**Yield: 24 servings**

**Per serving with frosting:**
Calories...... 182
Protein (g)... 3
Fat (g)....... 2.5
Sat. Fat (g).. 1
Choles. (mg).. 0
Fiber (g) .... 1.5
Sodium (mg)... 173
%Cal-Fat...... 10%

# Chocolate Angel Food Cake

12 egg whites
1 1/2 teaspoons cream of tartar
2 teaspoons vanilla
1 cup sugar
1 cup sifted cake flour
1/3 cup unsweetened cocoa
    powder
3/4 cup sugar
1/4 teaspoon ground cinnamon
Amaretto Custard Sauce
    (Recipe, page 385)

**Yield: 16 servings**

**Per serving:**
Calories...... 123
Protein (g)... 3
Fat (g)....... 0.4
Sat. Fat (g).. 0.2
Choles. (mg).. 0
Fiber (g)..... 0.3
Sodium (mg)... 38
%Cal-Fat...... 3%

Preheat oven to 375 degrees.

With an electric mixer, beat egg whites until foamy. Add cream of tartar. Beat until soft peaks form. Add vanilla, and gradually add 1 cup sugar. Beat until stiff peaks form.

Sift together flour, cocoa, 3/4 cup sugar and cinnamon. Fold into whites. Spoon batter into ungreased 10-inch tube pan.

Bake at 375 degrees for 35 to 40 minutes or until done.

Invert cake pan immediately and cool for 40 minutes. Loosen cake from sides and remove.

To serve, cut cake into slices. Top each slice with Amaretto Custard Sauce. If desired, sprinkle lightly with finely grated dark chocolate and garnish with thin chocolate wafer.

Preparation time: 20 minutes
Cooking time: 35–40 minutes

# Amaretto Fudge Cake

Preheat oven to 325 degrees.

Spray a 9-inch springform pan with vegetable cooking spray. Combine the first six ingredients (dry ingredients) in a large mixing bowl. Mix well. Add remaining ingredients except chocolate chips and raisins. Beat at high speed for 2 minutes. Batter will be very thin.

Pour into springform pan. Sprinkle chocolate chips and raisins, if desired, evenly over top. (Most of them will sink to the bottom.) Bake at 325 degrees 50 to 60 minutes, or until top of cake is firm to the touch.

Cool at least 30 minutes. Loosen edges of cake with knife before removing sides of springform pan. Cover to keep moist.

*This cake resembles a chocolate cheesecake in its rich fudginess. The top may crack slightly, similar to a cheesecake.*

Preparation time: 25–30 minutes
Cooking time: 50–60 minutes

*1 3/4 cups all-purpose flour*
*1 1/2 cups sugar*
*3/4 cup cocoa powder*
*1 1/2 teaspoons baking soda*
*1 1/2 teaspoons baking powder*
*1/2 teaspoon salt*
*4 egg whites*
*2/3 cup skim milk*
*1/3 cup Amaretto liqueur*
*1/2 cup applesauce*
*2 teaspoons vanilla*
*1 teaspoon almond extract*
*3/4 cup boiling water*
*1/4 cup mini-chocolate chips (2 ounces)*
*1/2 cup dark raisins (optional)*

### Yield: 12 servings

**Per serving:**
Calories...... 227
Protein (g)... 4
Fat (g)....... 1.8
Sat. Fat (g).. 0.8
Choles. (mg).. 0
Fiber (g)..... 1.8
Sodium (mg)... 297
%Cal-Fat...... 8%

# New Orleans Bread Pudding

1 10-ounce loaf stale French
  bread (very hard)
1 12-ounce can evaporated
  skim milk
2 1/2 cups skim milk
4 egg substitutes (1 cup),
  slightly beaten
2 cups sugar
2 tablespoons vanilla extract
1 teaspoon cinnamon
3/4 cup golden raisins
1 apple, peeled and diced
1 tablespoon tub margarine,
  melted
Hard Sauce (optional) *
  (Recipe, page 384)

**Yield: 15 servings**

*Per serving:*
Calories...... 240
Protein (g)... 7
Fat (g)....... 1.9
Sat. Fat (g).. 0.4
Choles. (mg).. 3
Fiber (g)..... 1
Sodium (mg)... 199
%Cal-Fat...... 7%

Preheat oven to 350 degrees.

In large mixing bowl, crumble bread into bite-size pieces. Pour evaporated milk and skim milk over bread. Soak until bread is completely softened.

Meanwhile, combine eggs, sugar, vanilla, cinnamon, raisins and diced apple. Add to bread mixture.

Spread melted margarine in bottom of 9 x 13-inch baking pan. Add bread pudding mixture, and bake until it is firm to the touch and the top is golden brown, approximately 40 to 45 minutes.

Cool slightly and cut into 3-inch squares. Serve either warm or cold. Place on individual dessert dishes. Drizzle Hard Sauce over top, if desired. Store in refrigerator.

*The hard sauce converts a simple bread pudding into a rich, elegant dessert.*

Preparation time: 25–35 minutes
Cooking time: 40–45 minutes

# Carrot Cake

Preheat oven to 375 degrees.

Grate carrots. Set aside.

Combine sugar, flours, baking soda, baking powder, salt, cinnamon and allspice in a large mixing bowl. Blend together well.

To same mixing bowl, add egg whites, milk, applesauce, vanilla and boiling water. Beat at high speed for 2 minutes. Fold in grated carrots.

Spray 10-inch bundt pan with vegetable cooking spray. Pour in batter. Bake at 375 degrees 40 to 50 minutes, or until toothpick inserted in center comes out clean. Remove from oven and cool slightly. Loosen edges of cake and invert onto serving plate. After cake is cooled completely, frost with Cream Cheese Frosting.

*Cream Cheese Frosting:* Mix together all ingredients except walnuts. Add small amount of skim milk if necessary for proper spreading consistency.

Spread frosting on cake. Immediately sprinkle walnuts over top. (If you wait even a few minutes before sprinkling walnuts, frosting will be set, and the nuts will slip off.)

Preparation time: 35–40 minutes
Cooking time: 35–40 minutes

*1 1/2 cups sugar*
*1 1/2 cups all-purpose flour*
*1 cup whole wheat flour*
*1 1/2 teaspoons baking soda*
*1 1/2 teaspoons baking powder*
*1/2 teaspoon salt*
*2 teaspoons cinnamon*
*1 teaspoon allspice*
*4 egg whites*
*3/4 cup skim milk*
*1/2 cup natural applesauce*
*2 teaspoons vanilla*
*3/4 cup boiling water*
*2 cups finely shredded carrots*
  *(2 to 3 carrots)*

*Cream Cheese Frosting:*
*3 ounces light cream cheese*
*1 tablespoon tub margarine*
*1 teaspoon vanilla*
*2 cups powdered sugar*
*3 tablespoons chopped walnuts*

## Yield: 24 servings

*Per serving:*
Calories...... 156
Protein (g)... 3
Fat (g)....... 1.8
Sat. Fat (g).. 0.7
Choles. (mg).. 4
Fiber (g)..... 1.3
Sodium (mg)... 148
%Cal-Fat...... 11%

# Steamed Date-Nut Pudding

2 cups all-purpose flour
1 cup sugar
1 teaspoon baking soda
1 teaspoon baking powder
2 egg whites, slightly beaten
1 cup skim milk
1 1/2 teaspoons lemon juice
3/4 cup chopped dates
1/2 cup chopped pecans
Brandy Sauce (Recipe, page 384)

*Yield: 8 to 10 servings*

*Per serving:*
Calories...... 277
Protein (g)... 5
Fat (g)....... 4.8
Sat. Fat (g).. 0.5
Choles. (mg).. 0
Fiber (g)..... 2.3
Sodium (mg)... 154
%Cal-Fat...... 15%

Combine flour, sugar, baking soda and baking powder in a large mixing bowl. Add slightly beaten egg whites and skim milk, stirring until dry ingredients are moistened. Stir in lemon juice, dates and pecans. (If chopping your own dates, mix with 1 tablespoon flour, to avoid sticking together.)

Spray a 1 1/2-quart pudding mold* with a vegetable cooking spray. Pour batter into mold and cover tightly with lid; or pour batter into a well-greased heat-proof bowl and cover with a double layer of aluminum foil. Secure with string.

Position mold on a 1-inch rack in a large kettle placed over medium heat. Add boiling water, filling kettle one-third full. Cover and steam 2 1/4 hours. Water should boil gently during this time. Add more boiling water if necessary.

Lift mold from kettle. Remove lid to allow steam to escape. After 15 minutes, loosen sides with knife and invert onto serving dish. Garnish with twisted lemon slices and serve warm or cold. To serve, place slice of pudding cake on dessert plate and top with Brandy Sauce.

*A pudding mold is a metal dome-shaped mold with a lid that fastens down with clamps. It comes in various sizes and can be purchased at most kitchen accessory stores.*

Preparation time: 20 minutes
Cooking time: 2 1/4 hours

# Mock Cherry Cheesecake

Preheat oven to 350 degrees. Line outside of 9-inch springform pan with aluminum foil, shiny side out. (This is to slow down cooking process and minimize cracking of top.)

Combine all ingredients, except cherry pie filling, in large blender or food processor. Process on high until smooth and slightly foamy.

Pour into prepared springform pan. Bake at 350 degrees for 60 to 70 minutes, or until cheesecake is set (firm in center) and top is golden brown. Cool to room temperature.

Carefully remove sides from springform pan. Spoon cherry pie filling over cheesecake to within 1/2-inch of outside edge. Cover and refrigerate until ready to serve.

*The batter is very thin so springform pan may leak slightly. This should not be a problem because the aluminum foil will catch any drips that may occur.*

Preparation time: 10–15 minutes
Cooking time: 50–60 minutes

2 cups sugar
6 egg substitutes (1 1/2 cups)
2 teaspoons vanilla
3/4 cup self-rising flour
1 1/2 tablespoons yellow cornmeal
17 ounces evaporated skim milk
1/4 cup lemon juice
2 tablespoons light margarine, melted
1 21-ounce can cherry pie filling

**Yield: 12 to 14 servings**

**Per serving:**
Calories...... 260
Protein (g)... 8
Fat (g)....... 2.6
Sat. Fat (g).. 1
Choles. (mg).. 2
Fiber (g)..... 0.5
Sodium (mg)... 221
%Cal-Fat...... 9%

# Lemon Custard Delight

1 cup sugar
3 tablespoons self-rising flour
1 cup skim milk
2 teaspoons canola oil
2 teaspoons egg substitute
2 drops yellow food coloring
1/4 teaspoon salt
Juice and grated zest of 1
   lemon *
2 egg whites

**Yield: 6 servings**

**Per serving:**
Calories...... 179
Protein (g)... 3
Fat (g)....... 1.7
Sat. Fat (g).. 0.2
Choles. (mg).. 0
Fiber (g)..... 0.2
Sodium (mg)... 182
%Cal-Fat...... 8%

Preheat oven to 350 degrees.

In a medium-size bowl, combine sugar and flour. Mix well with a wire whisk. Add milk, canola oil, egg substitute, food coloring, salt, grated zest and lemon juice. Mix well with wire whisk.

In separate bowl, beat egg whites until stiff. Gently fold whites into lemon mixture until lumps have disappeared. Spoon mixture into 6 3-inch ramekins.

Set ramekins in a 9 x 13-inch pan and add hot water until it is halfway up the sides of the ramekins. Carefully place in oven and bake for 30 to 35 minutes or until a knife blade can be inserted into the center of ramekin and come out clean. Remove from oven. Cool 30 minutes. Invert ramekins onto a dessert plate. Serve immediately or make ahead and chill. Garnish with a twisted lemon slice and a sprig of fresh mint.

*A zest of lemon is a small piece of the lemon peel. This dessert forms a light fluffy cake on the bottom and a rich "creamy" custard on top.*

Preparation time: 25–30 minutes
Cooking time: 30–35 minutes

# Hamilton Pie

Preheat oven to 325 degrees. Spray 9-inch pie pan with vegetable cooking spray, covering surface well.

In large mixing bowl, beat egg whites until soft peaks form. Add vanilla. Gradually add sugar and continue beating until very stiff peaks form. Set aside.

Crush soda crackers with rolling pin. Transfer cracker crumbs to medium-size mixing bowl. Add baking powder to crumbs and mix well. Carefully fold crumb mixture into egg whites.

Pour into pie plate and bake at 325 degrees for 25 minutes, or until top is light golden brown. Cool completely.

Meanwhile wash raspberries. To serve, cut pie into eighths and place on individual plates. Top with whipping cream (about 1/4 cup per serving) and raspberries. Spoon approximately 2 teaspoons liqueur over each serving. Serve immediately.

*A light, elegant dessert, which also tastes excellent with blackberries, blueberries or strawberries.*

*\*Chambord is a raspberry-flavored liqueur.*

Preparation time: 20 minutes
Cooking time: 25 minutes

5 egg whites
1 teaspoon vanilla
1 cup sugar
1 package (36 crackers) nonfat soda crackers
1 teaspoon baking powder
1 can pressurized light whipping cream
3 cups fresh raspberries
4 to 6 tablespoons Chambord* or Amaretto liqueur

*Yield: 8 servings*

*Per serving:*
Calories...... 227
Protein (g)... 4
Fat (g)....... 3
Sat. Fat (g).. 1.6
Choles. (mg).. 8
Fiber (g)..... 1.4
Sodium (mg)... 202
%Cal-Fat...... 12%

# *Strawberry Shortcake*

*1 pint fresh strawberries, sliced*
*2 tablespoons sugar*
*1 1/4 cups all-purpose flour*
*2 tablespoons sugar*
*1 1/2 teaspoons baking powder*
*1/4 teaspoon salt*
*2 tablespoons light margarine*
*1 egg substitute (1/4 cup)*
*2 tablespoons skim milk*
*3 tablespoons natural*
*  applesauce*
*1 teaspoon finely shredded*
*  lemon peel (optional)*
*Vanilla frozen yogurt, nonfat*
*  or low-fat (optional)*

### *Yield: Serves 4*

*Per serving:*
Calories...... 221
Protein (g)... 6
Fat (g)....... 5.4
Sat. Fat (g).. 1.1
Choles. (mg).. 0
Fiber (g)..... 2.7
Sodium (mg)... 363
%Cal-Fat...... 22%

Preheat oven to 450 degrees.

Wash and slice strawberries. Sprinkle 2 tablespoons sugar over top and toss lightly. Sprinkle with 1 tablespoon water. Set aside.

Combine flour, 2 tablespoons sugar, baking powder and salt. Stir to blend. Cut in margarine with a pastry cutter until the consistency of course crumbs. Add egg substitute, milk, applesauce and lemon peel. Mix together, just until blended. Do not overmix.

Divide dough into 4 equal portions. On a floured surface, roll each portion into a ball and flatten into a circle about 1/2-inch thick. Place on lightly greased cookie sheet and bake at 450 degrees for 8 to 10 minutes, or until golden. Remove from baking sheet and cool. Slit each biscuit.

Assemble 4 individual shortcakes. Place lower halves of biscuits on plates, followed by 1/2 of strawberries, then upper halves of biscuits, followed by remaining strawberries.

Top with vanilla frozen yogurt, if desired.

Preparation time: 20–30 minutes
Cooking time: 8–10 minutes

# Frozen Yogurt Charlotte

Let frozen yogurt thaw at room temperature approximately 20 minutes.

Meanwhile, split ladyfingers and lay flat, placing split side upward. Brush Amaretto over ladyfingers. Line bottom and sides of a 10-inch springform pan with ladyfingers, with cut side facing up or inward.

Sprinkle 6 tablespoons of wafer crumbs over the ladyfingers placed on bottom of pan.

Carefully spoon black cherry frozen yogurt over ladyfingers, spreading to the sides.

Combine vanilla frozen yogurt with 1 tablespoon rum. Spoon over black cherry frozen yogurt. Sprinkle with remaining 2 tablespoons wafer crumbs. Garnish with bing cherries, if desired.

Freeze until ready to serve. Remove sides from springform pan before serving.

*Remove from freezer 10 to 15 minutes before serving, for greater ease in slicing.*

Preparation time: 30–35 minutes
Additional time: 4 hours to freeze

24 ladyfingers, split (2 packages)
1/4 cup Amaretto liqueur
1/2 cup chocolate wafer crumbs, divided
1 1/2 quarts black cherry low-fat frozen yogurt
1 1/2 quarts vanilla low-fat frozen yogurt
1 tablespoon rum
Fresh bing cherries for garnish, if desired

**Yield: 14 to 16 servings**

**Per serving:**
Calories...... 254
Protein (g)... 6
Fat (g)....... 4.7
Sat. Fat (g).. 0
Choles. (mg).. 11
Fiber (g)..... 0.1
Sodium (mg)... 116
%Cal-Fat...... 17%

# Ice Cream Cake Roll with Blueberry Sauce

*2 egg substitutes (1/2 cup)*
*1 tablespoon canola oil*
*1/4 cup sugar*
*1 teaspoon vanilla*
*4 egg whites*
*1/2 cup sugar*
*3/4 cup all-purpose flour*
*1 teaspoon baking powder*
*1/4 teaspoon salt*
*1 quart vanilla ice milk or
  nonfat ice cream*
*Blueberry Sauce (Recipe, page
  371)*

**Yield: 10 1-inch slices**

**Per serving:**
Calories...... 297
Protein (g)... 6
Fat (g)....... 4.2
Sat. Fat (g).. 1.7
Choles. (mg).. 7
Fiber (g)..... 1
Sodium (mg)... 170
%Cal-Fat...... 13%

Preheat oven to 350 degrees.

Grease a 15 1/2 x 10 1/2 x 1-inch jelly-roll pan. Line with waxed paper and grease again.

With an electric mixer, beat egg substitutes and oil until well mixed; gradually add 1/4 cup sugar and beat until mixture is frothy. Add vanilla and set aside.

Beat egg whites until soft peaks form. Gradually add 1/2 cup sugar and beat until stiff peaks form. Fold egg substitute mixture into whites.

Sift together flour, baking powder and salt. Fold into egg mixture. Spread batter evenly in jelly-roll pan.

Bake at 350 degrees for 10 to 12 minutes or until done.

Immediately invert cake onto a clean linen towel that has been liberally sprinkled with sifted confectioners sugar. Remove waxed paper. Trim cake if edges are brown.

Starting at narrow end, roll cake and towel together. Cool completely on wire rack.

Meanwhile, soften ice milk by letting it stand at room temperature for 15 to 20 minutes.

Unroll cake in towel. Press carefully to flatten. Spread slightly softened ice milk up to 1/2-inch from outside edges of cake. Roll up. Spoon in ice milk at outside edges of roll where needed, to make ice milk flush with outside edge. Wrap with clear plastic wrap or aluminum foil and freeze until firm.

So serve, cut 1-inch slices from roll, place on dessert plates, and top with warmed Blueberry Sauce.

Preparation time: 35–45 minutes
Cooking time: 10–12 minutes
Additional time: 4 hours to freeze

# Blueberry Sauce

In saucepan, combine sugar, cornstarch, allspice and salt. With a wire whisk, gradually stir in boiling water. Cook and stir until mixture thickens and boils. Cook 2 minutes more.

Add fresh blueberries and return to boiling. Remove from heat. Stir in lemon juice. Serve either warm or chilled.

*Instead of fresh blueberries, you may use one 10-ounce package frozen unsweetened blueberries, thawed and drained. Follow instructions as given above except increase cornstarch to 3 tablespoons.*

Preparation time: 15 minutes

*1 cup sugar*
*2 1/2 tablespoons corn starch*
*1/4 teaspoon allspice*
*Dash salt*
*1 cup boiling water*
*1 pint fresh blueberries, washed*
*3 tablespoons lemon juice*

*Yield: 3 cups sauce*

*Per serving:*
Calories...... 43
Protein (g)... 0
Fat (g)....... 0
Sat. Fat (g).. 0
Choles. (mg).. 0
Fiber (g)..... 0.3
Sodium (mg)... 1
%Cal-Fat...... 1%

# Bananas Foster

Cut bananas in half crosswise; then slit down the middle. Set aside.

In sauté pan, melt margarine with brown sugar. Heat until mixture begins to boil. Add bananas and sauté until tender but still firm, about 1 1/2 to 2 minutes. Sprinkle with cinnamon.

Pour liqueur and rum or brandy over bananas. Heat until liqueur becomes very hot and ignite with a match.

As soon as flames disappear, serve immediately over frozen yogurt or nonfat ice cream.

*Because of the spectacular flames from the ignited alcohol, this is an impressive dessert to serve. Since the flames shoot up fairly high, do not ignite near anything flammable.*

Preparation time: 15–20 minutes

*4 bananas*
*2 tablespoons tub margarine*
*1/4 cup firmly packed brown sugar*
*Cinnamon*
*1/4 cup banana liqueur*
*1/4 cup light rum or brandy*
*4 large scoops low-fat vanilla frozen yogurt, or nonfat ice cream*

*Yield: 4 servings*

*Per serving:*
Calories...... 434
Protein (g)... 6
Fat (g)....... 6.5
Sat. Fat (g).. 1.5
Choles. (mg).. 0
Fiber (g)..... 2
Sodium (mg)... 155
%Cal-Fat...... 13%

# Blueberry Meringue Tortes

*Individual Meringue Shells:*
*3 egg whites*
*1 teaspoon vanilla*
*1/4 teaspoon cream of tartar*
*1 cup sugar*
*1/4 cup finely chopped*
  *almonds, toasted*

*6 cups low-fat or nonfat frozen*
  *yogurt (3/4 cup/serving)*
*Blueberry Sauce (Recipe, page*
  *371)*
*Mint sprigs (optional)*

**Yield: 8 servings**

**Per serving:**
Calories...... 435
Protein (g)... 8
Fat (g)....... 6.4
Sat. Fat (g).. 2.1
Choles. (mg).. 11
Fiber (g)..... 2
Sodium (mg)... 125
%Cal-Fat...... 13%

Preheat oven to 250 degrees.

Place egg whites in large mixing bowl. Add vanilla, cream of tartar and dash salt. Beat until soft peaks form. Gradually add sugar, beating until very stiff peaks form. Stir in chopped almonds.

Cover baking sheet with waxed paper. Draw 8 circles, 3 1/2 inches in diameter, on waxed paper. Spread circles with approximately 1/3 cup meringue, using the back of a spoon to shape into individual shells.

Bake at 250 degrees for 45 to 60 minutes. Shells should be firm and dry, but still white. Turn off oven. Let shells dry in closed oven for 1 hour. Remove from paper while still warm.

Meanwhile make Blueberry Sauce. Cool slightly.

To serve, fill shells with frozen yogurt and spoon Blueberry Sauce over top. Garnish with mint sprigs, if desired.

*Fresh strawberries and other fruits in season may be substituted for the Blueberry Sauce.*

Preparation time: 35–40 minutes
Cooking time: 45–60 minutes

# Strawberry Russe

Spray vegetable cooking spray on bottom only of 10-inch springform pan.

Split ladyfingers and lay flat. Sprinkle cut side with liqueur. Place ladyfingers, cut sides facing up and inward, around sides and in bottom of springform pan.

In small saucepan, soften gelatin in cold water. Stir over low heat until completely dissolved. Remove from heat.

Chop up strawberries in food processor, keeping mixture slightly lumpy. Transfer to a large bowl. Stir in sugar, lemon juice and gelatin mixture. Whisk until foamy. Refrigerate until mixture thickens slightly, about 10 to 20 minutes.

Meanwhile, in mixing bowl, beat egg whites until stiff peaks form. Fold into strawberry mixture.

In small bowl, beat whipping cream until stiff peaks form. Fold into strawberry mixture.

Pour into springform pan. Refrigerate at least 4 hours. Before serving, carefully remove sides of pan. Garnish with fresh strawberries, if available.

Preparation time: 35–40 minutes
Refrigeration time: 4 hours

*20 ladyfingers, split*
*1/4 cup orange-flavored liqueur*
*2 envelopes unflavored gelatin*
*1/2 cup cold water*
*2 1/2 cups fresh strawberries, hulls removed, or 20-ounce pkg. frozen strawberries without syrup, thawed*
*3/4 cup sugar*
*4 tablespoons lemon juice*
*4 egg whites*
*1/2 cup whipping cream*

*Yield: 12 servings*

*Per serving:*
Calories...... 153
Protein (g)... 3
Fat (g)....... 3.8
Sat. Fat (g).. 2.3
Choles. (mg).. 14
Fiber (g)..... 1
Sodium (mg)... 57
%Cal-Fat...... 22%

# Brownie Baked Alaska

1 quart vanilla ice milk or
   nonfat ice cream
1 cup sugar
1 1/4 cups all-purpose flour
1/2 cup cocoa powder
1 teaspoon baking soda
1/2 teaspoon baking powder
1/4 teaspoon salt
3 egg whites
2/3 cup skim milk
1/3 cup applesauce
1/2 cup boiling water
1 1/4 teaspoons vanilla
1/4 cup chopped walnuts

*Meringue Topping:*
5 egg whites
1 cup sugar

### Yield: 10 to 12 servings

*Per serving:*
Calories...... 351
Protein (g)... 9
Fat (g)....... 6
Sat. Fat (g).. 2.8
Choles. (mg).. 12
Fiber (g)..... 1.8
Sodium (mg)... 291
%Cal-Fat...... 15%

Line an 8-inch cake pan with waxed paper, leaving an overhang around the edges. Pack slightly softened nonfat ice cream or ice milk into pan. Cover with foil. Freeze until firm (at least 3 to 4 hours).

Meanwhile, make brownie cake. Preheat oven to 375 degrees.

Prepare 8-inch cake pan by spraying with vegetable cooking spray. Combine sugar, flour, cocoa powder, baking soda, baking powder and salt in large mixing bowl. Mix well. Add remaining ingredients except walnuts. Beat at high speed for two minutes. Batter will be thin. Fold in walnuts.

Pour into prepared cake pan. Bake at 375 degrees 30 to 35 minutes, or until toothpick inserted in center of cake comes out clean. Cool 20 minutes before removing from pan. Wrap in plastic wrap to maintain moisture. Refrigerate until ready to assemble.

*To assemble:* Preheat oven to 500 degrees.

Prepare meringue topping: Beat egg whites until soft peaks form. Gradually beat in sugar. Continue beating until stiff peaks form. Set aside.

Place brownie cake on ovenproof serving dish. Invert frozen ice cream onto brownie layer, tugging at waxed paper to loosen from pan. Remove waxed paper. Spread meringue topping over top and sides, making sure the edges are sealed.

Bake at 500 degrees for 2 minutes or until meringue peaks are lightly browned. Serve immediately.

*If you have difficulty removing frozen ice cream from container, dip container in lukewarm water for 30 to 60 seconds to loosen.*

Preparation time: 50–60 minutes
Cooking time: 35–40 minutes
Additional time: 4 hours to freeze

# Fresh Pineapple with Orange Liqueur

Cut leaves from pineapple. Next, cut lengthwise into four equal parts. Remove core from center of pineapple wedges; cut fruit away from rind into bite-size pieces, leaving it in the shell to serve. With a pastry brush, generously coat fruit pieces with orange liqueur.

Slice orange, crosswise, into four 1/4-inch slices. Cut a radius into the slice, twist and place in center of pineapple wedge. Next, place 2 strawberry halves on either side of orange slice. Chill before serving.

*A colorful, light dessert, ideal for lunch or brunch.*

Preparation time: 10–15 minutes

*1 ripe fresh pineapple, including shell*
*1/2 cup Triple Sec orange liqueur*
*1 orange*
*4 fresh strawberries*

*Yield: 4 servings*

*Per serving:*
Calories...... 135
Protein (g)... 1
Fat (g)....... 0.7
Sat. Fat (g).. 0
Choles. (mg).. 0
Fiber (g)..... 2.4
Sodium (mg)... 3
%Cal-Fat...... 5%

# Peach-Raspberry Supreme

Drain and rinse peach halves. Pat dry and set aside.

Defrost frozen raspberries. Drain liquid. Put drained raspberries in food processor. Add liqueur. Add 1 tablespoon sugar if no sugar is added to frozen raspberries. Process on and off until well chopped. Sauce will be thick.

Place each peach half on a small serving dish. (Stemmed glassware looks very elegant for this dessert.) Pour raspberry sauce over top, covering entire peach half. If desired, top with a small scoop of vanilla frozen yogurt or ice milk.

*For a variation, place a slice of pound cake or angel food cake as a foundation for this dessert. It is delicious.*

Preparation time: 10–15 minutes

*32-ounce can large peach halves, rinsed and drained*
*2 10-ounce packages frozen raspberries, defrosted and drained*
*2 tablespoons Kirsch liqueur (cherry flavored)*
*Vanilla frozen yogurt or ice milk (optional)*

*Yield: 8 servings*

*Per serving:*
Calories...... 156
Protein (g)... 1
Fat (g)....... 0
Sat. Fat (g).. 0
Choles. (mg).. 0
Fiber (g)..... 4.4
Sodium (mg)... 8
%Cal-Fat...... 1%

# Peaches in Wine

4 ripe peaches, peeled and sliced
1 1/2 cups Burgundy wine
1/2 cup sugar
1/2 teaspoon whole cloves
Lemon zest (narrow strips of
    lemon peel)

**Yield: 4 to 6 servings**

**Per serving:**
Calories...... 215
Protein (g)... 0
Fat (g)....... 0
Sat. Fat (g).. 0
Choles. (mg).. 0
Fiber (g)..... 1
Sodium (mg)... 7
%Cal-Fat...... 0%

Peel peaches and slice into small slices. Place in medium-size bowl.

In small bowl, combine wine, sugar, cloves and lemon zest. Mix until sugar begins to dissolve. Pour over peaches. Cover.

Marinate for at least 2 hours before serving. Stir occasionally. Refrigerate until ready to serve.

*This tastes best if prepared the same day it is served. Marinating fruit between 3 and 6 hours is ideal. For best results, use fresh peaches at their peak of ripeness, neither too soft nor too hard.*

Preparation time: 15–20 minutes
Marinating time: 3–6 hours

# Custard Pie

1 3/4 cups sugar
4 egg substitutes (1 cup)
1 teaspoon vanilla
1/2 cup self-rising flour
1 12-ounce can evaporated
    skim milk
1 1/2 tablespoons light
    margarine, melted

**Yield: 1 9-inch pie, or 8 to 10 servings**

**Per serving:**
Calories...... 239
Protein (g)... 7
Fat (g)....... 2.5
Sat. Fat (g).. 0.9
Choles. (mg).. 2
Fiber (g)..... 0.2
Sodium (mg)... 205
%Cal-Fat...... 9%

Preheat oven to 350 degrees.

Lightly spray 9-inch pie pan with vegetable cooking spray.

Combine all ingredients in blender or food processor. Process on high until smooth and slightly foamy.

Pour into pie pan. Bake at 350 degrees for 50 to 60 minutes, or until golden brown on top.

Preparation time: 10–15 minutes
Cooking time: 50–60 minutes

# Granola Apple Cobbler

Preheat oven to 350 degrees.

Peel apples and cut into thin slices. Place in 8-inch square baking dish. Add chopped dates.

In small mixing bowl, combine sugar, flour, cinnamon and nutmeg. Pour over apples and mix well.

Prepare topping: Combine oats, flour and brown sugar in mixing bowl. With a pastry cutter, cut in margarine until mixture is crumbly. Sprinkle over apples. Bake at 350 degrees for 45 minutes, or until apples are tender and topping is crisp. Serve warm or at room temperature.

To serve, spoon apple cobbler into individual bowls. Top with scoop of vanilla frozen yogurt or ice milk.

Preparation time: 20 minutes
Cooking time: 45 minutes

5 cups apples, peeled and sliced
 (4 to 6 apples)
1/2 cup chopped dates
3/4 cup sugar
2 tablespoons all-purpose flour
1/2 teaspoon ground cinnamon
1/4 teaspoon nutmeg

Topping:
1/2 cup rolled oats
1/2 cup whole wheat flour
1/4 cup firmly packed brown
 sugar
3 tablespoons light margarine
Low-fat vanilla frozen yogurt
 or ice milk

**Yield: 8 servings**

**Per serving:**
Calories...... 353
Protein (g)... 6
Fat (g)....... 5
Sat. Fat (g).. 1
Choles. (mg).. 0
Fiber (g)..... 3.5
Sodium (mg)... 58
%Cal-Fat...... 13%

# Frosted Apple Cookies

1 cup all-purpose flour
1 cup whole wheat flour
1 teaspoon baking soda
1/4 teaspoon salt
1 teaspoon ground cinnamon
1/2 teaspoon ground nutmeg
2/3 cup firmly packed brown
  sugar
1/2 cup skim milk
2 egg whites, slightly beaten
1/4 cup canola oil
1 cup raisins
1/4 cup chopped pecans
1 unpeeled apple, cored and
  finely chopped

Vanilla Frosting:
1 1/2 cups powdered sugar
2 1/2 tablespoons skim milk
1 tablespoon soft tub
  margarine
1/2 teaspoon vanilla extract

**Yield: 4 1/2 dozen**

**Per 2 cookies with frosting:**
Calories...... 125
Protein (g)... 2
Fat (g)....... 3.3
Sat. Fat (g).. 0.4
Choles. (mg).. 0
Fiber (g)..... 1.2
Sodium (mg)... 65
%Cal-Fat...... 23%

Preheat oven to 400 degrees.

Combine first seven ingredients in large mixing bowl. Set aside.

In small bowl, combine milk, egg whites and canola oil. Add to ingredients in large bowl, mixing well. Fold in raisins, pecans and chopped apple.

Drop dough by rounded teaspoonfuls, 1 1/2 inches apart, onto greased cookie sheets.

Bake at 400 degrees for 12 to 15 minutes. Cool. Frost with Vanilla Frosting.

*Vanilla Frosting:* Combine all ingredients in medium-size mixing bowl and beat until smooth. Makes enough frosting for 4 1/2 dozen cookies.

Preparation time: 35–45 minutes
Cooking time: 25–30 minutes

# Baked Rice Pudding

Prepare rice according to package directions. Set aside.

Preheat oven to 400 degrees.

In large mixing bowl, combine egg substitutes and egg whites. Beat with wire whisk until slightly frothy. Beat in sugar. Add remaining ingredients including rice, and stir until well mixed.

Pour into a 2 1/2-quart casserole dish. Bake, uncovered, at 400 degrees for 45 minutes or until custard is set. Serve warm or cold.

Preparation time: 15 minutes
Cooking time: 1 hour, 15 minutes

*4 egg substitutes (1 cup)*
*2 egg whites*
*3/4 cup sugar*
*1 3/4 cups skim milk*
*2 cups cooked white or brown rice*
*1 teaspoon cinnamon*
*1/4 teaspoon nutmeg*
*1/3 cup raisins (optional)*

**Yield: 6 to 8 servings**

**Per serving:**
Calories...... 215
Protein (g)... 9
Fat (g)....... 1.5
Sat. Fat (g).. 0.4
Choles. (mg).. 1
Fiber (g)..... 0.3
Sodium (mg)... 112
%Cal-Fat...... 6%

# Rice Pudding (Stovetop)

Cook rice according to package directions.

Heat milk in large saucepan until warm.

Meanwhile, with wire whisk, lightly beat together sugar, cornstarch and egg substitutes in bowl.

Add cooked rice and sugar mixture to warm milk. Add vanilla and cinnamon. Bring to a boil over medium heat, stirring frequently. Simmer until pudding thickens, about 2 minutes.

Serve warm or cold. Add raisins just before serving, if desired.

Preparation time: 15–20 minutes
Cooking time: 25 minutes

*1 1/2 cups brown or white rice (uncooked)*
*1 quart skim milk (4 cups)*
*1/2 to 3/4 cup sugar*
*3 tablespoons cornstarch*
*4 egg substitutes (1 cup)*
*2 teaspoons vanilla*
*1 teaspoon cinnamon*
*Raisins (optional)*

**Yield: 8 to 10 servings**

**Per serving:**
Calories...... 256
Protein (g)... 10
Fat (g)....... 2
Sat. Fat (g).. 0.5
Choles. (mg).. 2
Fiber (g)..... 1.6
Sodium (mg)... 109
%Cal-Fat...... 7%

# Oatmeal Crispies

*3 egg whites*
*Dash of salt*
*1/2 teaspoon vanilla*
*1/2 cup granulated sugar*
*1 1/2 cups corn flakes*
*1 cup oatmeal*
*1/3 cup chopped nuts (walnuts
or pecans)*

*Yield: 3 1/2 dozen cookies*

*For 2 cookies:*
Calories...... 53
Protein (g)... 2
Fat (g)....... 1.4
Sat. Fat (g).. 0.1
Choles. (mg).. 0
Fiber (g)..... 0.6
Sodium (mg)... 43
%Cal-Fat...... 23%

Preheat oven to 350 degrees.

Combine egg whites, salt and vanilla in large mixing bowl. Beat until soft peaks form. Gradually add sugar; beat until stiff. Stir in corn flakes, oatmeal and nuts.

Drop batter from a teaspoon onto a cookie sheet sprayed with vegetable cooking spray.

Bake at 350 degrees for 18 to 20 minutes. Cool for 10 minutes and remove from cookie sheet.

*These taste best if eaten soon after they are baked. They lose some of their crispness after a few hours.*

Preparation time: 25 minutes
Cooking time: 35–40 minutes

# Lemon-Glazed Spice Bars

Preheat oven to 350 degrees.

Combine first six ingredients in large mixing bowl, mixing well. Add oil, egg whites, lemon juice, vanilla and pecans. Mix thoroughly.

Spoon batter into 9 x 13 x 2-inch nonstick baking pan.

Bake at 350 degrees for 25 minutes. Cool slightly.

Spread glaze over top while still warm. Cool. Cut into 2 x 2-inch bars.

*Lemon Glaze:* Combine all ingredients in medium-size mixing bowl, mixing until smooth. Spread evenly over spice bars.

Preparation time: 25 minutes
Cooking time: 25 minutes

*1 cup all-purpose flour*
*1 teaspoon baking powder*
*1/2 teaspoon ground cinnamon*
*1/4 teaspoon ground cardamom*
*1 cup quick-cooking oats, uncooked*
*3/4 cup firmly packed brown sugar*
*1/3 cup canola oil*
*2 egg whites, slightly beaten*
*1 tablespoon lemon juice*
*1/2 teaspoon vanilla*
*1/4 cup chopped pecans*

*Lemon glaze:*
*1 1/2 cups powdered sugar*
*1 tablespoon lemon juice*
*1/4 teaspoon ground cinnamon*
*3 tablespoons skim milk*

**Yield: 4 1/2 dozen**

**Per serving:**
Calories...... 52
Protein (g)... 1
Fat (g)....... 1.8
Sat. Fat (g).. 0.1
Choles. (mg).. 0
Fiber (g)..... 0.3
Sodium (mg)... 10
%Cal-Fat...... 31%

# Low-Fat Lemon Bars

1 3/4 cups all-purpose flour
1/2 cup oatmeal (uncooked)
1/2 cup powdered sugar
1/4 teaspoon salt
1/2 cup canola oil
4 egg substitutes (1 cup)
1 3/4 cups sugar
1/4 cup flour
5 tablespoons fresh-squeezed
  lemon juice
Powdered sugar

**Yield: 28 lemon bars, 2 inches x 2 inches, or 54 bars 1 x 2 inches**

Per 2 x 2-inch serving:
Calories...... 133
Protein (g)... 2
Fat (g)....... 4.4
Sat. Fat (g).. 0.4
Choles. (mg).. 0
Fiber (g)..... 0.4
Sodium (mg)... 35
%Cal-Fat...... 29%

Preheat oven to 350 degrees.

Combine first four ingredients in medium-size bowl. Gradually pour in cooking oil, stirring until well blended. (Small lumps will be present. Large lumps can be broken up with fingers.) Press flour mixture firmly into bottom of 9 x 13-inch nonstick pan. Bake for 15 minutes at 350 degrees.

Meanwhile, in a medium-size bowl, combine egg substitutes, sugar, flour and lemon juice. Beat with a wire whisk. Pour over hot pastry. Bake an additional 20 minutes at 350 degrees.

Remove from oven. Sprinkle with powdered sugar. Cut after cooled. Refrigerate until ready to serve.

*These bars have less than half the fat of the classic lemon bar recipe, and the oil used is much less saturated than butter or margarine. These work out great when finger foods are preferable for dessert—picnics, buffet lunches and cocktail parties.*

Preparation time: 15–20 minutes
Cooking time: 35 minutes

# Guilt-Free Tiramisu

Add skim milk to pudding mix and prepare according to package directions. Set aside and cool to room temperature.

In the meantime, sprinkle unflavored gelatine over 1/4 cup cold water. To dissolve gelatin, heat according to package directions. Set aside and cool.

While pudding and gelatin are cooling, prepare coffee, either perked, drip or instant. Combine coffee and Kahlua liqueur in a small bowl. Set aside.

Place ricotta cheese in food processor and process until smooth and creamy. Add to cooled pudding. Add gelatin mixture.* Stir in sugar, vanilla and rum. Set aside.

Split ladyfingers and place one layer, cut side up, in 8-inch square glass pan. Drizzle half of coffee mixture over top of ladyfingers. Pour half of pudding mixture over ladyfingers, spreading evenly. Place second layer of ladyfingers over pudding, drizzle with remaining coffee mixture, and spread remaining pudding over top. Sprinkle lightly with grated chocolate or hot chocolate mix.

Chill at least 3 hours or overnight before serving.

*If you prefer a less firm filling, use only half of the dissolved gelatin mixture.*

Preparation time: 20–25 minutes
Cooking time: 10 minutes

1 3-ounce package cook &
  serve vanilla pudding mix
2 cups skim milk
1 envelope Knox unflavored
  gelatine*
1/4 cup cold water
1/4 cup strong brewed or
  instant coffee
1/4 cup Kahlua liqueur
1 cup light ricotta cheese
1/4 cup plus 1 tablespoon sugar
1 teaspoon vanilla
2 tablespoons light rum
4 1/2 ounces (2 3-ounce
  packages) ladyfingers, split
2 teaspoons finely grated
  chocolate or hot chocolate mix

**Yield: 9 servings**

**Per serving:**
Calories..... 204
Protein (g).. 6
Fat (g)...... 2.7
Sat. Fat (g). 0.7
Choles. (mg). 5
Fiber (g).... 0
Sodium (mg).. 225
%Cal-Fat..... 12%

# Brandy Sauce

1/2 cup sugar
1 tablespoon cornstarch
1/4 teaspoon salt
2 cups skim milk
2 egg substitutes (1/2 cup)
1 teaspoon cooking oil
1/2 teaspoon vanilla
1/4 cup brandy

**Yield: 2 1/2 cups sauce**

**Per 2 tablespoons:**
Calories...... 43
Protein (g)... 2
Fat (g)....... 0.5
Sat. Fat (g).. 0.1
Choles. (mg).. 0
Fiber (g)..... 0
Sodium (mg)... 51
%Cal-Fat...... 11%

Combine sugar, cornstarch and salt in heavy saucepan. Stir in milk, egg substitute and cooking oil. Cook over medium heat, stirring frequently, until mixture begins to boil. Boil 1 minute longer, stirring constantly.

Remove from heat. Stir in vanilla and brandy.

Serve warm or cold.

*If time is limited, packaged vanilla pudding mix (3-ounce) may be used instead. Follow package directions, and after it is cooked, add brandy.*

Preparation time: 20 minutes

# Hard Sauce

1 tablespoon tub margarine
1 cup powdered sugar
2 tablespoons brandy
Water

**Yield: Approximately 1/2 cup sauce**

**Per 1 teaspoon:**
Calories...... 35
Protein (g)... 0
Fat (g)....... 0.6
Sat. Fat (g).. 0.1
Choles. (mg).. 0
Fiber (g)..... 0
Sodium (mg)... 10
%Cal-Fat...... 15%

In a small mixing bowl, combine margarine, powdered sugar and brandy. Mix until smooth. Add a small amount of water, if necessary, to make a thin syrup, thin enough to spoon over desserts.

*This is a very rich sauce, so only 1 to 2 teaspoons per serving is generally sufficient. If you prefer more, you will want to double the recipe.*

Preparation time: 10 minutes

# Amaretto Custard Sauce

Combine sugar and cornstarch in double boiler, placed over medium-high heat. Stir in milk and egg substitute, stirring frequently until mixture thickens to a pudding consistency.

Remove from heat and stir in vanilla and Amaretto. Serve either warm or chilled.

*This is a smooth and flavorful sauce, especially good spooned over slices of unfrosted cake. In preparing the sauce, a heavy saucepan (placed over medium heat) may be used instead of a double boiler, but the double boiler is much better for preventing scorching.*

Preparation time: 20 minutes

1/2 cup sugar
2 tablespoons cornstarch
2 cups skim milk
2 egg substitutes (1/2 cup)
1/4 teaspoon vanilla
1/4 cup Amaretto liqueur

**Yield: 2 1/2 cups sauce**

**Per 2 tablespoons:**
Calories...... 46
Protein (g)... 2
Fat (g)....... 0.3
Sat. Fat (g).. 0.1
Choles. (mg).. 0
Fiber (g)..... 0
Sodium (mg)... 24
%Cal-Fat...... 5%

# Yogurt Dessert Topping

Mix together yogurt, brown sugar and cinnamon. Serve over fruit desserts in place of whipped cream.

Preparation time: 5 minutes

2 cups nonfat or low-fat plain
  yogurt
1/4 cup firmly packed brown
  sugar
1/4 teaspoon cinnamon

**Yield: 2 cups dessert topping**

**Per serving:**
Calories...... 29
Protein (g)... 2
Fat (g)....... 0
Sat. Fat (g).. 0
Choles. (mg).. 0
Fiber (g)..... 0
Sodium (mg)... 23
%Cal-Fat...... 2%

# Appendix: Nutrition Information on Foods From Fast Food Restaurants

| | Cal | Pro | Fat | S. Fat | Chol | Na | %Fat |
|---|---|---|---|---|---|---|---|
| **BURGER KING** | | | | | | | |
| Apple Pie, Dutch | 308 | 3 | 15 | 3 | 0 | 228 | 44% |
| *Broiler Chicken Sandwich | 267 | 22 | 10 | 2 | 45 | 728 | 32% |
| Bacon Dbl Cheeseburger | 470 | 32 | 28 | 14 | 105 | 800 | 54% |
| Cheeseburger | 318 | 17 | 15 | 7 | 50 | 661 | 42% |
| Chicken Sandwich (Fried) | 685 | 26 | 40 | 8 | 82 | 1417 | 53% |
| Chicken Tenders (6) | 236 | 16 | 13 | 3 | 46 | 541 | 50% |
| Croissan'wich, Egg, Cheese | 353 | 13 | 23 | 8 | 222 | 780 | 59% |
| Croissan'wich, Sausage, Egg, Cheese | 534 | 21 | 40 | 13 | 268 | 985 | 67% |
| Fish Sandwich, Big | 710 | 24 | 43 | 8 | 60 | 1110 | 55% |
| French Fries, medium | 372 | 5 | 20 | 5 | 0 | 238 | 48% |
| French Toast Sticks | 440 | 4 | 27 | 7 | 0 | 490 | 55% |
| *Hamburger | 272 | 15 | 10 | 4 | 37 | 505 | 35% |
| Mini Muffins, Blueberry | 292 | 4 | 14 | 3 | 72 | 244 | 43% |
| *Potato, Baked | 210 | 5 | 0 | 0 | 0 | 15 | 0% |
| Salad, Chef | 178 | 17 | 9 | 4 | 103 | 568 | 46% |
| *Salad, Chunky Chicken | 142 | 20 | 4 | 1 | 49 | 443 | 25% |
| *Salad, Side | 25 | 1 | 0 | 0 | 0 | 27 | 0% |
| Shake, Vanilla | 310 | 9 | 6 | 4 | 20 | 230 | 17% |
| Shrimp, Butterfly | 300 | 15 | 17 | 5 | 105 | 610 | 51% |
| Whopper | 614 | 27 | 36 | 12 | 90 | 865 | 53% |
| Whopper w/ Cheese | 706 | 32 | 44 | 16 | 115 | 1177 | 56% |
| Whopper, Dbl w/ Cheese | 935 | 51 | 61 | 24 | 194 | 1245 | 59% |

\* Indicates best choices.
Abbreviations used in this table: Cal = Calories; Pro = protein (g); Fat = total fat (g); S. Fat = Saturated fat (g); Chol = cholesterol (mg); Na = sodium (mg); % Fat = percentage of calories from fat.

|                          | Cal | Pro | Fat | S. Fat | Chol | Na   | %Fat |
|--------------------------|-----|-----|-----|--------|------|------|------|
| **DOMINO'S PIZZA (2 SLICES, THIN CRUST, 16")** | | | | | | | |
| *Cheese Pizza            | 376 | 22  | 10  | 5      | 19   | 483  | 24%  |
| Deluxe Pizza             | 498 | 27  | 20  | 9      | 40   | 954  | 37%  |
| Dbl Cheese/Pepperoni     | 545 | 32  | 25  | 13     | 48   | 1042 | 42%  |
| Pepperoni Pizza          | 460 | 24  | 17  | 8      | 28   | 825  | 34%  |
| Sausage/Mushroom Pizza   | 430 | 24  | 16  | 8      | 28   | 552  | 33%  |
| Veggie Pizza             | 498 | 31  | 18  | 10     | 36   | 1035 | 33%  |
| **HARDEE'S**             | | | | | | | |
| Bacon Cheeseburger       | 610 | 34  | 36  | 15     | 50   | 950  | 53%  |
| Big Deluxe Burger        | 500 | 27  | 30  | 12     | 70   | 760  | 54%  |
| Biscuit, Ham, Egg, Cheese| 500 | 16  | 27  | 10     | 170  | 1620 | 49%  |
| Biscuit, Rise N' Shine   | 390 | 5   | 21  | 6      | 0    | 1000 | 48%  |
| Biscuit, Sausage         | 510 | 13  | 31  | 10     | 25   | 1360 | 55%  |
| Cheeseburger             | 320 | 16  | 14  | 7      | 30   | 710  | 39%  |
| *Chicken Fillet Sand.    | 400 | 19  | 14  | 3      | 55   | 1100 | 32%  |
| Chicken, Frisco Grilled  | 620 | 35  | 34  | 10     | 95   | 1730 | 49%  |
| *Cool Twist Cone, Vanilla| 180 | 5   | 4   | 3      | 15   | 100  | 20%  |
| Cool Twist Sunday, Fudge | 320 | 7   | 10  | 5      | 25   | 270  | 28%  |
| Crispy Curls (Fries)     | 300 | 4   | 16  | 3      | 0    | 840  | 48%  |
| Fisherman's Fillet       | 500 | 23  | 24  | 6      | 70   | 1030 | 43%  |
| French Fries, small      | 230 | 3   | 11  | 2      | 0    | 85   | 43%  |
| Fried Chicken Breast     | 370 | 29  | 15  | 4      | 75   | 1190 | 36%  |
| Fried Chicken Leg        | 170 | 12  | 7   | 2      | 40   | 570  | 37%  |
| *Hamburger               | 270 | 13  | 10  | 4      | 20   | 490  | 33%  |
| Hot Dog, All Beef        | 450 | 17  | 20  | 6      | 35   | 1090 | 40%  |
| Hot Ham N' Cheese        | 530 | 18  | 30  | 9      | 65   | 1710 | 51%  |
| Muffin, Blueberry        | 400 | 7   | 17  | 4      | 65   | 310  | 37%  |
| *Pancakes (3)            | 280 | 8   | 2   | 1      | 15   | 890  | 6%   |
| Roast Beef, Big          | 360 | 24  | 15  | 6      | 65   | 1050 | 38%  |
| *Roast Beef, Regular     | 270 | 15  | 11  | 5      | 25   | 780  | 37%  |
| Salad, Chef              | 200 | 22  | 13  | 8      | 45   | 930  | 59%  |
| Salad, Garden            | 210 | 14  | 14  | 8      | 105  | 270  | 60%  |
| *Salad, Side             | 20  | 2   | 0   | 0      | 0    | 15   | 0%   |
| Shake, Vanilla           | 400 | 13  | 9   | 6      | 25   | 210  | 20%  |
| **KENTUCKY FRIED CHICKEN** | | | | | | | |
| *Baked Beans             | 133 | 6   | 2   | 1      | 1    | 492  | 11%  |
| Buttermilk Biscuit       | 235 | 0   | 12  | 3      | 1    | 530  | 45%  |
| Chick Littles Sandwich   | 169 | 6   | 10  | 2      | 18   | 331  | 54%  |

|  | Cal | Pro | Fat | S.Fat | Chol | Na | %Fat |
|---|---|---|---|---|---|---|---|
| Cole Slaw | 119 | 2 | 7 | 1 | 5 | 197 | 50% |
| Col.'s Chicken Sandwich | 482 | 21 | 27 | 6 | 47 | 1060 | 51% |
| Corn on the Cob | 222 | 5 | 12 | 2 | 0 | 76 | 47% |
| Cornbread(1) | 228 | 3 | 13 | 2 | 42 | 194 | 51% |
| Extra Crsp Center Breast | 342 | 26 | 20 | 5 | 75 | 790 | 52% |
| Extra Crsp Drumstick | 190 | 14 | 12 | 3 | 71 | 324 | 57% |
| Extra Crsp Side Breast | 400 | 22 | 27 | 6 | 81 | 748 | 59% |
| Extra Crsp Thigh | 406 | 20 | 30 | 8 | 129 | 688 | 66% |
| Extra Crsp Wing | 254 | 12 | 19 | 4 | 67 | 320 | 66% |
| Kentucky Nuggets (6) | 276 | 17 | 17 | 4 | 71 | 840 | 57% |
| *Mshd Potatoes w/ Gravy | 71 | 2 | 2 | 0 | 0 | 339 | 20% |
| Orig Rec Center Breast | 283 | 28 | 15 | 4 | 93 | 672 | 49% |
| Orig Rec Drumstick | 146 | 13 | 8 | 2 | 67 | 275 | 52% |
| Orig Rec Side Breast | 267 | 19 | 16 | 4 | 77 | 604 | 56% |
| Orig Rec Thigh | 294 | 18 | 20 | 5 | 123 | 619 | 60% |
| Orig Rec Wing | 178 | 12 | 12 | 3 | 64 | 372 | 59% |
| Parfait, Strwbry Shtcake | 230 | 2 | 9 | 5 | 20 | 162 | 34% |
| Potato Salad | 180 | 2 | 11 | 2 | 14 | 423 | 55% |
| *Rice, Garden | 75 | 2 | 1 | 0 | 0 | 576 | 11% |
| Rotis Chick, whitemeat | 335 | 40 | 19 | 5 | 157 | 1014 | 50% |
| *Rotis Chick, whitemeat, no skin, wing | 199 | 37 | 6 | 2 | 97 | 667 | 27% |
| *Red Beans & Rice | 114 | 4 | 3 | 1 | 4 | 315 | 23% |
| *Vegetable Medley | 126 | 1 | 4 | 1 | 0 | 240 | 31% |

## McDONALD'S

|  | Cal | Pro | Fat | S.Fat | Chol | Na | %Fat |
|---|---|---|---|---|---|---|---|
| Apple Pie | 280 | 2 | 15 | 2 | 0 | 90 | 52% |
| Big Mac | 500 | 25 | 26 | 9 | 100 | 890 | 47% |
| Biscuit with Sausage | 420 | 12 | 28 | 8 | 44 | 1040 | 60% |
| Biscuit w/ Saus & Egg | 500 | 19 | 33 | 10 | 270 | 1210 | 59% |
| Cheeseburger | 305 | 15 | 13 | 5 | 50 | 710 | 38% |
| *Chicken Sand, Mcgrilled | 390 | 30 | 12 | 4 | 80 | 800 | 31% |
| McChicken Sandwich | 470 | 19 | 25 | 5 | 60 | 830 | 48% |
| *Chicken Fajitas | 185 | 11 | 8 | 2 | 35 | 310 | 39% |
| Chicken McNuggets (6) | 270 | 20 | 15 | 4 | 56 | 580 | 50% |
| Danish, Cinnamon Raisin | 440 | 6 | 21 | 5 | 34 | 430 | 43% |
| Egg McMuffin | 280 | 18 | 11 | 4 | 235 | 710 | 38% |
| *English Muffin | 170 | 5 | 4 | 1 | 0 | 285 | 21% |
| Filet-O-Fish | 370 | 14 | 18 | 4 | 50 | 730 | 44% |
| French Fries, medium | 320 | 4 | 17 | 4 | 0 | 150 | 48% |

|  | Cal | Pro | Fat | S.Fat | Chol | Na | %Fat |
|---|---|---|---|---|---|---|---|
| *Frozen Yogurt Cone | 105 | 4 | 1 | 0 | 3 | 80 | 7% |
| *Hamburger | 255 | 12 | 9 | 3 | 37 | 490 | 32% |
| *Hotcakes w/ marg & syrp | 435 | 8 | 12 | 2 | 8 | 640 | 25% |
| *Hotcakes, plain | 245 | 8 | 4 | 1 | 10 | 570 | 14% |
| *McLean Deluxe | 320 | 22 | 10 | 4 | 60 | 670 | 28% |
| Milk Shake, Vanilla | 310 | 11 | 5 | 3 | 10 | 170 | 15% |
| *Muffin, Apple Bran | 180 | 5 | 0 | 0 | 0 | 170 | 0% |
| Quarter Pdnr w/ Cheese | 510 | 28 | 28 | 11 | 115 | 1090 | 49% |
| Salad, Chef | 170 | 17 | 9 | 4 | 111 | 400 | 48% |
| *Salad, Chunky Chicken | 150 | 25 | 4 | 1 | 78 | 230 | 24% |

### PIZZA HUT (2 SLICES, MEDIUM PIZZA)

|  | Cal | Pro | Fat | S.Fat | Chol | Na | %Fat |
|---|---|---|---|---|---|---|---|
| Pan Pizza, Cheese | 492 | 30 | 18 | 9 | 34 | 940 | 33% |
| Pan Pizza, Pepperoni | 540 | 29 | 22 | 9 | 42 | 1127 | 37% |
| Pan Pizza, Supreme | 589 | 32 | 30 | 14 | 48 | 1363 | 46% |
| Personal Pan Pepperoni | 675 | 37 | 29 | 12 | 53 | 1335 | 39% |
| Personal Pan Supreme | 647 | 33 | 28 | 11 | 49 | 1313 | 39% |
| Thin n' Crspy, Cheese | 398 | 28 | 17 | 10 | 33 | 867 | 38% |
| Thin n' Crspy, Pepperoni | 413 | 26 | 20 | 11 | 46 | 986 | 44% |
| Thin n' Crspy, Supreme | 459 | 28 | 22 | 11 | 42 | 1328 | 43% |

### TACO BELL

|  | Cal | Pro | Fat | S.Fat | Chol | Na | %Fat |
|---|---|---|---|---|---|---|---|
| *Burrito, Bean | 381 | 15 | 14 | 2 | 9 | 1148 | 33% |
| Burrito, Beef | 431 | 25 | 21 | 8 | 57 | 1311 | 44% |
| *Burrito, Chicken | 334 | 17 | 12 | 4 | 52 | 880 | 32% |
| Burrito Supreme | 440 | 20 | 22 | - | 33 | 1181 | 45% |
| Mexican Pizza | 575 | 21 | 37 | 11 | 52 | 1031 | 58% |
| Meximelt, Chicken | 257 | 14 | 15 | 7 | 48 | 779 | 53% |
| Nachos w/ Cheese | 346 | 7 | 18 | 6 | 9 | 399 | 47% |
| Nachos Supreme | 367 | 12 | 27 | - | 18 | 471 | 66% |
| Pintos 'N Cheese | 190 | 9 | 9 | - | 16 | 642 | 43% |
| Salad Dres, Ranch (2.5oz) | 236 | 2 | 25 | 5 | 35 | 571 | 95% |
| *Salsa (1/3oz.) | 18 | 1 | 0 | 0 | 0 | 376 | 0% |
| Taco, Hard, Beef | 183 | 10 | 11 | 5 | 32 | 276 | 54% |
| Taco Salad, w/ Shell | 905 | 34 | 61 | 19 | 80 | 910 | 61% |
| Taco Salad, no Shell | 484 | 28 | 31 | 14 | 80 | 680 | 58% |
| Taco, Soft, Beef | 225 | 12 | 12 | 5 | 32 | 554 | 48% |
| Taco, Soft, Chicken | 213 | 14 | 10 | 4 | 52 | 615 | 42% |
| Taco Supreme | 230 | 11 | 15 | 8 | 32 | 276 | 59% |
| *Tostada (Bean) | 167 | 6 | 7 | 2 | 9 | 324 | 38% |

|  | Cal | Pro | Fat | S.Fat | Chol | Na | %Fat |
|---|---|---|---|---|---|---|---|
| **WENDY'S** | | | | | | | |
| *Baked Potato, Brocli/Cheese | 450 | 8 | 14 | 2 | - | 455 | 28% |
| Baked Potato w/ Cheese | 550 | 14 | 24 | 8 | 30 | 640 | 39% |
| *Baked Potato, Plain | 270 | 6 | 0 | 0 | 0 | 20 | 0% |
| Big Classic Burger | 480 | 27 | 23 | 7 | 75 | 850 | 43% |
| Big Classic, Dbl, w/ Cheese | 820 | 50 | 51 | 14 | 170 | 1555 | 56% |
| Cheeseburger, Jr. | 320 | 18 | 13 | 5 | 45 | 760 | 37% |
| Cheeseburger, Double | 590 | 47 | 33 | 14 | 145 | 970 | 50% |
| Chicken Club Sandwich | 506 | 30 | 25 | 5 | 70 | 930 | 44% |
| Chicken Salad (1/4 cup) | 140 | 7 | 10 | 2 | 0 | 270 | 64% |
| Chicken Nuggets (6 pc.) | 280 | 14 | 20 | 4 | 50 | 600 | 64% |
| Chicken Salad, Grilled | 200 | 25 | 8 | 1 | 55 | 690 | 36% |
| Chicken Sandwich, Fried | 430 | 26 | 19 | 3 | 60 | 725 | 40% |
| *Chicken Sandwich, Grilled | 290 | 24 | 7 | 1 | 60 | 670 | 22% |
| *Chile, small | 190 | 19 | 6 | 2 | 40 | 670 | 28% |
| Chocolate Chip Cookie | 275 | 3 | 13 | 4 | 15 | 256 | 43% |
| Choc. Pudding (1/4 cup) | 80 | 1 | 3 | - | 0 | 70 | 34% |
| *Cottage Cheese (1/2 cup) | 108 | 13 | 4 | 3 | 15 | 425 | 33% |
| Fish Filet Sandwich | 460 | 18 | 25 | 5 | 55 | 780 | 49% |
| *Flour Tortilla (1) | 110 | 3 | 3 | 0 | - | 220 | 25% |
| French Fries, small | 240 | 3 | 12 | 2 | 0 | 145 | 45% |
| Frosty Dessert, medium | 460 | 12 | 13 | 7 | 55 | 286 | 25% |
| Hamburger, Double | 520 | 43 | 27 | 11 | 130 | 710 | 47% |
| Hamburger, Plain | 340 | 24 | 15 | 6 | 65 | 500 | 40% |
| Hamburger w/ Everything | 420 | 25 | 21 | 7 | 70 | 890 | 45% |
| *Hamburger, Jr. | 260 | 15 | 9 | 3 | 34 | 570 | 31% |
| *Refried Beans (1/4 cup) | 70 | 4 | 2 | 1 | 0 | 215 | 26% |
| Salad, Seafood (1/4 cup) | 70 | 3 | 4 | 1 | 0 | 300 | 51% |
| *Salad, 3 Bean (1/4c.) | 60 | 1 | 0 | 0 | - | 20 | 0% |

Note: Use low-fat salad dressings on salads. Fat content on some sandwiches can be further reduced by omitting cheese, mayonnaise or special sauces.

Note: A dash (-) means that data was not available.

Copyright 1991, CSPI. Reprinted from *The Completely Revised and Updated Fast-Food Guide*, which is available from CSPI, 1875 Conn. Ave., N.W. #300, Washington, DC 20009, for $7.95.

Updated with nutrition information supplied by Burger King, Hardee's, McDonald's, Kentucky Fried Chicken, Taco Bell and Wendy's.

# Bibliography

"A Barbecue Handbook," *USDA's Food News for Consumers*, U.S. Department of Agriculture, Summer, 1991.

"The Basic Four Food Guide," *Mayo Clinic Nutrition Letter*, Vol. 3, October 1990, pp. 4–5.

Bendich, Adrianne, and Lawrence J. Machlin, "Safety of Oral Intake of Vitamin E," *American Journal of Clinical Nutrition*, Vol. 48, 1988, pp. 612–619.

Blankenhorn, David H., "Beneficial Effects of Combined Colestipol-Niacin Therapy on Coronary Atherosclerosis and Coronary Venous Bypass Grafts," *The Journal of the American Medical Association*, Vol. 257, June 19, 1987, pp. 3233–3240.

"Breast Cancer," *Nutrition Action Healthletter*, Vol. 15, No. 2, March 1988, p. 1.

"But Is Your Cholesterol Level What They Say It Is?" *Tufts University Diet and Nutrition Letter*, Vol. 6, February 1989, p. 7.

"Can Taking Supplements Help You Ward Off Disease?" *Tufts University Diet & Nutrition Letter*, Vol. 9, No. 2, April 1991, pp. 3–5.

"Cancer-Free Colons," *Nutrition Action Healthletter*, Vol. 19, No. 10, December 1992, p. 4.

Castelli, W. P. "Epidemiology of Coronary Heart Disease: The Framingham Study," *The American Journal of Medicine*, February 27, 1984, pp. 4–12.

"Caffeine," *Mayo Clinic Nutrition Letter*, Vol. 3, October 1990, pp. 6–7.

"Chinese Restaurant Syndrome, Putting a Mysterious Ailment into Perspective," *Mayo Clinic Nutrition Letter*, Vol. 3, January 1990, pp. 4–5.

*Cholesterol, Current Concepts for Clinicians*, National Cholesterol Education Program, U.S. Department of Health and Human Services, National Institutes of Health, October 1, 1988.

Connor, Sonja L., et. al., "The Cholesterol-Saturated Fat Index for Coronary Prevention: Background, Use, and a Comprehensive Table of Foods," *Journal of the American Dietetic Association*, Vol. 89, No. 6, June 1989, pp. 807–816.

Connor, Sonja L. and William E. Connor, M.D., *The New American Diet*, New York: Simon and Schuster Inc., 1986.

Cooper, Kenneth H., *Controlling Cholesterol*, New York: Bantam Books, 1988.

*Diet, Nutrition, and Cancer*, by the Committee on Diet, Nutrition, and Cancer, National Research Council, Washington, D.C.: National Academy Press, 1982.

"A Different Kind of Open-Heart Procedure," *Tufts University Diet and Nutrition Letter*, Vol. 8, No. 11, January 1991, p. 3.

"Eat to Swim … Bike … Run …," *Nutrition Action Healthletter*, Vol. 15, June/July 1988, pp. 1, 4–6.

"'Eat Your Vegetables' as Sound Today as Ever," Tufts University Diet and Nutrition Letter, Vol. 7, October 1989, pp. 1–2.

"Eating Out," *Mayo Clinic Nutrition Letter*, Vol. 2, February 1989, pp. 4–5.

*Eating Smart*, American Cancer Society, Inc., 1987.

"The Effects of Nonpharmacologic Interventions on Blood Pressure of Persons with High Normal Levels," The Trials of Hypertension Prevention Collaborative Research Group, Bethesda, Md., *The Journal of the American Medical Association*, Vol. 267, No. 9, March 4, 1992, pp. 1213–1220.

Enos, Major William F., et. al., "Coronary Disease among United States Soldiers Killed in Action in Korea," *The Journal of the American Medical Association*, Vol. 152, July 18, 1953, pp. 1090–1093.

"Facts About … Exercise," The National Heart, Lung and Blood Institute, National Institutes of Health.

"Fast Food," *Mayo Clinic Nutrition Letter*, Vol. 2, July 1989, pp. 4–5.

"Final Report on the Aspirin Component of the Ongoing Physicians' Health Study," *The New England Journal of Medicine*, Vol. 321, No. 3, July 20, 1989, pp. 129–135.

"Five a Day," *Tufts University Diet and Nutrition Letter*, Vol. 6, February 1989, p. 2.

"Focus on Food Labeling," *FDA Consumer*, Food and Drug Administration, May 1993.

"For Your Heart's Sake, More B Vitamins," *Tufts University Diet & Nutrition Letter*, Vol. 11, No. 12, February 1994, pp. 1–2.

Gambino, Raymond, "NIH Consensus Development Conference on Triglycerides, High-Density Lipoprotein, and Coronary Heart Disease," *Lab Report*, Vol. 14, No. 3, March 1992, pp. 17–19.

Ganz, Patricia, and Anne Coscarelli Schag, "Nutrition and Breast Cancer," *Oncology*, Vol. 7, No. 12, December 1993, pp. 71–80.

"Genetic Factors Help Shape Your Shape," *Mayo Clinic Nutrition Letter*, Vol. 3, September 1990, p. 7.

Glueck, Charles J., "Pediatric Primary Prevention of Atherosclerosis," *The New England Journal of Medicine*, Vol. 314, January 16, 1986, pp. 175–177.

Hamilton, Eva, May Nunnelley, Eleanor Ross Whitney and Frances Sienkiewicz Sizer, *Nutrition: Concepts and Controversies*, St. Paul: West Publishing Co., 1985.

"Have You been Doing the Other Kind of Exercise?" *Tufts University Diet & Nutrition Letter*, Vol. 11, No. 5, July 1993, pp. 3–6.

Heinonen, Olli, and Demetrius Albanes, "The Effect of Vitamin E and Beta-Carotene on the Incidence of Lung Cancer and other Cancers in Male Smokers," *The New England Journal of Medicine*, Vol. 330, No. 15, April 14, 1994, pp. 1029–1035.

"High Blood Pressure," *Scientific American Medicine*, Vol. 1, October 1988, pp. 1–10.

"Hyperlipoproteinemia," *Scientific American Medicine*, Vol. 9, August 1986, pp. 1–4.

Infante-Rivard, Clair, et. al., "Fetal Loss Associated with Caffeine Intake before and during Pregnancy," *The Journal of the American Medical Association*, Vol. 270, No. 24, December 1993, pp. 2940–2943.

Ingersoll, Bruce, "U.S. Is Ready to Limit What Food Processors Can Claim on Labels," *The Wall Street Journal*, November 6, 1991, p. 1+.

"It's Never Too Late to Start Exercising," *Tufts University Diet and Nutrition Letter*, Vol. 6, February 1989, p. 5.

"Label Language: Still Sounds a Lot Like Babel," *Tufts University Diet and Nutrition Letter*, Vol. 9, No. 8, October 1991, pp. 3–6.

Lefferts, Lisa Y., "Great Grilling," *Nutrition Action Healthletter*, Vol. 16, July/August 1989, pp. 5–7.

Liebman, Bonnie, "Roughing It: How Fiber Fights Cancer," *Nutrition Action Healthletter*, June 1984, pp. 5–9.

— — —, "CSPI's Poultry Primer," *Nutrition Action Healthletter*, November 1986, pp. 8–9.

— — —, and Anne Montgomery, "Dining Out in Beverly Hills, Seattle, Houston," *Nutrition Action Healthletter*, Vol. 14, No. 6, July/August 1987, p. 10.

— — —, and Anne Montgomery, "Preventing Cancer," *Nutrition Action Healthletter*, Vol. 14, No. 6, July/August 1987, pp. 1, 4–6.

— — —, and Robert Davis, "Eating for Your 80s," *Nutrition Action Healthletter*, Vol. 14, November 1987, pp. 1, 4–7.

— — —, "Carrots Against Cancer?" *Nutrition Action Healthletter*, Vol. 15, No. 10, December 1988, pp. 1, 5–7.

— — —, "Life in the Fat Lane," *Nutrition Action Healthletter*, Vol. 17, July/August 1990, pp. 8–9.

— — —, "The HDL/Triglycerides Trap," *Nutrition Action Healthletter*, Vol. 17, No. 7, September 1990, pp. 1, 4–6.

— — —, "Trans in Trouble," *Nutrition Action Healthletter*, Vol. 17, October 1990, p. 7.

— — —, "Antioxidants and Cancer," *Nutrition Action Healthletter*, Vol. 19, No. 6, July/August 1992, pp. 5–7.

— — —, "The Ultra Mega Vita Guide," *Nutrition Action Healthletter*, Vol. 20, No. 1, January/February 1993, pp. 7–8.

— — —, "The Heart Health-E Vitamin?" *Nutrition Action Healthletter*, Vol. 21, No. 1, January/February 1994, pp. 4, 8–10.

"Lowering the Risk for High Blood Pressure," *Tufts University Diet and Nutrition Letter*, Vol. 5, No. 3, May 1987, pp. 3–6.

Luepker, Russell, et. al., "Isolated Low HDL-Cholesterol As a Risk Factor for Coronary Heart Disease," Abstracts from the 66th Scientific Sessions, *Circulation* (Suppl.), Vol. 88, No. 4, October 1993, p. 511.

Naito, Herbert K., "Effect of Cholesterol Lowering on CHD Risk," *Consultant*, Vol. 28, June 1988, pp. 15–24.

——, "New Concerns on Detection and Treatment of Hypercholesterolemia," *Physicians Market Place*, Vol. 21, November 1987, p. 2.

——, "New Guidelines and Recommendations on the Detection, Evaluation, and Treatment of Patients with Undesirable Cholesterol Levels," *American Journal of Clinical Pathology*, Vol. 90, September 1988, pp. 358–361.

"New RDAs Call for More Calcium, Less Sodium," *Tufts University Diet and Nutrition Letter*, Vol. 7, January 1990, pp. 1–2.

Newman III, William P., et. al., "Relation of Serum Lipoprotein Levels and Systolic Blood Pressure to Early Atherosclerosis," *The New England Journal of Medicine*, Vol. 314, January 16, 1986, pp. 138–144.

"Nutrition and Aging," *Nutrition Action Healthletter*, Vol. 19, No. 4, May 1992, pp. 5–7.

Ornish, Dean, "Can Life-Style Changes Reverse Coronary Heart Disease?" *The Lancet*, Vol. 336, July 21, 1990, pp. 129–133.

"Osteoporosis: Alternatives to Estrogen," *Harvard Health Letter*, Vol. 19, No. 5, March 1994, pp. 6–8.

"Pesticide Residues: Forbidden Fruit?" *Harvard Health Letter*, Vol. 19, No. 3, January 1994, pp. 6–8.

Physicians' Health Study Research Group and Steering Committee, "Final Report on the Aspirin Component of the Ongoing Physicians' Health Study," *The New England Journal of Medicine*, Vol. 321, No. 3, July 20, 1989, pp. 129–135.

Piscatella, Joseph C., *Don't Eat Your Heart Out Cookbook*, New York: Workman Publishing Co. Inc., 1983.

"Prevention: A Toast to the Heart," *Harvard Health Letter*, Vol. 19, No. 5, March 1994, pp. 4–5.

"Pumping Immunity," *Nutrition Action Healthletter*, Vol. 20, No. 3, April 1993, pp. 5–7.

"A Quick Consumer Guide to Safe Food Handling," U.S. Department of Agriculture, Food Safety and Inspection Service, September 1990.

"Recommendations for Treatment of Hyperlipidemia in Adults," (A Joint Statement of the Nutrition Committee and the Council on Arteriosclerosis), American Heart Association Special Report, Circulation 69, No. 5, 1984.

*Recommended Dietary Allowances*, Washington, D.C.: National Academy of Sciences, 1980.

—— 10th Edition, National Research Council, Washington, D.C.: National Academy Press, 1989.

"Report of the Expert Panel on Detection, Evaluation and Treatment of High Blood Cholesterol in Adults," National Cholesterol Education Program, National Heart, Lung and Blood Institute, *Archives of Internal Medicine*, Vol. 145, 1988, pp. 36–69.

"Report of the Expert Panel on Detection, Evaluation and Treatment of High Blood Cholesterol in Adults," National Cholesterol Education Program, National Institutes of Health, U.S. Government Printing Office, 1989.

Rimm, Eric B., et. al., "Vitamin E Consumption and the Risk of Coronary Disease in Men," *The New England Journal of Medicine*, Vol. 328, No. 20, May 20, 1993.

Rosenthal, Elizabeth, "Salt in Diet Might Be OK, Research Suggests," New York Times News Service, printed in *The News and Observer*, Raleigh, NC, December 31, 1991.

Ryan, Donna H., MD, and Barry M. Starr, "Vitamins in Prevention and Treatment of Cancer," *Contemporary Oncology*, January/February, 1992, pp. 45+.

Schardt, David, "Lifting Weight Myths," *Nutrition Action Healthletter*, Vol. 20, No. 8, October 1993, pp. 8–9.

———, "These Feet Were Made for Walking ..." *Nutrition Action Healthletter*, Vol. 20, No. 10, December 1993, pp. 5–7.

Schuler, Gerhard, et. al., "Regular Physical Exercise and Low-Fat Diet: Effects of Progression of Coronary Artery Disease," *Circulation*, Volume 86, 1992, pp. 1–11.

Selhub, Jacob, et. al., "Vitamin Status and Intake as Primary Determinants of Homocysteinemia in An Elderly Population," *Journal of the American Medical Association*, Vol. 270, No. 22, December 8, 1993, pp 2693–2698, 2726–2727.

"Smart Loser's Guide to Choosing a Weight Loss Program," *Tufts University Diet and Nutrition Letter*, Vol. 8, August 1990, pp. 3–6.

"Some Calories Count More Than Others," *Tufts University Diet and Nutrition Letter*, Vol. 6, November 1988, p. 2.

Stampfer, Meir, et. al., "Vitamin E Consumption and the Risk of Coronary Disease in Women," *The New England Journal of Medicine*, Vol. 328, No. 20, May 20, 1993, pp 1444–1448.

——— "Fat, Alcohol, and Selenium and Breast Cancer Risk," *Contemporary Oncology*, July 1993, pp. 28–39.

Statland, Bernard E., "Vitamins and Minerals: Passing Fads or Keys to Health?" *Medical Laboratory Observer*, December 1993, pp. 21–28.

Steinberg, Daniel, et. al., "Antioxidants in the Prevention of Human Atherosclerosis," *Circulation*, Vol. 85, No. 6, June 1992, pp. 2338–2344.

Strong, Jack P., M.D., "Coronary Atherosclerosis in Soldiers, A Clue to the Natural History of Atherosclerosis in the Young," *The Journal of the American Medical Association*, Vol. 256, November 28, 1986, pp. 2863–2866.

Strong, William B., "Cholesterol Screening for Children Is Warranted," *Clinical Chemistry News*, April 1989.

"Sugar Substitutes—Can They Help You Control Weight Safely?" *Mayo Clinic Nutrition Letter*, Vol. 3, August 1990, pp. 3–4.

"Tackling High Blood Pressure," *Nutrition Action Healthletter*, Vol. 16, May 1989, p. 1.

"Washing Away Sodium," *Nutrition Action Healthletter*, Vol. 16, June 1989, p. 13.

"What is Simplesse, The New Fat Substitute," *Mayo Clinic Nutrition Letter*, Vol. 3, April 1990, p. 8.

# General Index

## a

Aerobic exercise. *See* Exercise, aerobic
Alcohol:
    blood pressure and, 7, 9, 56, 114
    calories per gram, 28
    definition of one drink, 56
    triglycerides and, 113–14
American Heart Association, 31–32, 40,
    111–12, 136
    recommendations on cholesterol con-
      sumption, 32
    recommendations on fat consumption,
      31, 111–12
Angiotensin Converting Enzyme:
    (ACE) inhibitors, 59
Antioxidant supplements, 12, 100–3, 105–6
    animal studies and, 12, 101
    cancer and, 102–3
    cataracts and, 103
    heart disease and, 101–2
    typical supplemental intakes of, 105–6
    *See also* Beta carotene, Vitamin C and
      Vitamin E supplements
Antioxidants, 11–13, 100–3, 105–6
    how they function, 12–13, 100–1
    supplements of, *See* Antioxidant
      supplements
    *See also* Beta carotene, Vitamin C and
      Vitamin E
Applesauce (use in baking), 54
Artery spasm, 2
Artichoke Relish, 38
Artificial Sweeteners. *See* Sweeteners,
    artificial
Aspartic acid, 70
Aspertame, 70

Aspirin:
    colon cancer and, 103
    heart attacks and, 103
Atherosclerosis, 2–7
    and cholesterol levels, 4–5
    development of, 3–4
    high blood pressure and, 7–8
    incidence of, 2
Athletes, diet tips for, 98–99
Au gratin, 137

## b

Barley, 83
Beans:
    baked, vegetarian, 54
    benefits of, 84
    fiber in, 14, 52–53, 79, 84
    increasing intake of, 84
    as protein source, 53, 84, 89
    recommended daily servings of, 87
    as source of iron, 53
    as source of omega-fatty acids, 23
Bearnaise sauce, 137
Bechamel sauce, 137
Beta blockers, 59
Beta carotene, 11–12, 72–73, 101–2
Beta-carotene supplements, 100–3, 105–6
    cancer and, 102
    cataracts and, 103
    heart disease and, 102
    smokers and, 12, 102
Blackened (meat or fish), 137–38
Blankenhorn, David, 6
Blood Pressure, 7–9, 55–65, 117, 119–20
    dietary influences on, 8–9, 55–58, 119–20
    medical tests for, 109, 117, 119

Fricasseed, 137
Fructose, 28, 69
Fruit sauces, nonfat, 54
Fruits:
  increasing intake of, 85
  nutrients in, 75
  pesticides and herbicides in, 74–75
  preserving nutrients in, 76–78
  recommended daily intake of, 73

# g

Glucose, 69
Grains, 81–84
  corn products, 83
  increasing intake of, 84–85
  protein in, 89
  rice, 82, 89
  types of, 82–84
  wheat, 82–83
  whole vs. refined, 81
Gravy, nonfat, 53
Greek restaurants, 141
Greenwald, Peter, 9
Grilling, outdoor, 144–45
  safety tips, 144

# h

HDL cholesterol, *See* Cholesterol, blood, HDL
Hardee's, 42–45, 143, 388
Harvard School of Public Health, 101, 103
Health Management Resources (HMR) diet, 125–26
Heart attack, 2–4
  blood cholesterol and, 4–5, 7–8
  estrogen and, 5
  high blood pressure and, 7–8
  risk factors cumulative, 7–8
  risk factors for, 111
  smoking and, 8
Heart disease, *See* Coronary heart disease
Hemorrhoids, 13–14
Herbicide residues, 74–75
  children and, 74
  how to minimize, 74–75

Heredity:
  heart disease risk factor, 111
  weight control and, 123–24
Heterocyclicamines (HAs), 138, 145
High-fructose corn syrup, 28. 69
Hollandaise sauce, 137
Hominy, 83
Homocysteine, 104
Honey, 28, 69
Hummous, 38
Hydrogenated fats, 19–20
Hypertension, *See* Blood pressure, high
Hypertension, labile, 119

# j

Japanese restaurants, 141
Jenny Craig diet, 127

# k

Kentucky Fried Chicken, 45, 143, 388–89
Keys, Ancel, 5

# l

LDL cholesterol, *See* Cholesterol, blood, LDL
Lactose, 28, 69
Lipoprotein analysis, 110–11
Lipoproteins, 17
  *See also* Cholesterol, blood, HDL and LDL
Liquids, in diet, 14, 88, 131
  recommended daily intake of, 14, 88, 131

# m

Magnesium, 84, 108
Margarine, 20, 35–36
  CSI of, 35–36
  trans fatty acids in, 20
McDonalds, 42, 45, 143, 389–90

Vitamin E supplements, 100–6
    cancer studies and, 102–3
    cataracts and, 103
    heart disease studies and, 101
Vitamin/Mineral supplements, 12, 100–8
    antioxidant supplements, *See* Antioxidant
        supplements
    calcium supplements, *See* Calcium
        supplements
    chromium, 108
    dissolution test, 104–5
    elderly and, 103–5, 107–8
    how to choose, 104–8
    iron, 108
    generic vs. name brand, 104
    magnesium, 108
    natural vs. synthetic, 104
    selenium, 106
    specific vitamin needs, 106–8
    vitamin D, *See* Vitamin D
    women and, 105–8
    *See also* Vitamin C, Vitamin E and Beta-
        carotene supplements
Vitamins, deficiencies of, 104, 106–8

## W

Weight control, 121–35
    complex carbohydrates and, 73
    dietary fat and, 16, 121–22
    exercise and, 91, 122–23, 134–35
    heredity and, 123–28
    types of diets for, 125–28
    vitamin/mineral supplements and, 129
Weight lifting, 95–97, 99, 151

Weight loss:
    blood pressure and, 9, 16, 56, 114, 121
    body's reaction to, 124–25
    cholesterol levels and, 113–14, 121
    choosing best diet program for, 128–29
    diets, liquid, 125–26
    diets, real food, 127–28
    exercise and, 91, 122–23, 125, 134–35
    fifteen-day meal plan for, 132–33
    health benefits of, 121
    lifelong commitment to, 128–29
    recommended rate of, 124
    snacks and, 131
    suggested plan for, 129–35
    yo-yo dieting, 126, 129
    *See also* Weight control
Weight Loss Clinic diet plan, 127–28
Weight table, Metropolitan Life Insurance
    Co., 15
Weight training, *See* Exercise, strength
    training
Weight Watchers, Inc., 121, 127–28
Wendy's, 143, 391
Wheat:
    berries, 83
    germ, 82–83, 85–86
    grains, types of, 82–83
    kernel of, 81
Wild rice, 82
Wine, 152

## Y

Yogurt:
    in fruit salads, 54
    in tuna salad, 53

# Recipe Index